Feeding and Swallowing Disorders in Infancy

Assessment and Management

by
Lynn S. Wolf, M.O.T., OTR
and
Robin P. Glass, M.S., OTR

Illustrations drawn under contract
by A. Brian Carr

HAMMILL INSTITUTE ON DISABILITIES
8700 SHOAL CREEK BOULEVARD
AUSTIN, TEXAS 78757-6897
512/451-3521   FAX 512/451-3728

H HAMMILL INSTITUTE ON DISABILITIES

8700 SHOAL CREEK BOULEVARD
AUSTIN, TEXAS 78757-6897
512/451-3521   FAX 512/451-3728
ORDER NUMBER 1005

ISBN-13: 978-160251005-0
ISBN-10: 160251005-9

Previously published by Therapy Skill Builders, a division of The Psychological Corporation, under ISBN 0761641904.

Printed in the United States of America

 4 5 6 7   16 15 14 13

About the Authors

Lynn S. Wolf, M.O.T., OTR, is a pediatric occupational therapist at Children's Hospital and Medical Center in Seattle, Washington, where she is a clinical specialist in infants. In this position she has gained many years of experience working with neonates and infants with feeding problems. She also has a faculty appointment in the Department of Pediatrics at the University of Washington, which includes research and clinical training responsibilities. Ms. Wolf's training includes a master's degree in occupational therapy from the University of Washington and certification in neurodevelopmental therapy (NDT) through the Neuro-Developmental Treatment Association, Inc. She has also completed advanced NDT courses in feeding and infant treatment. In addition to her clinical practice, Ms. Wolf has a number of research publications in the area of pediatric occupational therapy and has presented many continuing education workshops focusing on infant feeding and swallowing.

Robin Pritkin Glass, M.S., OTR, is a pediatric occupational therapist and clinical infant specialist at Children's Hospital and Medical Center in Seattle, Washington. She received her bachelor of science degree in occupational therapy from Columbia University and her master of science degree in occupational therapy from the University of Washington. In addition to her clinical responsibilities, she holds a clinical assistant professor appointment in the Department of Rehabilitation Medicine at the University of Washington. In this role she has been involved in the clinical training of undergraduate and graduate students in neonatal occupational therapy, as well as clinical research in the area of infant feeding. Ms. Glass is certified in neurodevelopmental therapy by the Neuro-Developmental Treatment Association, Inc., and has taken advanced NDT courses in feeding and infant treatment. Since 1977, she has published a number of articles and given national, regional, and local presentations on various aspects of feeding and swallowing in infancy.

Trademark Credits

Aldactone® is a registered trademark of G. D. Searle and Co.

Corecto® is a registered trademark of Corecto Corporation.

Degree® is a registered trademark of Degree Baby Products, Inc.

Diuril® is a registered trademark of Merck Co., Inc.

Enfamil® is a registered trademark of Mead Johnson and Company.

Evenflo® is a registered trademark of Questor Corporation.

Gerber® is a registered trademark of Gerber Products Company.

Inderal® is a registered trademark of American Home Products Corp.

Lasix® is a registered trademark of Hoechst Aktiengesellschft.

Maalox® is a registered trademark of William H. Rorer, Inc.

Mead Johnson® is a registered trademark of Mead Johnson and Company.

Medela® is a registered trademark of Medela A G.

Natural nipple® is a registered trademark of Mead Johnson and Company.

NUK® is a registered trademark of Mapa GmbH, Gummi-und Plastikwerke.

Playtex® is a registered trademark of International Playtex, Inc.

Reglan® is a registered trademark of Societe d'Etudes Scientifiques et Industrielles de l'Ile-de-France.

Riopan® is a registered trademark of Byk-Gulden, Inc.

Ross® is a registered trademark of Abbott Laboratories.

Similac Natural Care® is a registered trademark of Abbott Laboratories.

SMA® is a registered trademark of American Home Products Corp.

Soother™ is a trademark of Abbott Laboratories.

Tagamet® is a registered trademark of Smithline Corporation.

Volu-feed® is a registered trademark of Abbott Laboratories.

Wyeth® is a registered trademark of American Home Products Corp.

Zantac® is a registered trademark of Glaxo Group Limited.

Contents

Acknowledgments

Our thanks and appreciation are wholeheartedly extended to the many people who have provided professional expertise, review of various portions of the manuscript, and encouragement to complete this project.

Barbara E. Anderson, RN, BSN
Craniofacial Program Clinical Nurse Specialist
Children's Hospital and Medical Center
Seattle, Washington

Jane Case-Smith, Ed.D., OTR
Chief of Occupational Therapy
Nisonger Center
Ohio University
Columbus, Ohio

Denis Christie, M.D.
Associate Professor
University of Washington, School of Medicine
Division Head of Gastroenterology
Children's Hospital and Medical Center
Seattle, Washington

Sterling K. Clarren, M.D.
Aldrich Professor of Pediatrics
Head, Division of Embryology, Teratology, and Congenital Defects
University of Washington, School of Medicine
Seattle, Washington

Karen Corlett, RN, BSN
Cardiovascular Surgery Clinical Nurse Specialist
Children's Hospital and Medical Center
Seattle, Washington

Nora Davis, M.D.
Assistant Professor, Department of Pediatrics
University of Washington, School of Medicine
Attending Physician, Neurodevelopmental Clinic and
  Director of Apnea Program
Children's Hospital and Medical Center
Seattle, Washington

Amy Faherty, M.S., CCC-SP
Speech and Language Services
Children's Hospital and Medical Center
Seattle, Washington

Sandra N. Jolley, ARNP, M.S.
Pediatric Nurse Practitioner
Lactation Specialist
Seattle, Washington

Susan G. Marshall, M.D.
Assistant Professor, Department of Pediatrics
University of Washington, School of Medicine
Attending Physician, Division of Pulmonary Medicine
Children's Hospital and Medical Center
Seattle, Washington

Gayle McCreary, PT, MPH
Department of Occupational and Physical Therapy
Children's Hospital and Medical Center
Seattle, Washington

Karen Quinn, OTR
Department of Occupational and Physical Therapy
Children's Hospital and Medical Center
Seattle, Washington

Gay Lloyd Pinder, M.Ed., CCC-S/LP
Speech Language Pathologist
Children's Therapy Center of Kent
Seattle, Washington

Robert Sawin, M.D.
Assistant Professor of Surgery
University of Washington, School of Medicine
Attending Surgeon
Children's Hospital and Medical Center
Seattle, Washington

Judy Thorpe, RN, BSN
Pediatric Surgery Clinical Nurse Specialist
Children's Hospital and Medical Center
Seattle, Washington

A special thank you is reserved for Nora Davis, M.D., who has freely shared her professional knowledge and offered many challenging ideas over the years.

A project of this scope could never have been completed without the flexibility and support of our co-workers. Sincere thanks is extended to our colleagues Gayle McCreary, MPH, PT, and Kristie Bjornson, MS, PT, and to Arlene Libby, OTR, the manager of Occupational Therapy, Children's Hospital and Medical Center, Seattle, Washington.

Special thanks to our illustrator, A. Brian Carr, ABC Designs, Seattle, Washington.

The most important thank you is saved for our families—Greg and Rachel Glass and Steve, Ellie, and Kailey Wolf. Without their love, support, and immense flexibility this book would never have been possible.

Foreword

The clinical area of infant feeding impairments is evolving rapidly. Its evolution is impelled by an increasing incidence of dysphagic infants who have survived embryopathy, prematurity, or genetic or other early pathologic mechanisms. Resources for feeding evaluation are becoming more effective. But a principal reason for this evolution is the greater effectiveness of feeding therapy. This unique book describes the insights and skills in evaluation and care of dysphagic infants that are being demonstrated by a growing number of occupational, physical, and speech therapists and nurses.

The book describes infant feeding evaluation and therapy in a medical context. The pertinent pediatric entities (prematurity and bronchopulmonary dysplasia, clefts and other malformations, various neurologic impairments) and evaluation methods (videofluoroscopy, endoscopy, and esophageal pH recording and manometry) are well reviewed.

The distinction of the book is in its descriptions of feeding impairments and their therapy. Its information is specific: examples of individual infants and well-detailed problem-driven models and treatment strategies. The information is reinforced by illustrations, lists, and classifications. Therapists and all clinicians who deal with feeding-impaired infants will be helped by this book.

The writing is perceptive. There are many examples of mothers' concerns and problems. Subtle interactions within the clinical team, as its members gain insight into the causes and mechanisms of feeding impairments, are also highlighted. I suspect that iatrogenic problems of oral hypersensitivity and feeding resistance are few in this company.

The book is timely as the field of infant dysphagia is evolving. Techniques that enhance both feeding and nutrition are discussed. These include: prefeeding oral area stimulation, adaptations of nutrient density and volume, adaptation of head positioning, and choice of nipples. Even breastfeeding can be adapted. The feeding specialists described here are essential in the arena of infant care.

James F. Bosma, M.D.

Introduction

Feeding specialists encompass a variety of disciplines—occupational, physical, or speech therapists; nurses in inpatient or outpatient settings; physicians. Historically, these professionals have dealt with feeding problems from a functional or rehabilitative perspective (modifying utensils and providing adaptive equipment) or from a neuromuscular perspective (modifying oral tone, movement, position, and/or alignment) that is exemplified by a neurodevelopmental treatment approach. As feeding specialists work with younger and sicker infants, especially those who have received neonatal intensive care, the theoretical constructs underlying evaluation and treatment need to change. Basing our interventions on only these two frames of reference would be limiting.

In small or sick infants there is often no clear underlying neuromuscular pathology—either none is present or it is not yet evident. Infants with immature central nervous systems often respond to the stress of their environment or medical condition with behaviors or movements that appear similar to those observed when there is frank central nervous system damage. Yet the etiology and underlying mechanism for these behaviors is very different, and the infant therefore would not necessarily respond to a purely neurodevelopmental or rehabilitative approach.

Furthermore, young infants feed primarily by sucking. This method of feeding, although extremely efficient, involves a much more complex interaction of multiple systems than do other, more mature feeding skills. The dynamic and intricate coordination between sucking, swallowing, and breathing superimposed on a background of the infant's behavioral state make infant feeding a complicated, multidimensional task. Dysfunction in one component of this system can have far-reaching effects on the other components. A uni-dimensional assessment or treatment approach, therefore, would be unable to deal fully with problems in this complex system.

A framework to address infant feeding problems needs to consider the range of feeding-related problems that can be observed:

- A "healthy" baby who is not sucking well
- A full-term baby who becomes cyanotic and bradycardic with feedings
- A baby with congenital heart disease who is unable to finish feedings
- A preterm baby who becomes cyanotic and bradycardic with feedings
- A baby with bronchopulmonary dysplasia with a tracheostomy who will not allow a bottle in its mouth
- A baby with meningomyelocele who suddenly stops feeding well
- A baby who is unable to suck well at the breast and gains weight poorly
- An infant who spits up frequently

Due to the breadth of possible infant feeding difficulties, any approach to the assessment and management of these infant feeding problems must

- be applicable to the broad range of feeding problems;
- reflect an understanding of infant sucking, swallowing, and breathing mechanisms and their complex interaction, including the influence of an immature central nervous system;
- take into consideration that infants communicate their responses to the events surrounding feeding through state-behavior physiologic and/or motoric behaviors;
- reflect the potentially broad group of medical specialists, tests, and procedures that may be required for comprehensive assessment and management of these problems; and
- consider the interaction between known medical diagnoses and the feeding process.

This book seeks to present such a comprehensive, multidimensional approach to feeding problems. The goal is to assist the feeding specialist in acquiring the knowledge and skills to take an active and effective part in the process of assessment and management of infant feeding.

1 Functional Anatomy and Physiology of the Suck/Swallow/Breathe Triad

Throughout this text it will be apparent that three processes—sucking, swallowing, and breathing—are the cornerstones of infant feeding. Not only are these processes related functionally as they come together in bottle- and breast-feeding, but they are related anatomically. The anatomical structures responsible for sucking, swallowing, and breathing are physically in close proximity and overlap in function, with some structures having roles in the life-sustaining processes of both feeding and respiration. The close proximity of these structures, the interrelated nature of their functions, and the dual role some structures play in providing oxygen and nourishment to the body often underlie the feeding problems of infants.

Thus, professionals working with infants who have feeding problems need a thorough understanding of the functions and their interrelationship. This chapter will provide a background by reviewing the anatomy and neural control of the region; by discussing the individual functions of sucking, swallowing, and respiration; and by considering issues in coordination of these functions during infant feeding by breast or bottle.

Anatomy

Structures

The nose, mouth, pharynx, airways, and esophagus provide a conduit for the passage of both air (into and out of the lungs) and food (traveling to the stomach). At the proximal end of this conduit are two distinct channels, the oral and the nasal cavities (see figure 1-1). These come together in a combined channel, the pharynx, which divides into two distinct sections, the esophagus and the trachea. Although air may pass through the food passages with little impact, when food inappropriately enters the air passages, particularly the trachea, significant consequences may result. (Anatomy is shown in figure 1-2.)

Nasal cavity: The nasal cavity is the primary inlet for air, helping to clean and moisturize it before the air enters the lungs. Anteriorly, the nasal cavity is bounded by the cartilaginous portions of the nose, with air entering through the nares. Inferiorly, the palatine process of the maxilla and palatine bone provide a rigid boundary between the nasal and oral cavities. Tissue extending beyond this bony hard palate forms the soft palate. Superiorly, the rigid boundaries consist of portions of the nasal, frontal, ethmoid, and sphenoid bones. Internally, the nasal cavity is divided vertically into two sections by the nasal septum, ethmoid bone, and vomer. Nasal conchae (turbinates) run horizontally through each section and direct airflow through the nasal cavity. At the posterior aspect, each side of the nasal cavity narrows to form the choanae, which mark the junction with the pharynx. The nasal cavity is completely sealed from the oropharynx and the oral cavity when the soft palate is fully elevated.[2,15]

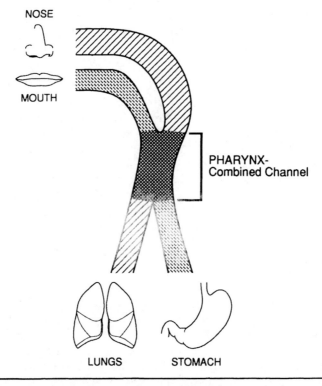

Figure 1-1 The pharynx is the crossroad for the overlapping channels that move air and food.

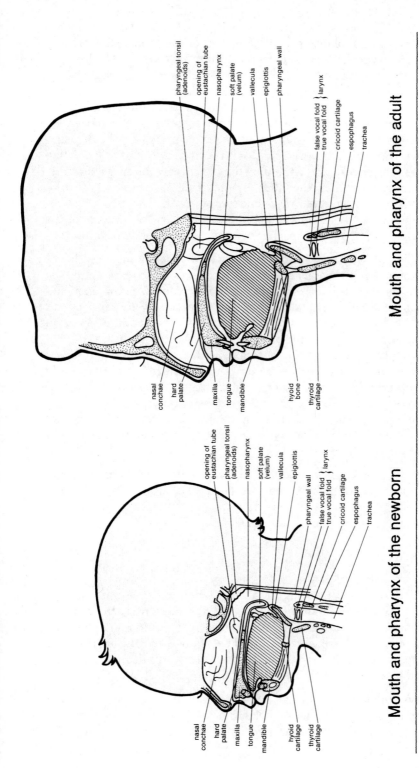

Mouth and pharynx of the newborn

Mouth and pharynx of the adult

Figure 1-2 Anatomy of the head and neck as it relates to feeding in the infant and the adult.
From *Pre-Feeding Skills* by Marsha Dunn Klein and Suzanne Evans Morris,
The Psychological Corporation, 555 Academic Court, San Antonio, TX 78245. Reprinted with permission.

Oral cavity: The oral cavity, or mouth, has a major role in ingestion of food, as well as in vocalization and oral respiration. It is bounded by the roof, the floor, the lips, and the cheeks. The roof of the mouth consists of the palatine process of the maxilla and the palatine bone (hard palate), which transitions posteriorly into the soft palate and uvula. The floor of the mouth includes the bony mandible, spanned by the mylohyoid and geniohyoid muscles, along with the anterior belly of the digastric muscle. The orbicularis oris muscle and surrounding soft tissue define the lips. The cheeks are defined by the buccinator and masseter muscles, though in infancy the fat pads or sucking pads are a key feature of the cheeks. The tongue is a mobile component in the oral cavity, with attachments to the mandible, hyoid bone, and styloid process of the cranium by the genioglossus, hypoglossus, and styloglossus muscles.[1]

Pharynx: One of the functions of the pharynx is swallowing. Another is maintenance of pharyngeal patency which is crucial to respiration. The pharynx is a soft tube with contour and dimension determined posteriorly and laterally by the sleeve of pharyngeal constrictor muscles and anteriorly by the soft palate, tongue, and suspension of the laryngeal cartilages. The origins of the pharyngeal constrictors include the sphenoid, mandible, tendinous connections with the buccinator and fibers of the tongue musculature (superior portion), the hyoid bone (middle portion), and the thyroid and cricoid cartilages (inferior portion). Insertion of a portion of the pharyngeal constrictors is on the posterior median pharyngeal raphe. These anatomic connections with the structures of the mouth and larynx closely link the functions of respiration and feeding in the pharynx.[1,12,15]

The pharynx is often considered in three parts: the oropharynx, the nasopharynx, and the hypopharynx. The nasopharynx is the section of the pharynx between the nasal choanae and the elevated soft palate. The eustachian tubes originate in the nasopharynx.[3]

The faucial arches (also called palatine arches, tonsilar pillars, palatopharyngeal arches, or palatoglossal arches) are the "bridge" between the mouth and oropharynx. Here the soft palate and tongue appose to close the oral cavity during nasal respiration and the oral phase of feeding. This junction and the base of the tongue form the anterior boundary of the oropharynx. The oropharynx is composed of the area of the pharynx between the elevated soft palate and the epiglottis. It includes the epiglottis and the valleculae, which are bilateral "pockets" formed by the base of the tongue and the epiglottis.[9]

The hypopharynx or laryngeal pharynx extends from the base of the epiglottis to the cricopharyngeal sphincter. The anterior wall of the hypopharynx includes the laryngeal inlet and the cricoid cartilage. The piriform sinuses are bilateral "pockets" located laterally below the inlet of the larynx.

Larynx: The larynx is the gateway to the trachea. It is a primarily cartilaginous structure suspended by muscular and ligamentous attachments to the hyoid bone and cervical vertebrae. It includes structures that modify airflow for phonation and also protect the airway during swallowing. The primary airway protective mechanism is the epiglottis, which folds down to seal against the aryepiglottic folds and close the inlet to the larynx. The false vocal folds and true vocal folds within the larynx also adduct during swallowing, providing additional protection to the lungs. During swallowing these structures close in a distal to proximal progression (true vocal folds, false vocal folds, then the epiglottis) to protect the airway from aspiration of food substances.[2,14,18]

Trachea: The trachea is a semirigid tube composed of semicircular, cartilaginous rings connected to each other and to the larynx by ligamentous membranes. The posterior aspect is a membranous wall that abuts the soft tissue of the esophagus. As it descends, the trachea branches into the primary bronchi leading to each lung.

Esophagus: Superiorly, the esophagus begins at the cricopharyngeous muscle, the lower portion of the inferior pharyngeal constrictor. This muscle tonically maintains closure of the cricopharyngeal sphincter (upper esophageal sphincter, UES, or pharyngoesophageal segment, PE segment). When a swallow is triggered, this sphincter relaxes and allows passage of the bolus into the esophagus. The esophagus is a thin, muscular tube that distends as food boluses are propelled through it by peristaltic movements. The esophagus is in close proximity to the trachea until the tracheal bifurcation. It is also adjacent to the aorta, from the aortic arch to the diaphragm. The esophagus passes through the diaphragm and terminates in the stomach at the lower esophageal sphincter (LES, cardiac sphincter, or gastroesophageal sphincter). This is technically not a sphincter but is actually a segment of esophageal and diaphragmatic muscle that creates a region of high intraluminal pressure, which is relaxed during esophageal peristalsis.[15]

Craniocervical Relationships

A discussion of anatomy in this region must include mention of the anatomic relationship between the cavities for feeding, breathing, and swallowing and other craniocervical structures. There are numerous muscular connections between the structures of the mouth, pharynx, and larynx and the skull and shoulder girdle. These structural connections are the basis for the reciprocal influences between feeding, swallowing, and breathing and head and neck posture. Although numerous interconnections exist, the hyoid bone plays a key role in this relationship. It is the site for muscular interface between the mandible, tongue, temporal bone, cervical vertebrae, laryngeal cartilages, sternum, and scapulae (see figure 1-3).

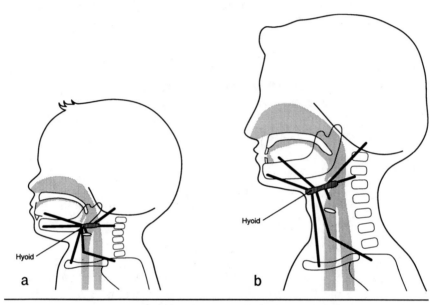

Figure 1-3 Muscular attachments to the hyoid provide an anatomic link between the structures of sucking, swallowing, and breathing and craniocervical posture.

Movement of Air and Food

In this system of chambered organs, muscular activity and changing pressure gradients combine to move air and food.[4] To accommodate the transport of these two substances through the same and adjacent structures in a safe manner, a system of "valves" channels food and air in the proper direction at the proper time.[17] The resting position of these valves favors respiration, with most valves changing position to allow swallowing. The primary valving mechanisms include the following.

Lips: Closing the lips physically aids in keeping food in the mouth during eating, but it also allows changes in intra-oral pressure. These pressure changes facilitate bolus organization and movement, which plays a role in initiating swallowing.

Soft palate/tongue: The soft palate and tongue work together to form a valve between the oral cavity and the pharynx. The soft palate approximates the tongue except during swallowing, oral breathing, and vocalization. Tongue movement can also assist in maintaining closure of this valve. When apposed to the tongue, the soft palate retains food in the mouth until a swallow is initiated. In this position it also channels air from the nasal pharynx directly through the pharynx and into the larynx/trachea. During swallowing, the soft palate is elevated against the posterior pharyngeal wall, and the tongue forms a deep median groove, directing food into the pharynx. The apposition of the elevated soft palate and the pharyngeal constrictors seals the nasopharynx and prevents food from entering the nasal passages.[7]

Epiglottis: At rest the epiglottis is elevated and allows air to freely flow into the larynx and trachea. During swallowing it folds down against the aryepiglottic folds to seal the larynx, and ultimately the lungs, against the entry of food substances.

Cricopharyngeal sphincter: By remaining tonically closed, this sphincter keeps previously swallowed food in the esophagus and prevents it from reentering the pharynx, where it could interfere with respiration. In addition it plays a role in preventing air from filling the esophagus during inspiration.[13]

Maturational Considerations

During the early months of life, many changes occur in the anatomic relationships of the oral, pharyngeal, and laryngeal areas. In addition, there are changes in the composition and control of the various structures. Although mechanical stability is required to carry out the functions of respiration and feeding, as the baby grows there is a shift in the method by which stabilization is achieved. At birth, *positional stability* is provided by the close proximity of various structures and the infant's large amount of subcutaneous fat. As the infant matures, greater *postural stability* is provided. While the structures move farther apart, they are supported by increased amounts of connective tissue, cartilage, and more highly specialized muscle control.[1,3,17]

At birth the mouth is a "potential cavity" (see figure 1-2a).[11,16] It is fully filled by the tongue, which is in loose approximation with the cheeks, hard palate, and soft palate. The tongue has a large area of contact with the soft palate, separating the mouth from the pharynx. The tongue tip protrudes past the alveolar ridge to maintain contact with the lower lip. These close approximations are felt to contribute to tongue stability in the newborn.[1] Relatively large amounts of subcutaneous fat, including the fat pads or sucking pads, provide the firm consistency and puffy profile of the infant's cheeks. Bosma describes this subcutaneous fat as providing a functional "exoskeleton" to support oral and pharyngeal function.[1] As the temporomandibular joint is quite mobile in the newborn, secondary to poorly developed connective tissue and capsular ligaments, this exoskeleton provides stabilization for mandibular movement.[1]

As the infant matures, the oral cavity enlarges, particularly with mandibular growth and dental eruption (see figure 1-2b). The tongue descends and moves back into the mouth, with the tip now behind the alveolar ridges. This creates an open "masticatory space" and allows room for the development of the large variety of tongue movements used in mature feeding skills and speech.[3,17] As the sucking pads and other adipose tissue of the cheeks diminish, mandibular stability is provided by increased muscular control and development of more rigid connective tissue. This reduction in the mass of the cheeks allows greater and more active mobility of the lips and cheeks.[3,11]

The pharyngeal area of the newborn is also characterized by close approximation of structures. The soft palate is relatively large and has a large area of contact with the tongue, bringing the uvula close to the tip of the epiglottis. The faucial arches of the newborn converge laterally about the epiglottis to create a closed area for bolus accumulation in the valleculae.[1] The hyoid and larynx are closely positioned and quite near the mandible.

With maturation, there is a cephalocaudal elongation of the pharynx. The hyoid, epiglottis, and larynx descend in relationship to the soft palate and mandible. The separation of the soft palate and epiglottis allows a portion of the tongue to become a surface in the anterior wall of the pharynx. Along with developing greater relative distances between them, the hyoid and larynx develop greater mobility. In this new arrangement, the larynx must use the increased mobility to elevate further and allow the epiglottis to seal completely during swallowing (see figure 1-3b, page 8).[12]

The larynx of the infant functions as a mobile and well-muscled general sphincter. The epiglottis is lax, the arytenoid cartilages are prominent, and the aryepiglottic folds are broad. The contour of the lumen of the larynx is primarily determined by muscular action. This arrangement may allow small amounts of fluid to enter the laryngeal vestibule, particularly if the infant is crying when fluids are introduced orally. These liquids, however, are expressed easily into the pharynx during subsequent swallows.[1,2]

Neural Control

In addition to anatomic interrelation of the structures involved with sucking, swallowing, and breathing, the neural control of these functions shows considerable overlap. At the level of peripheral innervation, the oral, nasal, pharyngeal, laryngeal, and respiratory structures are primarily innervated by branches of cranial nerves V, VII, IX, X, and XII and branches of the upper cervical nerve roots. Table 1-1 outlines the specific motor and sensory functions of these nerves, and figure 1-4 demonstrates their overlapping functions.

For example, the motor fibers of the trigeminal nerve (CN V) innervate the muscles of the lower jaw for sucking and the palatal elevators to initiate swallowing. The sensory fibers provide feedback from the mouth during sucking, the soft palate during swallowing, and the nose during respiration. Branches of the vagus and glossopharyngeal nerves (CN X and CN IX) provide extensive innervation to the structures of swallowing and respiration and to a lesser degree to the mouth. These nerves supply primary motor and sensory innervation to the pharynx, larynx, and trachea, as well as some sensory and motor input to the esophagus and sensory innervation to the tongue. In addition, the vagus nerve provides autonomic fibers to the heart, lungs, and digestive structures, further relating sucking, swallowing, and respiration to other visceral functions.

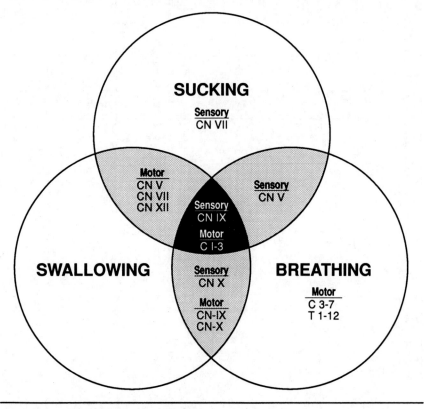

Figure 1-4 Overlapping function of the cranial nerves involved in sucking, swallowing, and breathing.

Table 1-1 Sensory and Motor Functions of Cranial and Cervical Nerves Involved in Sucking, Swallowing, and Respiration

Cranial Nerve	Motor		Sensory	
	Efferent Function	Brain-Stem Representation	Afferent Function	Brain-Stem Representation
Trigeminal N. CN V	– muscles of mastication – lower jaw – palatal elevators	trigeminal motor nucleus	scalp, face, teeth, tongue, membranes of mouth, palate, nose, nasal sinuses	trigeminal sensory nucleus
Facial N. CN VII	muscles of the face including: buccinator stylohyoid posterior belly of digastric	facial nucleus	– taste to anterior 2/3 of tongue – middle ear	geniculate ganglion to the NTS
Glossopharyngeal N. CN IX	pharynx	nucleus ambiguus	– pharynx – posterior 1/3 of tongue (taste) – carotid sinus	superior and inferior ganglion to the NTS
Vagus N. CN X	pharynx, larynx, esophagus, and parasympathetic function: autonomic fibers to the heart, lungs, esophagus, stomach, and other abdominal viscera	nucleus ambiguus - - - - - - - - - dorsal motor nucleus	pharynx, larynx, trachea, lungs	superior and inferior ganglion to the NTS

Table 1-1 *(continued)*

Cranial Nerve	Motor		Sensory	
	Efferent Function	Brain-Stem Representation	Afferent Function	Brain-Stem Representation
Accessory N. CN XI	joins vagus in distribution to pharynx and larynx - - - - - - sternocleidomastoid and trapezius	nucleus ambiguus - - - - - - NA: Spinal column origin	none	
Hypoglossal N. CN XII	tongue	hypoglossal nucleus	none	
Cervical Nerves 1-3	paramedian muscles between mandible, hyoid, and shoulder girdle	NA: Spinal column origin	dermatones of head, neck, shoulder	NA: Spinal column origin
Cervical Nerves 3-5	diaphragm	NA: Spinal column origin	dermatones of neck, shoulder, anterior arm	NA: Spinal column origin

The upper cervical nerves also play an important role in these three functions. Although they provide motor innervation to a relatively small number of muscles in this area, they are the muscles that link the mandible, hyoid, and shoulder girdle. These muscles, therefore, are a key to providing stability and maintenance of craniocervical posture during sucking, swallowing, and breathing.

In the brain stem, particularly the medulla, there are further structural interrelationships (see figure 1-5). Research on swallowing suggests that afferent input is primarily localized in the nucleus of the tractus solitarius (NTS), while efferent control is localized in the nucleus ambiguus (NA) as well as the trigeminal and hypoglossal nuclei.[7,8,9] In regard to respiration, afferent input is also received in the NTS. Efferent respiratory control is via premotoneurons in the medulla, which then project to spinal cord motoneurons and innervate the respiratory skeletal musculature. These premotoneurons are again felt to be located in areas of the NTS and NA.[6] During sucking, afferent input from the jaw, tongue, and oral mucosa via cranial nerves V, VII, and IX projects to the trigeminal sensory nucleus and the NTS. Additional patterns of facilitory and inhibitory interneuronal connections between the nuclei of the medulla are currently being explored.

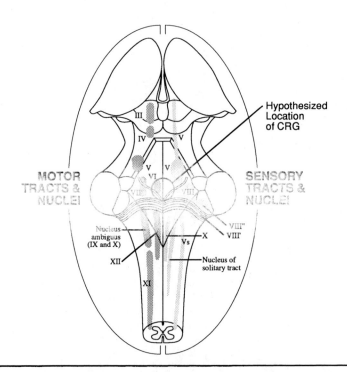

Figure 1-5 Brain-stem regions serving sucking, swallowing, and respiration.

FUNCTIONAL ANATOMY AND PHYSIOLOGY

Inherent in the activities of sucking, swallowing, and respiration are rhythmic patterns. Quiet respiration and non-nutritive sucking are each characterized by their own rhythmic pattern. In infant feeding, the rhythm of sucking must be highly coordinated with the rhythm of swallowing and breathing. Literature in the areas of oral control, deglutition, and respiratory control describes the presence of a "central rhythm generator" (CRG).[5,6,8,10] Although there is controversy over the exact neuronal populations and circuits, this CRG appears to be located in the medulla, adjacent to the NTS, NA, and reticular formation.[6,7,8] Its functions have been described as facilitating jaw depression/elevation in an alternating rhythmic pattern,[10] generating appropriate rhythmic patterns to drive oscillating inspiratory and expiratory neurons for respiration,[6] and perhaps initiating and sequencing swallowing.[8] It is also tempting to speculate that such a center would be responsible for inhibiting respiration during swallowing and thus aid in establishing the rhythm for coordinated sucking, swallowing, and breathing during feeding. Miller suggests that the CRG may react to "patterns" of synaptic activity and that its ability to respond to various patterns of synaptic activity may change with maturation.[5] Perhaps this is one factor that contributes to changes in respiratory and feeding rhythms with increasing age.

Pontine, subcortical, and cortical structures also play a role in sucking, swallowing, and breathing, primarily providing modifications to these functions as the infant matures. Via the higher structures, volitional inhibition and facilitation of sucking, swallowing, and breathing are possible to varying degrees. These responses can also be modified and integrated with other functions. The brain stem, however, is the region essential to the basic responses of sucking, swallowing, and breathing, particularly in infancy.

Sucking

Sucking plays a key role in the life of the young infant. Not only is it the primary means for receiving nutrition, but it can provide calming and pacification, and it is an initial method of exploring the environment. *Sucking, suckling, sucking act*—these are just a few of the terms found in the literature describing mouthing movements and the ingestion of food by the infant. Not only are there several terms, but the same term may be defined differently by each author. In this text *sucking* is the only term that will be used, and it will describe the rhythmic movements of the infant's mouth and tongue either on the bottle or breast to obtain nourishment or on a pacifier, hand, or other object to modulate state or explore the environment.

Sucking is observed in utero as early as 15 to 18 weeks gestation.[45,46,47] In the extrauterine environment, mouthing activity may be observed at 27 to

28 weeks, though in a disorganized and random pattern. These immature "sucks" are quite weak. By 32 weeks, stronger sucking is noted and a burst-pause pattern is emerging, though a stable rhythm to sucking is not established until 34 weeks. Sucking and the related components necessary for effective feeding are generally not reported to be present until 34 to 35 weeks gestation.[22,24,25] (Information on the development of sucking in the premature infant is found in chapter 6.)

Biomechanics of Sucking

Sucking pressure: Considering sucking as a pumping system and the mouth as a pump, the biomechanical principles of sucking can be described and applied to the evaluation and treatment of feeding problems in infants. A pump can be defined as a device that pushes or draws fluid out of something by differential pressure.

The key concept is that during infant feeding, fluid moves primarily because of changes in pressure. Two types of pressure can be created. *Positive pressure* or compression "pushes" fluid out of something, whereas *negative pressure* or suction "draws" fluid out. Both types of pressure can be generated within the infant's mouth. As the tongue compresses the nipple, positive pressure is created, which expels liquid (figure 1-6). With the oral cavity sealed, as the jaw and tongue drop down, the cavity is enlarged. This enlarging creates negative intra-oral pressure, or suction, which pulls fluid into the mouth (figure 1-7). To produce suction, the oral cavity must be fully sealed, or tongue and jaw movements will be ineffective in creating suction.

Early studies considered the role of these two types of pressure in infant feeding. Ardran and Kemp, in imaging studies of breast-and bottle-feeding, stressed the role of the tongue in squeezing or compressing the nipple to express milk into the mouth.[28,29] Colley and Creamer, on the other hand, emphasized the role of the tongue in creating negative intra-oral pressure, thus producing suction that stimulates fluid to flow through a bottle nipple.[40] It now appears that each type of pressure, positive and negative, plays a role in infant feeding.[19,24,34]

Ellison et al. have studied these components of sucking during the first hour of life.[26] In term newborns five minutes after birth, compression is the primary component of sucking, though over the first hour of life this changes rapidly. Not only does the total sucking pressure (compression plus suction pressure) increase roughly 16-fold, but by one hour of age nearly 90% of the pressure is created by the suction component.

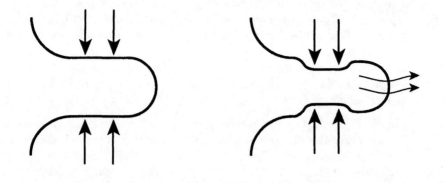

Figure 1-6 Positive pressure or compression "pushes" fluid out of the nipple.

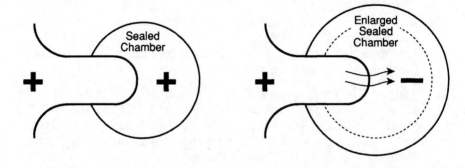

Figure 1-7 Negative pressure or suction "draws" fluid out of the nipple.

The young infant also shows great adaptability of these components. Sameroff has demonstrated that newborns are able to separate the suction and compression components of sucking based on the feeding condition.[41] A feeding apparatus was designed that could alternate between a suction-feeding condition and a compression-feeding condition. When fluid flow responded only to compression, the infant's suction diminished significantly. When fluid flow responded only to suction, suction increased, though compression was always present. This flexibility may aid the infant in feeding from both breast and bottle, as it appears that each type of pressure may be utilized differently in these two feeding situations.

It is likely that in bottle-feeding the development of adequate negative pressure and suction is crucial to efficient fluid flow. Although compression of the nipple delivers some fluid, infants who are able to compress the nipple but not develop suction (such as those with cleft lip or palate) generally cannot obtain adequate volume without modification to the bottle or nipple. Neither type of pressure is necessary to position the nipple or maintain the nipple in the mouth during bottle-feeding. Although some infants might "suck" the bottle nipple into the mouth, it can also be placed in the mouth, and its semirigid construction maintains it there.

On the breast, however, negative pressure and suction are prerequisite for drawing the nipple into the baby's mouth and maintaining its position. In breast-feeding it is not clear which pressure component is more important in actual milk delivery. Although mothers can obtain milk using only negative pressure (as with an electric breast pump) or only positive pressure (as with manual expression), the combination of these two types of pressure may be necessary for maximally effective breast-feeding.[26,44] (See chapter 8 for further information on breast-feeding.)

Motoric components: During sucking, the infant's mouth must also manage the bolus of food or fluid and move it appropriately to initiate the swallowing response. Each oral structure has specific roles to play so that the functions of sucking work effectively.

Tongue. The tongue plays a key role in all aspects of sucking. The tongue helps seal the oral cavity. Anteriorly, in conjunction with the lower lip, the tongue seals against the nipple. Posteriorly, the tongue seals against the soft palate until the palate is lifted during swallowing. With the nipple in the mouth, the anterior portion of the tongue elevates, compressing the nipple and producing positive pressure, which expresses some fluid. During sucking the posterior tongue also lowers, increasing the volume of the oral cavity. Because the oral cavity is sealed, negative intra-oral pressure, or suction, is created to pull fluid into the mouth.

The tongue also forms a "central groove" in the anterior-posterior direction. This configuration helps to stabilize the nipple and channels liquid toward the pharynx. Finally, the tongue assists in forming the fluid into a cohesive bolus and in maintaining the bolus in the mouth until the swallowing reflex is triggered.

Jaw. The jaw provides a stable base for movements of other structures. These include the tongue, lips, and cheeks. By moving slightly downward during sucking, the jaw also assists in enlarging the oral cavity to produce suction.

Lips. The lips work with the tongue to form the anterior seal around the nipple. They also help stabilize the nipple position in the mouth.

Cheeks. The cheeks provide stability, and in infants the fat pads are a key to this stability. If the cheeks are not stable, negative pressure will draw them into the mouth and there will be less pressure available to draw fluid from the nipple. The cheeks also provide lateral boundaries for food on the tongue, thus aiding in bolus formation.

Palate. The hard palate works with the tongue to compress the nipple and to maintain nipple position. The soft palate, with the tongue, creates the posterior seal for the oral cavity. It elevates during swallowing to allow passage of the bolus and to seal the nasal cavity and prevent nasal reflux of food.

Movement sequence during sucking: Working together, these structures produce the smooth, rhythmic movements that characterize sucking and allow the infant to take in adequate substance for nourishment. Imaging studies have helped describe the combined movements of these structures, though there are still portions of the movement sequence that are not fully understood. [3,27,30,31,39]

The tongue forms a trough, or central groove, along its longitudinal axis, which receives the nipple. Lateral portions of the tongue are felt to remain in contact with the palate during sucking. The lips and tongue then close around the nipple. The posterior tongue elevates slightly to maintain contact with the soft palate. Laterally the cheeks approximate the tongue and nipple. The medial portion of the tongue then produces a wavelike motion in the anterior-posterior direction. During this peristaltic movement, the nipple is initially compressed between the anterior portion of the tongue and the palate. As the posterior portion of the tongue is depressed, the sealed oral cavity is effectively enlarged, creating negative pressure and suction, propelling the bolus of fluid toward the pharynx. The mandible moves with the tongue in an alternating anterior-inferior, posterior-superior direction.

Morris describes changes in the mechanics of the sucking pattern during the first year of life,[17] although to date imaging studies have not reported such developmental changes. Imaging studies have included infants of varying ages, but none has specifically addressed the question of these developmental changes.[28,31,39] Because we know that the tongue becomes more mobile within the oral cavity and that patterns of mandibular stability change during the first year, it would not be surprising to find changes in the relationship between tongue and jaw movements, though further study is needed. Similarly, the differences in oral-motor patterns during sucking on the breast or bottle are not well documented. While some studies suggest that the tongue movements are distinctly different, others report no difference.[28-31] (See chapter 8 for further comparison of breast- and bottle-feeding.)

Sucking Characteristics

Nutritive and non-nutritive sucking: Two distinct patterns of infant sucking have been described.[32] Nutritive sucking (NS) is the process of obtaining nutrition, while non-nutritive sucking (NNS) occurs in the absence of nutrient flow and may be used to satisfy an infant's basic sucking urge or as a state regulatory mechanism. Many characteristics of sucking differ between NS and NNS (see table 1-2).

Table 1-2 Characteristics of Sucking

	Nutritive Sucking	Non-nutritive Sucking
Purpose	Obtain nourishment	State regulation, satisfy sucking desire, exploration
Rhythm	Initial continuous sucking burst, moving to intermittent sucking bursts with bursts becoming shorter and pauses longer over the course of the feeding	Repetitive pattern of bursts and pauses; stable number of sucks per burst and duration of pauses
Rate	One suck per second, constant over course of feeding	Two sucks per second
Suck: Swallow Ratio	Young infant—1:1, may be higher at end of feed Older infant—2 or 3:1	Very high ratio, 6:1 or 8:1

Sucking rhythm: Both NS and NNS occur in regular patterns of bursts punctuated by pauses. These patterns remain fairly constant in the mature infant and can provide a "sucking signature."[17] Non-nutritive sucking is characterized by a repetitive pattern of bursts and pauses (see figure 1-8). It is generally stable in regard to the number of sucks per burst and the duration of pauses, although it can vary somewhat with changes in state.[32,42] Wolff reports a mean of 7 to 8 sucks per burst and 6- to 7-second pauses between bursts in healthy term infants at 4 days of age.[32]

The nutritive sucking pattern is more complex but varies in a predictable way throughout the feeding period (see figure 1-8). Initially, there is an initial continuous sucking burst that lasts at least 30 seconds, and generally 60 to 80 seconds. The infant then transitions to a period of intermittent sucking. The duration of each sucking burst (and the number of sucks per burst) steadily declines while the length of the pauses steadily increases.[20,23,32,35,42] By the end of a feeding there may be only 2 to 3 sucks in a burst, followed by a 4- to 5-second pause.

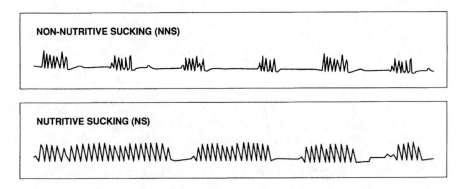

Figure 1-8 Non-nutritive and nutritive sucking patterns.

Sucking rate: Sucking rate is measured during sucking bursts only and does not consider the effect of pauses. It represents the length of time it takes the infant to complete one suck, rather than the actual number of sucks occurring in a given period of time. Although there is some variation in sucking rate among infants, this measurement is felt to be quite stable for an individual infant. During nutritive sucking, the rate averages about one suck per second and remains constant over the course of a feeding. While the length of each suck is the same at the beginning and end of a feeding, the actual number of sucks per minute decreases as the number and length of pauses increases at the end of feeding. The sucking rate is faster in non-nutritive sucking, averaging about 2 sucks per second.[32,42] Again, this value remains fairly constant for each infant. It is felt that the difference in sucking rate between NS and NNS is related to fluid flow. The nutritive sucking rate is slower to allow time for the swallow to occur.[21,33,42]

Swallowing pattern: There are differences in the swallowing pattern between NS and NNS. For the young infant, through most of a feeding session there is a 1:1 ratio of sucking to swallowing. In other words, almost every suck is followed by a swallow. At the end of the feeding, this ratio becomes higher (2:1 or 3:1), with the infant taking 2 to 3 sucks before swallowing.[30] Older infants frequently take several sucks before swallowing. In NNS, the suck:swallow ratio is quite high; there may be 6 to 8 sucks before a swallow, even in the young infant.

These variations in the suck:swallow ratio appear to be dependent on factors such as the rate of flow of liquid and the size of the oral cavity.[33,40] When the flow of liquid is high, swallowing follows each suck. When the flow of liquid is low, sucking pressure diminishes and the ratio increases. In NNS, with no liquid flow and only the need to handle oral secretions, the ratio is the highest.

The size of the oral cavity must also be considered. As the infant becomes several months of age the oral cavity enlarges. It is hypothesized that this allows the infant to hold a greater amount of fluid before needing to initiate a swallow. It may take 2 to 3 sucks to fill the mouth and trigger a swallowing response.

Sucking pressure: This is the characteristic of sucking that shows the most variability, with large differences among and within infants in regard to the type and amount of pressure that is generated. Additionally, the infant appears to have some control over sucking pressure.[41] The two types of pressure (compression and suction), as well as the infant's control in selecting compression versus suction, are discussed above.

In regard to the amount of pressure that is generated, suction pressures from -15 mm Hg to -130 mm Hg have been reported. Although numerous studies have measured sucking pressures, lack of consistency of measuring techniques makes comparison or compilation of data difficult.[26,33,36,37,38,41] It does appear that an infant can generate more pressure through negative intra-oral pressure (suction) than by positive pressure on the nipple (compression).[26] Sucking pressure will also vary based on state and behavioral factors. A sleepy infant will generate less pressure than an alert infant; a hungry infant will generate more pressure than one who is full. Finally, feeding characteristics can affect sucking pressure. Infants will suck harder for liquid that is sweet. They will also generate more pressure if it is difficult to obtain fluid, and conversely will decrease sucking pressure if the fluid flow is too fast.[41-43] Therefore, sucking pressure plays an important role in modulating fluid flow during nutritive sucking.

Fluid flow: The rate of fluid flow during sucking is the result of the amount of sucking pressure that is generated and the resistance to the flow of fluid. Resistance is influenced by factors such as nipple hole size, viscosity of fluid, and stiffness of nipple. (See chapter 7 for further discussion of this subject.) It can be calculated that a term neonate takes from 0.1 to 0.5 cc of fluid per suck.[35,41] This may increase with age.[37]

Etiologies of Sucking Abnormalities

In addition to specific problems in the oral area, dysfunction in any system relating to the feeding process (gastrointestinal, cardiorespiratory, swallowing) may lead to sucking refusal or abnormalities in sucking. This is due to the interrelationships among these processes. Although it is difficult to list all the possible causes for sucking dysfunction, several categories of oral causes for abnormalities in sucking can be described, including anatomic defects, poor muscular control, and pain. Some examples of specific problems in each category are described below.

Anatomic defects: The most frequently seen anatomic defects in the oral area are clefts of the lip and/or palate. Micrognathia (a recessed jaw and posteriorly placed tongue) may be seen independently or with a cleft, as in the Pierre-Robin malformation sequence. Some infants may have an excessively large tongue or macroglossia, and at times hemangiomas or masses are found in the tongue.

Poor muscular control: When there is poor muscular control in the oral area, it is generally secondary to some type of neurologic deficit. Such deficits include asphyxia, cranial hemorrhages, Down syndrome, and cerebral palsy.

Oral pain: If an infant is experiencing pain in the oral area, it may lead to sucking or feeding refusal. Some conditions that may cause pain or discomfort with feeding include oral infections, such as thrush or HSV lesions, or oral trauma/lacerations of any kind. It appears that infants' responses to oral pain and discomfort vary; only some infants develop feeding refusals and "sucking problems" in response to these conditions.

Swallowing

Swallowing is an extremely complex motor sequence involving the coordination of a large number of muscles in the mouth, pharynx, larynx, and the esophagus. Swallowing provides the mechanism by which food is transported from the environment to the alimentary tract for the survival of the infant.

In Utero Development of Swallowing

At approximately 26 days of fetal age, the respiratory and swallowing systems diverge to pursue independent development.[48] Since swallowing plays such a crucial role for the infant, it develops early[7,49] and has been described in fetuses as early as 12 to 14 weeks gestation.[7,45,46,47]

Swallowing by the fetus plays a significant role in the regulation of amniotic fluid volume in the normal pregnancy.[49] It is estimated that near term gestation, the normal fetus swallows approximately half of the total volume of amniotic fluid per day.[51] Polyhydramnios, a condition during pregnancy characterized by too much amniotic fluid, can be observed when there are anatomical defects that would affect swallowing, such as esophageal atresia,[34,52] or when a brain-stem lesion affecting swallowing occurs.[6] Thus, during pregnancy, an imbalance in the maternal-fetal regulation of amniotic fluid can be an indication of swallowing dysfunction.

Phases of Swallowing

The swallowing process is generally divided into a number of segments or phases to better describe the sequence of events. Researchers differ on the number of phases used to describe swallowing; however, three phases appear to be most commonly used: (1) the oral phase, (2) the pharyngeal phase, and (3) the esophageal phase. These phases, including sensory and motor innervation, will each be discussed separately.

Oral Phase
The oral phase of swallowing, also called the oral preparatory phase[5] or the lingual transport phase,[4] is involved in processing the food, so that it is small enough to progress through the pharynx and esophagus, and in propelling the food from the front of the mouth into the pharynx. In babies, the oral phase consists almost exclusively of sucking, as described in the preceding section. These oral activities are generally under voluntary control, with a foundation of subcortical reflexively mediated sucking in early infancy.[9,53]

An important function of the oral phase is the formulation of the food into a mass or bolus and holding the bolus in the mouth until it is released into the pharynx as the swallow is triggered. In infants, the transfer of liquids from the front of the mouth into the pharynx often appears to be one continuous motion. Although the sequence of events happens extremely quickly, it is important that the bolus be maintained as a cohesive mass so that liquid does not leak into the pharynx prior to triggering the swallow. Thus, the oral phase of swallowing, as reflected in the infant's oral-motor or sucking skills, sets the stage for the proper timing and coordination of the swallowing reflex.

Neural Control of the Oral Phase
Motor control: Three cranial nerves provide efferent control of the oral phase of swallowing. (See table 1-3.) Motoric control of the lips, cheeks, and mouth is accomplished by the facial nerve (CN VII). This nerve

supplies not only the musculature involved in the oral phase of swallowing but also those muscles controlling facial expression. The tongue movements of the oral phase are supplied by the hypoglossal nerve (CN XII). Jaw movements are controlled by the trigeminal nerve (CN V).

Sensory control (table 1-3): The oral region has many touch and pressure receptors that determine the shape, texture, and stereognostic qualities of the oral stimulus. This input is carried by the trigeminal nerve (CN V).[54] Sensory input about the position of the mandible, which is continually provided from the position of the temporomandibular joints and the length and tension of the muscles that elevate the mandible, is also carried through the trigeminal nerve (CN V). Taste is carried through cranial nerves VII and IX.[52] Peripheral sensory feedback from the palate and pharynx also assists with the tongue movements of the oral phase of swallowing.[55]

Table 1-3 Neural Control of the Oral Phase of Swallowing

Sensory		Motor
CN V (shape/texture)	Mouth	CN VII
CN VII, IX (taste)	Tongue	CN XII
CN V (position of TMJ)	Jaw	CN V

Initiation of the Swallowing Reflex

The demarcation between the oral and pharyngeal phases of swallowing occurs with the actual initiation of the swallowing reflex. The initiation of swallowing is dependent on sensory feedback from a number of areas, primarily at the faucial arches, but also from the uvula, soft palate, and posterior tongue and pharynx.[5]

Once the bolus reaches the faucial arches, however, swallowing is not automatically initiated. The threshold for elicitation of swallowing can be altered by input from higher cortical and hypothalamic regions, which integrate swallowing with visceral and somatic sensations,[5] or from the periphery by stimuli such as coldness.[56] In our clinical experience, changes in the speed of elicitation of the swallowing reflex can also be altered as a baby's medical status changes. For example, if an infant experiences an exacerbation of respiratory disease, the timing of the initiation of the swallow may be altered. Once the respiratory disease returns to baseline, the swallowing function may also return to baseline.

Control of Swallowing: Reflexive or Voluntary?

In trying to understand the motor control of swallowing, investigators have been faced with the question of the role of sensory information.[4] Swallowing has traditionally been thought of as a peripheral reflex dependent upon sensory information. The process of swallowing, with its interaction at all levels of the nervous system, however, is too complex to be considered simply a stereotyped reflex. On the one hand are the highly variable movements of the mouth, and on the other hand are the more invariable peristaltic movements of the esophagus.[4]

Kennedy and Kent describe swallowing as having at least three levels of organization.[4] The lowest level is the bolus and how it interacts with muscle forces in all phases of swallowing. The properties of the bolus in terms of size, shape, and consistency will affect muscular activity throughout all phases. The second level involves the subcortical pattern generators, reflexes, and other subcortical circuits that can generate the motor sequence of swallowing in the absence of sensory input. The third level includes descending cortical influences. These might include input from the stomach or vestibular system that may create conditions that either facilitate or inhibit the behavior of swallowing.

The complex nature of these three interacting levels seems to preclude characterizing the act of swallowing, or deglutition, as a two-dimensional phenomenon that is either voluntary or reflexive. The motor activities of swallowing can better be described by a continuum of variability.[4] There is significant variability in the oral phase during bolus preparation, somewhat less variability in the pharyngeal phase, and the least variability and greatest "repeatability" in the esophageal phase. Thus, the act of swallowing contains features of voluntary and reflexive behaviors throughout all phases.

Pharyngeal Phase

There appear to be three functional components of the pharyngeal phase of swallowing: (1) the closure of the nasal, laryngeal, and oral openings to prevent fluid leakage and to channel the direction of the bolus; (2) the opening of the cricopharyngeal sphincter; and (3) the creation of sufficient pharyngeal pressure gradient to transport the bolus from the oral cavity to the opening of the esophagus.[4]

Twenty-six muscles and six cranial nerves must be coordinated for the pharyngeal swallow to occur safely and efficiently. The pharyngeal phase of swallowing is initiated by the impact of the bolus on the sensory receptors of the soft palate, pharyngeal walls, faucial arches, and tongue. This tactile and pressure input activates the complex motor events of the pharyngeal phase. The duration of the pharyngeal phase is approximately one second.[5] The muscular activity of the pharyngeal phase appears to be a time-locked sequence. If the duration of this phase is lengthened, the activity of the muscles is elongated; however, the sequence remains constant.[58]

The pharyngeal phase begins with a "leading complex"[58] that raises the hyoid and contracts the posterior and lateral pharyngeal walls to help seal the nasopharynx. The bolus is propelled into the pharynx by the combined actions of the posterior portion of the tongue and the sequential contraction of the pharyngeal constrictors. This begins the pharyngeal peristaltic wave and the changing pressure gradients that propel the bolus through the pharynx.[4]

The larynx and hyoid continue to elevate while the laryngeal vestibule closes and the epiglottis tilts downward.[9] The epiglottis diverts the food to the sides long enough to insure sufficient closure of the larynx to prevent aspiration or pressure leakage.[59] The wave of pharyngeal constrictor contraction and pressure continues with the bolus passing through the hypopharynx and through the open cricopharyngeal sphincter. The pharyngeal airway opens again as the hyoid, larynx, soft palate, and tongue return to their resting positions. This sequence of events is graphically depicted in figure 1-9.

During the pharyngeal phase of swallowing, the bolus is propelled not only by the action of muscle contraction but also by the force of changing pressure gradients throughout the mouth, pharynx, and esophagus. Pressure gradients are created by the active contraction of pharyngeal muscles that sequentially narrow the pharyngeal lumen and by tonic contraction of muscles (such as the cricopharyngeus) that separate the pharynx into compartments and prevent pressure leakage. Several forces assist the pressure gradients in moving the food through the system: (1) the momentum of the bolus; (2) the translational force on the bolus from the posterior movement of the tongue; (3) peristaltic contractions; and (4) the force of gravity.[4] Momentum appears to be an important factor as the bolus is projected into the pharynx at a rapid rate.[60] The influence of the force of gravity can change not only with a change in the position of the body but also with the specific gravity of the materials that comprise the bolus.[61]

Neural Control of the Pharyngeal Phase

Motor control: The motoric innervation of the pharyngeal components of swallowing is through cranial nerves V, VII, IX, X, and XII, with some contributions from cervical cord segments C1-3 (see table 1-4, page 29). There is substantial overlap of motoric innervation, and this overlap underscores the importance of preserving function of the pharyngeal swallow. The entire sequence of movement and corresponding innervation[9] is summarized in table 1-5 (page 29).

Sensory control: Sensory innervation of the pharyngeal phase of swallowing is controlled primarily through cranial nerves V, IX, and X (see table 1-4). Most of the sensory input from the pharynx and larynx that elicits and guides swallowing is conveyed by the glossopharyngeal and vagus nerves (CN IX and X).[9,52] Sensations arising from the posterior

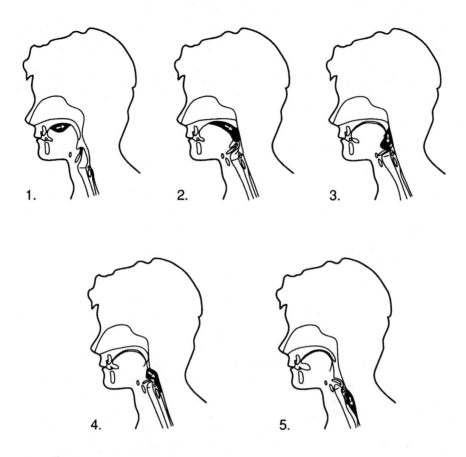

Figure 1-9 Steps in the pharyngeal phase of swallowing.

1. The initiation of the swallow occurs as the bolus is propelled backward by the tongue. Opposition of the tongue and soft palate prevent premature leakage of the bolus into the pharynx before the swallow is initiated.

2. As the swallow is initiated, the soft palate elevates and the posterior pharyngeal wall constricts to close the nasal cavity.

3. The larynx elevates and the epiglottis folds downward to cover the open airway. The true and false vocal folds also contract to provide additional airway protection. The bolus moves through the pharynx by the combined action of pharyngeal peristalsis and changing pressure gradients within the pharynx.

4. The bolus moves past the closed airway. The cricopharyngeus muscle relaxes and opens, allowing the bolus to pass into the esophagus.

5. Once the bolus is totally within the esophagus, the cricopharyngeus tonically closes to prevent reflux back into the pharynx. Peristalsis carries the bolus to the stomach.

tongue, uvula, and soft palate travel through the ninth cranial nerve, with a small portion of sensation to the palate and upper pharynx traveling through the trigeminal nerve (CN V).

Table 1-4 Neural Control of the Pharyngeal Phase of Swallowing

Sensory		Motor
CN V, IX	Palate	CN V, VII, IX, X
CN IX	Tongue	CN V, VII, XII
CN V, X	Pharynx	CN IX and X
CN X	Larynx	CN IX and X
	Cricopharyngeus	CN X

Table 1-5 Innervation of the Motor Sequence during the Pharyngeal Phase of Swallowing

- Backward movement of tongue to soft palate—CN V, VII, XII
- Movement of soft palate to tongue—CN V
- Palatal elevation and posterior pharyngeal wall constriction—CN V, IX, X
- Elevation of hyoid and tongue—CN VII, XII spinal cord segments C1-3
- Epiglottis descends, larynx elevates—CN IX, X
- Action of pharyngeal constrictors—CN IX, X
- Opening of cricopharyngeal sphincter—CN X
- After swallow, palate returns to resting position—CN V
- Tongue returns to resting position—CN XII, C1-3
- Larynx reopens and descends—CN IX, X, C1-3

Sensory receptors and fields: The pharynx and the larynx are richly supplied with chemoreceptors, slow-adapting stretch/pressure receptors (barroreceptors), and temperature receptors. The purpose of the receptors is to initiate and modify the swallow. Two concepts seem to underlie the sensory components of the pharyngeal swallow: (1) there are regions that are highly sensitive to specific kinds of sensory input, and (2) there is a broad area containing many receptive fields.[4] The large number of receptive sites for the elicitation of swallowing suggests that a group of sensory neurons must be stimulated to initiate

---

swallowing.[58] Combining stimuli from many sites over many nerves appears to be the most effective mechanism to trigger the swallow.[5]

The type of stimulus that initiates swallowing varies throughout the oropharyngeal and laryngeal regions. There is variability between regions in terms of sensitivity to the type of stimulus, intensity of stimulus needed to evoke a response, and distribution of receptor types within the receptive fields.[5] In the laryngeal region, liquids such as water appear to be the most effective stimuli to stimulate swallowing, while slow-adapting touch and pressure receptors appear to be more effective in the pharyngeal area.[62,64]

Esophageal Phase

The esophageal phase of swallowing is the final segment in the transfer of nutrients from the mouth to the stomach. It involves the coordinated relaxation of two sphincters, one at each end of the esophagus, and peristaltic action to propel the bolus.[65] At the rostral end of the esophagus is the upper esophageal sphincter (UES). At the caudal end is the lower esophageal sphincter (LES). The peristaltic contraction of the esophageal longitudinal and circular muscles alters the pressure of the esophageal lumen moving the bolus downward.[66]

The pharynx, cricopharyngeal sphincter, and the rostral end of the esophagus are composed of striated (voluntary) muscle, while the lower esophagus and LES are composed of smooth (involuntary) muscle.[67] Two types of esophageal peristalsis are observed, depending on whether the trigger for peristalsis is a pharyngeal swallow or a bolus within the esophagus. Primary peristalsis is associated with the pharyngeal phase of swallowing and involves the contraction of the entire esophagus, including both striated and smooth muscles. This type of peristalsis is dependent upon brain-stem motor output. Secondary peristalsis occurs independent of the pharyngeal swallow. It occurs when a bolus remains in the esophagus and consists primarily of smooth muscle action. Secondary peristalsis is dependent on local segmental ganglionic reflex arcs interconnected over the length of the esophagus, not on cortical control.[66,67]

Neural Control of the Esophageal Phase

Motor control: Motorically, the esophageal phase of swallowing begins with simultaneous inhibition of both smooth and striated muscles over the entire length of the esophagus. This is followed by descending excitatory signals, which activate the rostral to caudal motor sequence.[66] Both inhibitory and excitatory signals are carried by the vagus nerve (CN X). Descending motor impulses synapse through interneurons in the medulla of the brain stem, which can interact with cortical or subcortical nuclei that control the pharyngeal phase of swallowing. From these interactions the esophageal phase can be modified (see table 1-6).

Table 1-6 Neural Control of the Esophageal Phase of Swallowing

Sensory		Motor
CN X (superior laryngeal n.)	UES upper esophagus	CN X
CN X (recurrent laryngeal n.)	Lower esophagus	CN X
CN X (thoracic branches)	Distal esophagus LES	CN X

Sensory control: Sensory feedback during peristalsis is through the vagus nerve. The superior laryngeal nerve (SLN) innervates the upper esophageal sphincter and upper esophagus, the recurrent laryngeal nerve (RLN) innervates the lower esophagus, and the thoracic branches of the vagus nerve innervate the distal esophagus and the LES.[58] Touch to the esophageal mucosa or pressure to the deep mechanoreceptors can excite receptors and affect esophageal peristalsis. Sensory feedback from the bolus itself as it progresses through the esophagus is an important component in the initiation of esophageal peristalsis (see table 1-6).

Brain-Stem Organization of Swallowing

Many structural and functional systems are actively involved in the complex motor sequence of swallowing. These systems are directly controlled by centers in the medulla oblongata portion of the brain stem. Modulation of these brain-stem functions occurs through higher cortical centers or centers of the pons and limbic systems.[4] The organization of the swallowing motor sequence is dependent on activity of a neuronal network called the swallowing center in the medulla.[58,68] Some hypothesize that this motor sequence is centrally programmed and once initiated can be performed entirely without afferent feedback.[57,69]

The swallowing center can be divided into three levels or subsystems[58] (see figure 1-10). (1) An afferent level provides sensory input to this center. This level contains the fibers of the major nerves involved in the initiation of swallowing. (2) An efferent level conveys the motor commands from the center. (3) An organizing level composed of the interneuronal network programs the motoneurons for the whole motor sequence of swallowing through excitatory and inhibitory connections between neurons. There is still controversy over the exact location of this interneuronal network in the brain stem.[8]

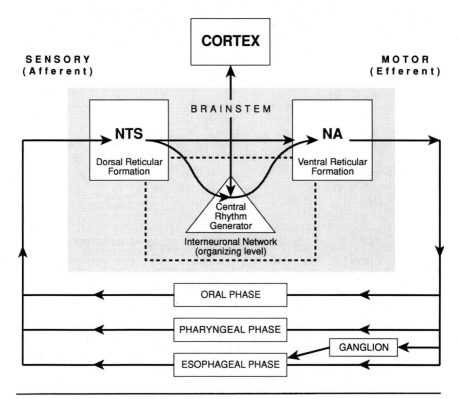

Figure 1-10 Organization of brain-stem control of swallowing.

Afferent system: The afferent nerve fibers of cranial nerves X (especially the SLN and the RLN), IX, and V, which are involved in the initiation of swallowing, converge into the solitary and trigeminal tracts and then progress to the nucleus tractus solitarius (NTS) in the brain stem. The swallowing neurons within the NTS and adjacent dorsal reticular formation play a main role in the initiation of swallowing. It is thought that this area serves not only as a relay station for sensory input but also as an integrative area for swallowing.[69] Swallowing interneurons are also located within the NTS and adjacent reticular formation and may constitute a major portion of the organizing level of the swallowing center.[8]

Efferent system: The efferent portion of the swallowing center, or output arm, is composed of motoneurons localized in the nucleus ambiguus (NA) and adjacent ventral reticular formation.[54,58,68] The swallowing neurons of this ventral group probably receive their input from the dorsal neurons and distribute the swallowing excitation to the various motoneurons involved in swallowing (cranial nerves V, VII, IX, X, XII).[8]

Organizing (interneuronal) system: The interneuronal network is thought to include portions of the dorsal region (NTS and adjacent reticular formation) and the ventral region (the NA and adjacent reticular formation).[8] These core interneurons have often been described as "central pattern generators" for the pattern of pharyngeal and esophageal muscle contraction.[58,69,70] It is hypothesized that each side of the brain stem has its own central pattern generator.[5] In addition, there may be separate centers responsible for generating patterns of pharyngeal and esophageal muscle contractions.[69]

Etiologies of Swallowing Dysfunction

When an infant presents with a swallowing disorder, there are multiple potential etiologies. These etiologies of swallowing have been categorized using a number of frameworks: whether they are congenital anatomical defects or neuromuscular abnormalities,[53,71,73] according to the phase of swallowing during which the problem occurs,[52,53,71,72] and in terms of functional suppression versus paralysis.[74]

Anatomic or Neuromuscular Abnormalities
Congenital anatomic defects that influence swallowing can occur anywhere in the mouth, palate, larynx, pharynx, or esophagus. These may include cleft lip and palate, micrognathia, laryngeal clefts, tracheoesophageal fistulas, esophageal lesions or dysmotility, vascular rings,[75] or trauma and foreign bodies. Neuromuscular abnormalities can include delays in maturation such as prematurity, brain damage from anoxic encephalopathy, congenital infections such as CMV or acquired infections such as AIDS,[76] hydrocephalus, vascular accident, or cerebral palsy. Other possibilities are myopathies such as Werdnig-Hoffman disease, syndromes like Prader-Willi,[77] chromosomal defects, cranial nerve palsies, or bulbar and pseudobulbar palsies such as Moebius syndrome.

Suppression versus Paralysis
Ardran and Kemp feel one must attempt to differentiate between swallowing difficulties that are due to functional suppression versus paralysis and neuromuscular causes.[74] These authors feel that most muscular contractions, including those involved in swallowing, can be suppressed either by failure to acquire the normal reflex or through voluntary suppression. Failure to acquire the normal reflex response can be secondary to cerebral damage or immaturity. Disuse, such as that observed in infants who are unable to feed for lengthy periods of time secondary to unrepaired congenital defects or other unusual environmental factors, may cause an infant to suppress the swallowing reflex. We have observed infants who fail to swallow while they are experiencing significant compromise in their pulmonary or cardiovascular system. With resolution or improvement in these conditions, swallowing function returns.

Swallowing Dysfunction According to Phases

In clinical practice, swallowing dysfunction is frequently classified according to the timing or phase during which aspiration occurs: before, during, or after the swallow. This system leads to a functional approach, since it may point directly to intervention strategies. Using this classification system, underlying neuromuscular, structural, or anatomic problems must still be considered.

Aspiration before the swallow: Dysfunction of the oral phase of swallowing, *particularly in bolus formation and retention, can result in aspiration* before the swallow. If the tongue is not able to form the bolus and maintain it in a cohesive mass in the mouth until the swallowing reflex is triggered, portions of the bolus may fall over the posterior portion of the tongue in a piecemeal fashion. Since the swallowing reflex has not yet been triggered, these portions of the bolus can fall into the unprotected larynx and be aspirated.[78] Delay in triggering the swallowing reflex, often in the presence of an intact oral phase, can result in pooling of the bolus in the vallecular and pyriform sinuses. This pooled material may then be aspirated prior to the swallow. The longer the delay in initiating the swallowing reflex, the greater the risk of aspirating all or a part of the bolus.[79]

Aspiration during the swallow: Aspiration during the swallow is usually caused by reduced or insufficient laryngeal elevation and closure.[80] Protection of the airway occurs at three levels that close in ascending order: the true vocal folds, the false vocal folds, and the aryepiglottic folds and the epiglottis. Aspiration during the swallow can occur if liquids or solids seep under the epiglottis and into the airway prior to sufficient closure by the larynx.

Some infants may have changes in the ability of the larynx to seal off the airway over the course of the feeding. As the feeding progresses and the infant fatigues, laryngeal elevation may become impaired. Thus, aspiration during the swallow may occur only toward the end of the feeding, as the infant tires, and not at the beginning of the feeding. Cumming and Reilly have termed this condition "fatigue aspiration."[59]

Aspiration after the swallow: Aspiration after the swallow is generally secondary to residual liquids or solids in the pharynx following the completion of the swallow. This material is then inhaled or aspirated into the airway. The residue may result from decreased pharyngeal peristalsis, failure to generate appropriate pressure gradients, reduced laryngeal elevation, or dysfunction of the cricopharyngeus muscle.[79] Also, if there is nasopharyngeal reflux during the swallow, the material left in the nasopharynx may trickle down the pharynx into the open airway and be aspirated after the swallow.[81]

Respiration

The purpose of the respiratory system in the infant is to maintain a balance of oxygen and carbon dioxide in the blood in order to meet the infant's changing metabolic needs during activities such as feeding, sleeping, or playing. This is accomplished through gas exchange in the lungs between the circulating blood and the alveoli. Rhythmic movement of the diaphragm and respiratory skeletal muscles expands and contracts the thorax to move air into and out of the lungs. Air moves through the nose, mouth, and upper airways (composed of the pharynx, larynx, and trachea), into the lower airways, (the bronchi and bronchioles), and then down to the alveoli, which serve as the final site of gas exchange (see figure 1-11).

The rhythmic drive for inspiration and exhalation originates in the brain stem. Chemoreceptors provide sensory information about oxygen/carbon dioxide status and acid/base balance in the blood. Mechanoreceptors (stretch receptors) in the upper and lower airways provide sensory information on the volume of air in the lungs and amount of resistance to airflow through the airways, thereby assisting with regulation of the rate and depth of respiration.

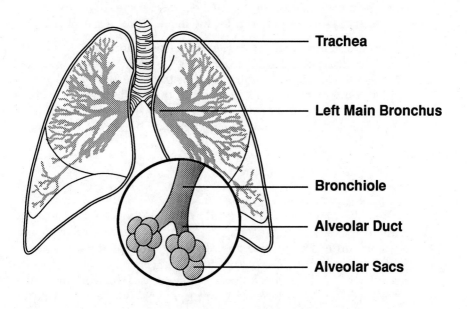

Trachea

Left Main Bronchus

Bronchiole

Alveolar Duct

Alveolar Sacs

Figure 1-11 Basic anatomy of the lower airways and lungs.

Mechanisms of Adjustment in the Respiratory System

The respiratory system has a number of mechanisms by which the rate of exchange of oxygen and carbon dioxide can be adjusted to meet the infant's varying metabolic needs. These include the respiratory rate, the depth of respirations, and changes in heart function associated with changes in respiratory drive.

Respiratory rate: Changes in the rate of respiration occur to maintain appropriate gas exchange. The frequency of breaths taken may increase or decrease, and changes in the length of the inspiratory and/or expiratory phases can occur. For example, if the alveoli have been damaged (such as with bronchopulmonary dysplasia), the number of sites available for gas exchange will be reduced. The baby may need to increase the rate of breathing to compensate for this loss of gas exchange sites.

Depth of respiration: The amount of air moved into and out of the lungs with a given breath is the tidal volume. Increases or decreases in tidal volume can occur separately or in conjunction with changes in respiratory rate. Tidal volume can be influenced by the strength of the baby's diaphragm and intercostal muscles, the resistance to airflow through the upper and lower airways during respiration, the structural integrity of the thorax, the compliance of the lung tissue, and the proportion of the lung alveoli that are healthy and available for gas exchange.

For example, if there is an increase in airway resistance, the baby would need to increase the depth of breathing to maintain the same tidal volume. If the depth of breathing remains the same, there is a decrease in tidal volume. As another example, if there is a decrease in lung compliance (that is, the lung parenchyma and airways become stiff due to respiratory disease), tidal volume decreases if there is no change in respiratory effort or depth. In this situation, an increase in respiratory rate would probably be needed to meet the infant's metabolic needs.[83]

Work of breathing: Changes can also occur in the amount of effort or work the infant expends with each breath. The work of breathing has two components: one is the work needed to activate muscles that cause the lungs to expand, and the other is the work needed to overcome resistance in the lung tissue and airways.[128] Respiratory disease or abnormalities in pulmonary structure or mechanics can lead to increased work of breathing. Exercise also increases the work of breathing as inspiratory muscles work to bring greater volumes of air into the lungs at higher rates. The work to feed may impose an even greater burden on the respiratory system of an infant who has increased work of breathing at rest.

Heart function: Heart rate and stroke volume (the amount of blood moved with each heartbeat) also change to modify oxygen and carbon dioxide levels in the blood. Changes in heart rate can be triggered through stimulation of the pulmonary mechanoreceptors, which are a vagally mediated reflex arc.[86] These changes allow the infant to pump more blood throughout the body (increasing the stroke volume) or move the blood through the heart and lungs more quickly to meet changing demands.

Respiratory drive: Complex interconnections between respiratory afferent and efferent signals are involved in regulating the "drive" to breathe. (These interconnections will be discussed more fully in the section on brain-stem control.) The peripheral arterial chemoreceptors provide the afferent input, which is responsible for the immediate increase in breathing when there are reduced oxygen or increased carbon dioxide levels in the blood. These chemoreceptors, located in the carotid and aortid bodies, respond to changes in oxygen and carbon dioxide arterial partial pressure (PaO_2 and $PaCO_2$), as well as changes in pH.

The carotid sinus will produce sensory output in response to decreased PaO_2, decreased pH, or increased $PaCO_2$. The aortic bodies will also respond to decreased PaO_2 and increased $PaCO_2$ but are generally not stimulated by a change in arterial pH.[84] In general, respiratory drive is more responsive to changes in carbon dioxide levels rather than oxygen levels. Therefore, changes in respiratory drive occur more frequently in response to changes in $PaCO_2$ and pH than to changes in PaO_2. Babies, however, have significant variability in their respiratory drive responses to CO_2 and may continue to hypoventilate even in the face of rising CO_2.[83] This lower responsivity to increasing blood CO_2 could potentially lead to apnea or hypoxemia.

The flow of air through the larynx and lower airways also influences respiratory drive. Central integration of input from the pulmonary stretch receptors (PSR), which lie in the smooth muscle of the lungs, is thought to be important in determining the rate and depth of breathing. PSRs are activated by lung distention. Their reflex effect is thought to be a slowing of inspiratory frequency by increasing expiratory time.[84] Drive receptors in the larynx assist in monitoring pressure changes in the upper airway to prevent partial airway obstruction leading to increased respiratory work.[85] These mechanoreceptors work in conjunction with the chemoreceptors to provide appropriate regulation and drive to the respiratory system.

Neural and Brain-Stem Control of Respiration

Similar to the neural and brain-stem control of swallowing, respiration has three levels: afferent control, brain-stem organization, and efferent control. Each level will be discussed separately. Their interaction and overall control of respiration is summarized schematically in figure 1-12.

Afferent (Sensory) Control

Nose: In infants, air generally enters the respiratory system through the nose. Sensory input from receptors located in the nasal mucosa travels to the nucleus tractus solitarius (NTS) in the brain stem. Input from these receptors causes changes in the size of the nasal lumen to improve respiration or trigger protective responses. Changes in air pressure and flow through the nose can also stimulate changes in rate and depth of respiration.[82]

Larynx: Sensory receptors at this level respond to mechanical (touch/pressure) and chemical (irritant) stimuli.[87] They again serve functions of airway protection and modulating airflow. Afferents from these receptors travel via the superior laryngeal nerve of the vagus (CN X) to the nucleus tractus solitarius (NTS).

Lungs: Various stretch and irritant receptors are located in the lungs. The pulmonary stretch receptors (PSRs), located within the smooth muscles of the lungs, carry input regarding lung volumes to the NTS via the vagus nerve. Irritant receptors respond to chemical irritants, such as cigarette smoke, and travel to the NTS via the vagus nerve. "J" receptors, located in the walls of the pulmonary capillaries, respond to increases in pulmonary interstitial fluid volume, such as that observed in pulmonary edema or congestion. They also send input via the vagus nerve to the NTS.[84]

Carotid and aortic bodies: These chemoreceptors transmit sensory information about pH, oxygen, and carbon dioxide content along the vagus and glossopharyngeal nerves.

Brain-Stem Organization

The nucleus tractus solitarius (NTS) in the medulla receives information about the effectiveness of gas exchange and mechanics of ventilation from the lungs, carotid and aortic bodies, and larynx through cranial nerves IX and X.[84] This afferent information then converges on an area in the medulla called the "central rhythm generator" (CRG).[84] The exact collection of neurons that make up the CRG and its precise location within the brain stem are still controversial issues. Premotor interneurons are concentrated in two bilateral sites in the tegmentum of the medulla called the dorsal respiratory group (DRG) and the ventral respiratory group (VRG). The DRG is located within the NTS, and the VRG is located within the nucleus

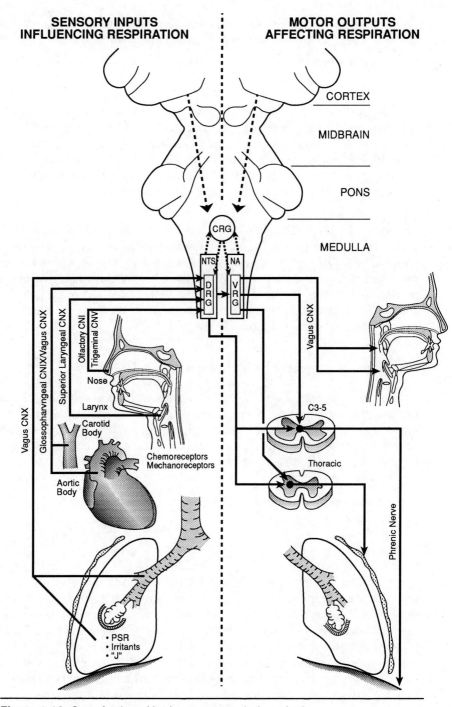

Figure 1-12 Organization of brain-stem control of respiration.

ambiguus (NA). Both the DRG and the VRG neurons project to the contralateral phrenic and intercostal motoneurons in the spinal cord.

The neurons of the DRG and VRG may not be involved in the development of the respiratory rhythm per se but may be driven by neurons within the CRG. Although the CRG may relay information about the basic respiratory rhythm, the DRG and VRG may integrate this with other pertinent afferent information to produce the appropriate pattern of respiratory outflow.[84] Sites rostral to the medulla in the limbic region and thalamus may also exert a modifying influence over respirations. These sites are not involved in respiratory rhythm but may stimulate changes in rate and depth of breathing to coordinate it with other motor and autonomic behaviors.

Efferent (Motor) Control
The spinal cord is the final common pathway for the control of respiration. The diaphragm is innervated by the phrenic nerve from spinal cord segments C3-C5. Other motoneurons at the thoracic and lumbar levels innervate the intercostal and abdominal muscles. The NA, through the motor portions of the vagus nerve, innervates the skeletal muscles of the pharynx and larynx to coordinate these with movements of the thoracic muscles to ensure appropriate and smooth airflow.

Respiratory Protective Mechanisms and Reflexes

The respiratory system has many mechanisms and reflexes involved in the two broad functions of airway maintenance (patency) and airway defense. These serve to keep the airway physically open, so that air is free to flow as efficiently as possible, and to keep the airway clear of foreign bodies or irritants that could cause infection, damage, or obstruction.

Airway Defense Reflexes
The reflexes involved in airway defense and protection keep foreign substances from entering the upper and lower airways by preventing further inhalation, or by expelling them should they enter the airway. These reflex responses arise from receptors located throughout the nose, nasopharynx, upper airway (pharynx and larynx), and the lungs. They are triggered by mechanical or chemical stimuli and result in a wide range of reflex responses, including cough, swallow, and cessation of respiration. In this context, any pause in respiration that is initiated by stimulation of these receptors is considered to be apnea, regardless of duration. Mechanisms such as laryngeal closure or central inhibition of respiratory effort may lead to such apnea. Although a brief apnea can be adaptive by keeping material out of the airway, it can become maladaptive if prolonged, as it can lead to hypoxia and possibly bradycardia. Table 1-7 summarizes these reflex responses by location, receptor, and response.

Table 1-7 Airway Defense Reflexes

Location	Receptor	Possible Response
Nose/Nasopharynx	Chemoreceptor e.g.: water irritant odors	Apnea
	Mechanoreceptor e.g.: touch to nasal mucosa	Sneeze Mucous secretion
Upper Airways		

• Pharynx	Chemoreceptor
	e.g.: residue of:
	e.g.:water
	  acid (GER)
	  milk
	  saline
		Swallowing
		Laryngeal adduction
		Apnea

• Larynx	Chemoreceptor
	e.g.: water
	  milk
	  saline
	  secretions
	  acid (GER)
		Apnea
		Cough
		Swallowing
		Bradycardia
		Bronchoconstriction
		Increased mucous secretion (in response to acid GER)

	Mechanoreceptor e.g.: touch/pressure	Bradycardia Laryngeal closure Cough Swallowing
Lungs	Chemoreceptors/ Mechanoreceptors	Mucociliary clearance Augmented breaths Cough Bronchoconstriction Bronchospasm (in response (to acid/GER)

Nose: Receptors in the nose respond to chemical stimuli (such as water or irritating odors) with a sneeze, an increase in mucous secretion, or apnea.[82] Mechanical stimulation to the nasal mucosa can also lead to a sneeze.[95] Generally these responses function to remove obstructive or irritant material from the nose.

Upper airway: In the pharynx and larynx, which form the upper airway, protective reflexes include cough, apnea, swallowing, laryngeal adduction, bronchoconstriction, mucous secretion, and bradycardia. Apnea and laryngeal adduction serve to prevent inhalation of substances that approach the airway, and swallowing assists in clearing the substance from the pharynx. Cough and mucous secretion assist with removal of the material; bronchoconstriction keeps the material from progressing further down into the airway. Mucus may provide a barrier that traps foreign material, which is then cleared from the airway by ciliary transport and/or through coughing or sneezing. Mucus itself can induce coughing.

The larynx is the site of some of the most potent receptors and contains a large variety of afferent end organs consistent with the richness of the reflex responses. Receptors in this area respond to chemical and mechanical stimuli. Chemical stimuli in the form of water, milk, saline, secretions, or acid (such as refluxed gastric acid) produce powerful reflex responses. The most typical response of the infant to stimulation of the laryngeal protective receptors is brief apnea and swallowing (to clear the material from the airway), followed by a cough.[97] In some infants, however, apneic response to liquids can be quite pronounced, leading to bradycardia.

The apneic response to fluids in the larynx diminishes with age and is superseded by coughing, the primary response in children and adults.[85,98] The maturation of this response in infants has been studied by monitoring coughing after several drops of saline were placed on the vocal cords. At birth to four days of age, only 20% of full-term infants responded by coughing, while 80% coughed at 30 days of age.[97] Thach feels that apnea of prematurity might result from an immaturity or abnormality of this airway protective mechanism.[101] Secretions collecting in the upper airways normally would stimulate sensory receptors and trigger coughing or swallowing. Since the immature response is apnea prior to a swallow, in apnea of prematurity the apneic response may be abnormally prolonged rather than leading to a swallow.[101] A similar pattern of prolonged airway protective responses and lengthy apnea has also been observed in conjunction with respiratory syncytial viral (RSV) infection in young infants.[75]

Water (as compared to milk or saline) appears to be the most potent stimulus of the laryngeal chemoreceptors that elicits this apneic response. The classic "diving reflex," which consists of a triad of effects including apnea, bradycardia, and peripheral vasoconstriction, is induced by water immersion.[97] Water also appears to be the most effective stimulus to elicit protective swallowing—that is, swallowing not elicited from the voluntary act of feeding but rather to clear liquids that impinge on the larynx.[87] Regurgitation can also introduce foreign substances into the larynx, leading to these protective responses. One study noted occurrences of both mixed and obstructive apnea immediately following overt regurgitation in young infants.[99]

Mechanical stimulation of the larynx and pharynx can produce protective responses similar to those produced by chemical stimulation. Swallowing can be induced by mechanical stimulation of the upper airway.[87] Mechanical stimulation of the epithelium of the epiglottis and the supraglottic area of the larynx results in immediate closure of the glottis.[96,98] Coughing can result from stimulation of the mechanoreceptors; however, the neurological control mechanisms, the musculoskeletal functions, and the lung mechanics involved in the cough are not fully developed at birth, and therefore the effectiveness of the cough may be less in the neonatal period.[103] Manipulations in and around the larynx can occasionally cause cardiac arrythmia or cardiac arrest.[85]

Lungs: Chemo- and mechanoreceptors that are responsible for protective reflexes are also located in the lungs. Mucociliary clearance, augmented breaths, or coughing can occur from stimulation of these receptors.[97] Stimulation of such receptors in the tracheobronchial airways can result in bronchoconstriction, which may make the airways less susceptible to collapse during forced expiratory efforts (like a cough) or may prevent particulate matter from entering the alveoli.[85] Irritants, such as cigarette smoke or microaspiration of refluxed gastric acid, can result in bronchospasm or increased respiratory rate.[104]

Airway Maintenance

Neuromuscular and structural mechanisms are involved in maintaining the patency of the airway—that is, maintaining the proper size or caliber of the airway lumen so that airflow is smooth and unobstructed with minimal resistance. All regions of the upper airway may change from their static size and shape either due to the characteristics of the airway wall or by the actions of the muscles controlling airway structures.

The term *airway stability* is commonly used to indicate the ability of the airway to resist collapse. This stability is dependent on a balance between airway-dilating forces and airway-constricting forces. Negative pressure within the airway lumen created during inspiration is a major airway-constricting force, whereas the activity of the airway muscles appears to be a major dilating force. A temporary imbalance between these two forces may account for the pharyngeal airway closures that occur during obstructive apnea.

Airway-constricting forces include airway suction created during inspiration and airway compression caused by neck flexion.[101] Structural abnormalities of the airway can also weaken its ability to resist collapse from changes in pressure or head position and may make the airway more prone to collapse. The magnitude of the intraluminal pressure changes depends on the elasticity of the airway walls, the distribution of resistance along the airway, and the magnitude of the forces that drive airflow.[105]

Airway-dilating forces include the elastic properties of the airway muscles and connective tissue, and the perfusion pressure from its vascular supply.[105] In addition, the active tonic and phasic contraction of the airway musculature plays a crucial role in resisting airway collapse. Tone in the upper airway muscles is regulated by several reflex mechanisms responsive to chemoreceptor or mechanoreceptor stimuli.[106] Studies have shown that the intrinsic elasticity of the infant's upper airway is insufficient to withstand the upper airway collapsing force of the inspiratory suction created during an average breath, implying that an active neuromuscular mechanism is necessary to maintain airway patency.[107] Tonic or phasic muscle contraction is therefore needed during respiration to allow the airway to resist collapse.

It is not clear whether muscle activity causes the airway to be more stable by making it stiffer or by making it larger.[105] Different regions of the airway have varying abilities to resist collapse, with the oropharynx relatively the most compliant (that is, easier to collapse) and the larynx the least compliant.[108] Sleep state and/or the presence of structural abnormalities like micrognathia can affect the airway's ability to resist collapse, making it easier to overcome the neuromuscular airway-dilating forces.[109] Once the airway collapses, greater pressure is needed to reopen the airway, suggesting that the walls of the closed airway tend to adhere. Surface forces may, therefore, impose an additional load to the airway-maintaining musculature in an infant who might be experiencing an obstructive apnea event.[107]

Airway stability in relation to head position: The patency of the airway can be affected by the relative degree of neck flexion or extension. With increasing neck flexion the airway is more prone to collapse; whereas it is more resistant to collapse with increasing neck extension[110] (see figure 1-13). With marked neck flexion, the airway may be placed at a mechanical disadvantage so that the airway dilating and stiffening mechanisms are less effective in resisting airway collapse. When the neck is extended, there may be a mechanical advantage favoring keeping the airway open. Some researchers feel that the size of the airway lumen is increased when the neck is extended, which may also be a factor in increasing resistance to collapse.[111] Other researchers feel that the change in airway stability in relationship to neck flexion or extension may be due to the placement of the axis of rotation. It is hypothesized that the axis of rotation for flexion and extension is behind the airway.[105] During neck flexion, therefore, the mass of tissue behind and below the jaw and hyoid may push into the airway, causing collapse.

Neck movements and neck/head stability are controlled by muscles that traverse the pharyngeal area. They have their origins and insertions between the mandible, the spinal column, the midfacial skeleton, and the shoulder girdle. Therefore, craniocervical posture and pharyngeal airway stability are interconnected. Bosma proposes that pharyngeal airway maintenance is the antecedent of craniocervical posture, that the development of craniocervical posture begins with stabilization around the pharyngeal airway in the infant, and that the airway continues to play a central role in postural mechanisms throughout the infant's life.[2] In light of the relationship between the postural and pharyngeal airway musculature and the changes in airway configuration in response to change in head position, the underlying mechanism for infants in respiratory distress to adopt an extended head and neck posture becomes clear. Not only will this extended position enlarge the airway, perhaps assisting airflow, but as the amount of negative inspiratory pressure increases with increasing work of breathing, these infants may seek a position of greater airway stability to oppose this heightened collapsing force.

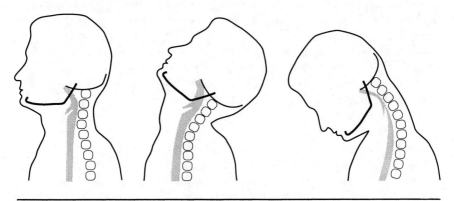

Figure 1-13 Influence of neck position on airway caliber.

Nasal versus Oral Breathing in Infants

Traditionally it was thought that infants were obligate nose breathers (i.e., that they were unable to breathe through their mouths) until a later, ill-defined age.[88] Recent studies, however, have shown this to be an inaccurate and incomplete view. Nasal breathing was thought to be obligate due to obstruction of the oropharynx by opposition of the soft palate and the tongue at rest. Rodenstein et al. studied 19 infants ranging in age from 1 day to 7½ months, while awake and asleep, to determine their ability to switch to mouth breathing in the face of acute nasal occlusion.[89] All infants were able to initiate mouth breathing after a mean of 7.8 +/- 6.4 seconds, by separating the soft palate and the tongue. Older and/or more awake infants would start to orally breathe sooner than younger and/or more asleep infants. The study concluded that although nasal breathing may be preferred in infants, it is not obligatory.

Miller et al. further supported these results in a study of 30 healthy term infants, aged 1 to 3 days, who were studied while asleep.[90] They found that several of the infants spontaneously breathed through their noses and mouths but the distribution of tidal volume still favored nose breathing (70% nasal to 30% oral). After nasal occlusion, 40 percent of the infants studied could initiate oral breathing after a mean delay of 6 +/- 3 seconds and sustain it for at least 1 minute. In evaluating the effectiveness of oral breathing in comparison to nasal breathing, they found that during this short study period there were no significant differences in heart rate, respiratory rate, tidal volume, or oxygen and carbon dioxide saturations; however, there was a significant decrease in minute ventilation during oral breathing.

The response of premature infants to nasal occlusion is slightly different from that of full-term babies and changes with increasing gestational age. Miller et al. studied the ventilatory response of 11 sleeping premature infants at 31 to 32 weeks, 33 to 34 weeks, and 35 to 36 weeks gestation during 15-second nasal occlusions.[91] They found that the percent of infants able to switch to oral breathing after no longer than 15 seconds significantly changed from 8% at 31-32 weeks to 26% at 33-34 weeks and was similar (28%) at 35-36 weeks. At 31-32 weeks, the babies who could switch to oral breathing had a discontinuous oral breathing pattern, with frequent periods of airflow occlusion. This gradually changed to a more continuous type of oral breathing, but even at 35-36 weeks only 35% of the preterm infants could sustain continuous oral breathing, compared to 78% at term. In contrast to term infants, there was a considerable increase in pulmonary resistance during mouth breathing and a significant decrease in respiratory rate, oxygen saturation, tidal volume, and minute ventilation. These researchers felt, therefore, that the consequence to the premature infant of continued oral breathing would be increased work of breathing, which could lead to diaphragmatic fatigue, hypercarbia, and hypoxia.

Thus, all infants, term and preterm, are able to breathe through their mouths to some degree when faced with nasal occlusion. To do so, however, requires the infant to carry out a series of complex motions. The baby must open the lips and generate sufficient muscle tone to overcome the adhesive forces between the palate and tongue, and maintain separation of these structures to allow airflow through the mouth.[92] Although infants can spontaneously breathe through the mouth, frequently it is done at a cost to the infant in terms of efficiency of breathing. Although this cost is more significant in preterm than in term infants, neither group may be able to effectively sustain oral breathing and may therefore develop progressive respiratory failure.[93] So, while infants are not *obligatory* nose breathers and can switch to oral breathing for short periods of time, nasal breathing is clearly preferred from a respiratory standpoint. It is still unclear at what age, if ever, a baby could sustain itself on oral breathing alone, without respiratory compromise.

Etiologies of Respiratory Failure

There are numerous disease processes and anomalies that can lead to respiratory failure and thus impact infant feeding. Redding et al. classified these respiratory disorders based on their anatomic "compartment," which relates to respiratory function.[112] The respiratory system can be divided into six anatomic compartments: the central nervous system, the upper airways, the lower airways, the lung parenchyma, the pleural space, and the bones and muscles surrounding the lungs. Disorders commonly seen in infancy, which might then impact feeding, will be discussed for each compartment.

Central nervous system: Any congenital defect or insult to the respiratory centers of the brain can lead to changes in ventilation. Frequently the pattern and depth of respiration is altered. These might include CNS depression due to narcotics, hemorrhages, severe Arnold Chiari malformation in an infant with meningomyelocele, or central hypoventilation syndrome.

Upper airways: These are the structures of the mouth, nose, pharynx, larynx, and extrathoracic trachea. Obstruction in these areas increases the resistance to airflow, thus increasing the work of breathing. The obstruction may be continual or intermittent. Examples include: choanal atresia; vocal cord anomalies or paralysis; edema from trauma (such as intubation and extubation); structural narrowing (e.g., subglottic stenosis); instability or spasms (e.g., tracheomalacia, laryngomalacia, laryngospasm); or glossoptossis associated with micrognathia.

Lower airways: These include the intrathoracic trachea, the bronchi, and bronchioli. Obstruction in this area may have a "fixed" dimension or may be dynamic. Again, these obstructions increase the work of breathing. Lower airway disorders include asthma, bronchitis and bronchiolitis, aspiration syndromes, and bronchospasm.

Lung parenchyma: The anatomic structures in this compartment include the bronchioles, alveoli, interstitium, and pulmonary vasculature. Disorders in the function of these structures may occur in association with some types of congenital heart disease, infant respiratory distress syndrome, and bronchopulmonary dysplasia (see chapter 6). When these structures are not functioning properly, gas exchange is impaired.

The pleurae: Reduced distensibility of the pleural surface and compression of the lung parenchyma may lead to respiratory failure; the normal expansion of the lungs is restricted. Cystic fibrosis is an example of a disorder resulting in these lung changes.

Thoracic cage and surroundings: Any disease process that reduces the effective movement of the thoracic cage or diaphragm will also reduce the excursion of the lungs and can result in respiratory failure. Examples include kyphoscoliosis and congenital anomalies of the ribs, respiratory muscle weakness from infant botulism or myopathies, and processes that restrict movement of the diaphragm (ascites, hepatic or splenic enlargement).

Coordination of Sucking, Swallowing, and Breathing

Clearly, sucking, swallowing, and breathing are complex tasks, even as each occurs in relative isolation from the others. In infant feeding they must act together, working smoothly and effectively, with highly accurate timing and coordination, to result in safe and efficient feeding. Unfortunately, the complexity of this process in infant feeding is often overlooked since it appears to happen so effortlessly in most infants. Although our knowledge of the individual functions of sucking, swallowing, and breathing is relatively complete, information about the coordination of these functions during infant feeding is sparse. Coordination of these activities, however, is essential to the prevention of aspiration of food and swallowing of air, and to efficient intake of nutrients.

Relationship between Breathing and Swallowing

For many years it was felt that infants were spared the task of having to coordinate breathing and swallowing during feeding. It was believed that sucking and swallowing occurred in isolation from breathing. The infant's anatomy was presumed to allow breathing during swallowing: fluid flowed down lateral food channels, passing safely around the open entrance of the relatively elevated larynx.[121,125,126]

Wilson et al. provide more detailed study of this question.[92] Infant respiratory effort and nasal airflow were measured during spontaneous swallowing in periods of regular respiration. The study found that swallowing always coincided with cessation of nasal airflow. In other words, infants stopped breathing briefly with every swallow. The mean length of the respiratory pause was about one second. This value did not vary with changes in respiratory rate and appeared stable among all infants. Weber et al. also reported that the swallows accompanying sucking interrupt respiration.[122] Such findings have led to the current view that sucking, swallowing, and breathing must be coordinated in infant feeding. These specific interrelationships will be discussed further and are summarized in figure 1-14.

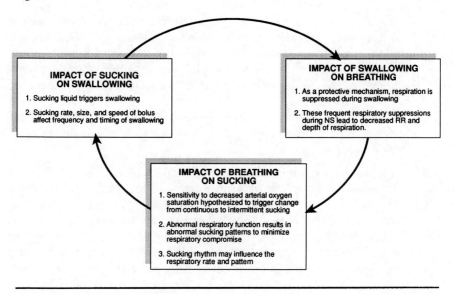

Figure 1-14 The interrelationship of sucking, swallowing, and breathing in infant feeding.

Impact of Swallowing on Breathing

Timing of swallowing within the respiratory cycle: Based on the concept that swallowing suppresses respiration, several authors have studied at what point in the ventilatory cycle this interruption occurs. Wilson et al. measured spontaneous swallows of oral secretions in premature infants and found that the swallow might occur at any point in the respiratory cycle.[92] When evaluating nutritive sucking in term infants, Weber and colleagues reported that swallowing occurred during inspiration or expiration in two-day-old infants.[122] In four- and five-day-old infants, during a regular suck-swallow pattern, swallowing reportedly occurred after expiration. Selley et al., however, disagree with Weber and associates' interpretation of their respiratory tracings.[123] Their results, using more sophisticated respiratory assessment, indicate that during rhythmic suck-swallow chains in the five- to eight-day-old term baby, swallowing consistently occurs after inspiration.

Obviously further study will be required before conclusions can be reached on this aspect of the coordination of swallowing and breathing. Several factors, however, should be considered. The relation of swallowing to the respiratory cycle may well be different during spontaneous swallowing of secretions than during nutritive sucking. Weber et al. note that when a smooth rhythm of sucking and swallowing is established, respirations become synchronized with sucking.[122] In such a case, it is more likely that swallowing would occur at a consistent point in the respiratory cycle. It is unlikely, however, that a smooth rhythm is maintained throughout the entire feeding. Clinically, some variation in the interface of swallowing and respiration appears typical. The other consideration is maturation. The variety of patterns found by Wilson et al. may reflect the immaturity of their premature subjects.[92] Maturational changes are reported by both the Weber and Selley groups,[122,123] and suggest greater stability of this timing with increasing age.

Effect of swallowing on breathing rate and pattern: Significant changes in ventilatory pattern occur during nipple-feeding. Since each swallow interrupts the respiratory cycle for approximately 1 second, decreasing the time available for breathing during nutritive sucking, alterations in the breathing pattern must occur.[27,33] These changes in breathing pattern are more pronounced during the initial continuous sucking phase than during the intermittent sucking phase that follows. During continuous sucking, term infants have a decrease in overall respiratory rate, lengthening of the expiratory phase, and shortening of the inspiratory phase, all leading to a reduction in minute ventilation. Minute ventilation returns to baseline during the intermittent sucking phase.[20] Comparison of breathing rate and pattern between NS and NNS suggests that the mechanism responsible for these reductions in ventilation is the repeated swallowing that occurs during nutritive sucking, since these changes in ventilation are not observed in the absence of fluid to swallow.

Impact of Breathing on Sucking

Interactions between breathing and sucking exist, although the relationship is less clearly understood and is less dramatic than the interplay between swallowing and breathing. Changes in sucking pattern are observed between the continuous and intermittent sucking phases. These changes involve an increase in the number and frequency of pauses during feeding, which results in a greater percentage of time available for breathing that is not interrupted by sucking or swallowing. It has been hypothesized that the type of ventilatory pattern seen during continuous sucking leads to changes in blood chemistry, which are then the trigger for the baby to change to an intermittent sucking pattern.[23] Non-nutritive sucking may also influence respiratory rate and pattern.[117,118,124]

The impact of respiration on sucking may be more dramatic, however, in the baby with a compromised respiratory system. In this case, the baby may not be able to tolerate the reduction in ventilation that occurs during the initial continuous sucking phase. This reduction in ventilation may potentially lead to further respiratory compromise or fatigue. To meet the challenge of feeding, the infant with respiratory compromise may use compensatory sucking patterns. Instead of having an initial continuous sucking phase, the infant may adopt a pattern of short sucking bursts punctuated by frequent pauses to breathe throughout the entire feeding. This would reduce the number of swallows per minute, allowing more opportunity for breathing, but could potentially decrease feeding efficiency.

Impact of Sucking on Swallowing

It is clear that the presence of a bolus in the oral cavity and oropharynx is the stimulus to initiate swallowing. During non-nutritive sucking (NNS), fluid accumulation is low and swallowing occurs infrequently. Although NNS may stimulate increased production of secretions, enough oral secretions must accumulate to trigger a swallow. This may be the reason that the suck to swallow ratio during NNS is 6-8:1. During nutritive sucking (NS), on the other hand, the suck/swallow ration is 1:1 at the beginning of the feeding and may decrease to 2:1 or 3:1 toward the end of the feeding.

A key factor in determining this ratio is the rate of fluid flow through the nipple.[33] During NNS, when there is no active fluid flow, just the accumulation of oral secretions, the ratio of sucking to swallowing is high. In the eagerly feeding infant, fluid is flowing rapidly. Therefore, a swallow must accompany each suck. As the infant fatigues over the course of the feeding and the rate of fluid flow declines, several sucks may be needed to accumulate a sufficiently large liquid bolus to initiate the swallow.

Therefore, sucking characteristics that increase the flow of fluid through the human or manufactured nipple will place a greater burden on the swallowing mechanism. These characteristics include sucking rate, sucking pressure, and resistance to fluid flow (which is a result of factors such as size of nipple hole or stiffness of nipple). If sucking pressure and

---

resistance to fluid flow are held constant, a higher sucking rate will result in an increase in the rate of swallowing. For example, an infant eagerly and continuously sucking at a rate of 60 sucks per minute will need to swallow 60 times to handle that rate of flow. If the infant is only sucking at a rate of 30 sucks per minute, 30 swallows would be required.

If sucking rate and resistance to fluid flow are constant, increasing sucking pressure will increase the bolus size and the speed with which it travels in the oral cavity. Although this may have little impact on swallowing, it is not clear at what point a bolus becomes so large, or moves so fast, that it causes disruption of swallowing. Clinical observation suggests that in some instances infants suck so vigorously that there is not time to organize the bolus adequately before the swallow is triggered, resulting in coughing and choking. There is also clearly a limit on the bolus size the infant can handle adequately during swallowing. Large boluses from excessively large nipple holes are known to produce coughing and choking. Perhaps for some infants, strong sucking pressure on a moderately sized nipple hole produces a large enough bolus to have the same effect.

It has been demonstrated that the infant has some control over sucking pressure; it can vary based on fluid flow, type of fluid, and degree of satiation.[32,41,119] This allows most infants to feed from a variety of nipples with different flow characteristics without difficulty. The maturational nature of this adaptability, however, is not well understood. Some infants, for reasons of immaturity or neuromotor dysfunction, may not be able to make appropriate adjustments in sucking pressure. This can also lead to disorganization of swallowing.

Maturational Considerations

Preterm infants: It is clear that in premature infants sucking patterns and respiratory patterns are maturing. Immature respiratory patterns are characterized by irregular periods of respiration, brief apnea, and apnea of prematurity. With maturity, nutritive and non-nutritive sucking become more rhythmic, with greater stability of the length of bursts and pauses. The rate of NNS increases slightly, and the strength of NS becomes greater. Although there is no evidence for maturational changes during isolated swallows, the coordination of sucking and swallowing is felt to improve as the infant matures.[119] The premature infant may, over time, become more effective at organizing the bolus to trigger a swallow, though to date there is no specific evidence for this. There is, however, evidence that the interface between swallowing and respiration improves with maturation.[23] This may then be reflected in better coordination between sucking and swallowing.

Studying premature infants, Wilson et al. found that spontaneous swallows that interrupted irregular breathing were more likely to be associated with prolonged airway closure than those occurring during smooth respiration.[92] Therefore, this suggests that premature infants who have more periods of irregular respiration may have prolonged airway closure associated with swallowing. This is indeed the finding of Mathew[115] and Guilleminault and Coons.[114] They found high rates of apnea (greater than 10 seconds) in premature infants during feeding. The number of apneic episodes was significantly greater during feeding than sleep, suggesting that some aspect of the feeding process was responsible. The coordination of breathing and swallowing is implicated, though immature laryngeal chemoreflexes may also be involved. Although premature infants show increasing coordination of sucking, swallowing, and breathing between 34 and 40 weeks, it is not unusual for discoordination to continue past term.[120] (Also see chapter 6.)

Term Infants: It is generally assumed that the functions underlying feeding are mature in the full-term infant, who is expected to feed without compromise. In the first few days of life, however, dysrhythmic sucking and poor coordination of sucking, swallowing, and breathing are common.[122,123] When infants are monitored closely, apnea and bradycardia are also seen.[113,116] Almost 20% of the full-term neonates Mathew studied demonstrated apnea ($\geq$ 20 seconds) or bradycardia. These episodes typically occurred early in the feeding (during continuous sucking) and were self-limiting.[116]

Although feeding patterns are reported to be smooth by 5 to 8 days of life,[122,123] changes in physiologic stability with feeding beyond the neonatal period have not been well studied. Guilleminault and Coons, however, report no episodes of apnea or other related respiratory compromise during feeding in a group of term infants who were 4 to 18 weeks of age.[114] Feeding is reported to become more efficient, and changes in sucking rates, suck/swallow ratios, and coordination of sucking, swallowing, and breathing are likely to be involved.

It is known that the respiratory rate tends to decrease with growth.[127] With a lower respiratory rate, the impact of sequential swallowing during feeding would be reduced. As the oral and pharyngeal cavities enlarge, the infant may also be able to handle a larger bolus of liquid during swallowing, thus allowing the fluid from several sucks to accumulate prior to a swallow. As the number of swallows is reduced, the impact on respiration would also diminish. These maturational changes deserve further study.

References

1. Bosma, J. F. 1972. Form and function in the infant's mouth and pharynx. In *Oral sensation and perception: The mouth of the infant*, edited by J. F. Bosma, 3-29. Springfield, IL: Charles C. Thomas.

2. _____. 1988. Functional anatomy of the upper airway during development. In *Respiratory function of the upper airway*, edited by O. P. Mathew and G. Sant'Ambrogio, 47-86. New York: Marcel Dekker, Inc.

3. _____. 1967. Human infant oral function. In *Oral sensation and perception*, edited by J. F. Bosma, 98-110. Springfield, IL: Charles C. Thomas.

4. Kennedy, J. G., and R. D. Kent. 1988. Physiologic substrates of normal deglutition. *Dysphagia* 3:24-27.

5. Miller, A. J. 1986. Neurophysiologic basis of swallowing. *Dysphagia* 1:91-100.

6. Brazy, J. E., H. C. Kinney, and W. J. Oakes. 1987. Central nervous system structural lesions causing apnea at birth. *The Journal of Pediatrics* 111:163-75.

7. Bosma, J. F. 1985. Postnatal ontogeny of performances of the pharynx, larynx and mouth. *American Review of Respiratory Disease* 131:S10-S15.

8. Jean, A. 1984. Brain stem organization of the swallowing network. *Brain Behavior* 25:109-16.

9. Donner, M. W., J. F. Bosma, and D. L. Robertson. 1985. Anatomy and physiology of the pharynx. *Gastrointestinal Radiology* 10:196-212.

10. Campbell, S. K. 1981. Neural control of somatic motor function. *Physical Therapy* 61:16-22.

11. Bosma, J. F. 1980. Physiology of the mouth. In *Otolaryngology*, edited by M. M. Paparella and D. A. Shumrick, 319-31. Philadelphia: W. B. Saunders Company.

12. Bosma, J. F., and M. W. Donner. 1980. Physiology of the pharynx. In *Otolaryngology*, edited by M. M. Paparella and D. A. Shumrick, 332-44. Philadelphia: W. B. Saunders Company.

13. Donner, M. W. 1980. Physiology of the esophagus. In *Otolaryngology*, edited by M. M. Paparella and D. A. Shumrick, 345-53. Philadelphia: W. B. Saunders Company.

14. Kirchner, J. A. 1980. Physiology of the larynx. In *Otolaryngology*, edited by M. M. Paparella and D. A. Shumrick, 366-76. Philadelphia: W. B. Saunders Company.

15. Caruso, V. G., and E. K. Sauerland. 1990. Embryology and anatomy. In *Pediatric otolaryngology*, edited by C. D. Bluestone and S. E. Stool, 807-15. Philadelphia: W. B. Saunders Company.

16. Schechter, G. L. 1990. Physiology of the mouth, pharynx and esophagus. In *Pediatric otolaryngology*, edited by C. D. Bluestone and S. E. Stool, 816-22. Philadelphia: W. B. Saunders Company.

17. Morris, S. E. 1982. *The normal acquisition of oral feeding skills: Implications for assessment and treatment.* Central Islip, NY: Therapeutic Media.

18. Meller, S. M. 1984. Functional anatomy of the larynx. *Otolaryngologic Clinics of North America* 17:3-12.

19. Anderson, G. C., and D. Vidyasagar. 1979. Development of sucking in premature infants from 1 to 7 days post birth. *Birth Defects: Original Articles Series* 15:145-71.

20. Mathew, O. P., M. L. Clark, M. L. Pronske, H. G. Luna-Solarzano, and M. D. Peterson. 1985. Breathing pattern and ventilation during oral feeding in term newborn infants. *The Journal of Pediatrics* 106:810-13.

21. Daniels, H., H. Devlieger, P. Casaer, and E. Eggermont. 1986. Nutritive and non-nutritive sucking in preterm infants. *Journal of Developmental Physiology* 8:117-21.

22. Casaer, P., H. Daniels, H. Devlieger, P. DeCock, and E. Eggermont. 1982. Feeding behavior in preterm neonates. *Early Human Development* 7:331-46.

23. Shivpuri, C. R., R. J. Martin, W. A. Carlo, and A. A. Fanaroff. 1983. Decreased ventilation in preterm infants during oral feeding. *The Journal of Pediatrics* 103:285-89.

24. Brake, S., W. P. Fifer, G. Alfasi, and A. Fleischman. 1988. The first nutritive sucking responses of premature newborns. *Infant Behavior and Development* 11:1-9.

25. Hack, M., M. M. Estabrook, and S. S. Robertson. 1985. Development of sucking rhythms in preterm infants. *Early Human Development* 11:133-40.

26. Ellison, S. L., D. Vidyasagar, G. C. Anderson. 1979. Sucking in the newborn infant during the first hour of life. *Journal of Nurse-Midwifery* 24:18-25.

27. Mathew, O. P. 1988. Regulation of breathing pattern during feeding: Role of suck, swallow, and nutrients. In *Respiratory function of the upper airway*, edited by O. P. Mathew and G. Sant'Ambrogio, 535-60. New York: Marcel Dekker, Inc.

28. Ardran, G. M., F. H. Kemp, and J. Lind. 1958. A cineradiographic study of breast-feeding. *British Journal of Radiology* 31:156-62.

29. Ardran, G. M., F. H. Kemp, and J. Lind. 1958. A cineradiographic study of bottle-feeding. *British Journal of Radiology* 31:11-22.

30. Weber, F., M. W. Woolridge, and J. D. Baum. 1986. An ultrasonographic study of the organization of sucking and swallowing by newborn infants. *Developmental Medicine and Child Neurology* 28:19-24.

31. Smith, W. L., A. Erenberg, and A. Nowak. 1988. Imaging evaluation of the human nipple during breast-feeding. *American Journal of Diseases in Children* 142:76-78.

32. Wolff, P. H. 1968. The serial organization of sucking in the young infant. *Pediatrics* 42:943-55.

33. Mathew, O. P., and J. Bhatia. 1989. Sucking and breathing patterns during breast- and bottle-feeding in term neonates. *American Journal of Disease in Children* 143:588-92.

34. Logan, W. J., and J. F. Bosma. 1967. Oral and pharyngeal dysphagia in infancy. *Pediatric Clinics of North America* 14:47-61.

35. Jain, L., E. Sivieri, S. Abbasi, and V. K. Bhutani. 1987. Energetics and mechanics of nutritive sucking in the preterm and term neonate. *Journal of Pediatrics* 111:894-98.

36. Kron, R. E., M. Stein, and K. E. Goddard. 1963. A method of measuring sucking behavior of newborn infants. *Psychosomatic Medicine.* 25:181-91.

37. Pollitt, E., B. Consolazio, and F. Goodkin. 1981. Changes in nutritive sucking during a feed in two-day and thirty-day-old infants. *Early Human Development* 5:201-10.

38. Dubignon, J., and D. Cooper. 1980. Good and poor feeding behavior in the neonatal period. *Infant Behavior and Development* 3:395-08.

39. Bosma, J. F., L. G. Hepburn, S. D. Josell, and K. Baker. 1990. Ultrasound demonstration of tongue motions during suckle feeding. *Developmental Medicine and Child Neurology* 32:223-29.

40. Colley, J. R. T., and B. Creamer. 1958. Sucking and swallowing in infants. *British Medical Journal* 2, no. 5093:422-23.

41. Sameroff, A. J. 1968. The components of sucking in the human newborn. *Journal of Experimental Child Psychology* 6:607-23.

42. Wolff, P. H. 1972. The interaction of state and non-nutritive sucking. In *Oral sensation and perception,* edited by J. F. Bosma, 293-312. Springfield, IL: Charles C. Thomas.

43. Crook, C. K., and L. P. Lipsitt. 1976. Neonatal nutritive sucking: Effects of taste stimulation upon sucking rhythm and heart rate. *Child Development* 47:518-22.

44. Lawrence, R. A. 1989. *Breast-feeding: A guide for the medical profession.* St. Louis, MO: C. V. Mosby Company.

45. Humphrey, T. 1964. Some correlations between the appearance of human fetal reflexes and the development of the nervous system. *Progress in Brain Research* 4:93-135.

46. Hooker, D. 1942. Fetal reflexes and instinctual processes. *Psychosomatic Medicine* 4:199-205.

47. Ianniruberto, A., and E. Tajani. 1981. Ultrasonographic study of fetal movements. *Seminars in Perinatology* 5:175-81.

48. Tucker, J. A. 1985. Perspective of the development of the air and food passages. *American Review of Respiratory Diseases* 131:S7-S9.

49. Pritchard, J. A. 1966. Fetal swallowing and amniotic fluid volume. *Obstetrics and Gynecology* 28:606-10.

50. Grand, R. J., J. B. Watkins, and F. M. Torti. 1976. Development of the human gastrointestinal tract. A review. *Gastroenterology* 7:796-810.

51. Diamant, N. E. 1985. Development of esophageal function. *American Review of Respiratory Diseases* 131:S29-S32.

52. Fisher, S. E., M. Painter, and G. Milmoe. 1981. Swallowing disorders in infancy. *Pediatric Clinics of North America* 28:845-53.

53. Kramer, S. S. 1985. Special swallowing problems in children. *Gastrointestinal Radiology* 10:241-50.

54. Dubner, R. B., B. J. Sessle, and A. T. Storey. 1978. *The Neural Basis of Oral and Facial Function*. New York: Plenum.

55. Thexton, A. J. 1973. Oral reflexes elicited by mechanical stimulation of palatal mucose in the cat. *Archives of Oral Biology* 18:971-80.

56. Lazzara, G. L., C. Lazarus, and J. A. Logemann. 1986. Impact of thermal stimulation on the triggering of the swallowing reflex. *Dysphagia* 1:73-77.

57. Doty, R. W., and J. F. Bosma. 1956. An electromyographic analysis of reflex deglutition. *Journal of Neurophysiology* 19:44-60.

58. Doty, R. W. 1968. Neural organization of deglutition. In *Handbook of physiology: Alimentary canal*, vol. 4, edited by C. F. Code, 1861-902. Washington, DC: American Physiological Society.

59. Cumming, W. A., and B. J. Reilly. 1972. Fatigue aspiration. *Radiology* 105:387-90.

60. Fisher, M., T. Hendrix, J. Hunt, and A. Murrills. 1978. Relation between volume swallowed and velocity of the bolus ejected from the pharynx into the esophagus. *Gastroenterology* 74:1238-240.

61. Ingervall, B., and B. Lantz. 1973. Significance of gravity on the passage of bolus through the human pharynx. *Archives of Oral Biology* 18:351-56.

62. Miller, F. R., and C. S. Sherrington, 1916. Some observations on the buccopharyngeal stage of reflex deglutition in the cat. *Quarterly Journal of Experimental Physiology* 9:147-86.

63. Storey, A. T. 1968. Laryngeal initiation of swallowing. *Experimental Neurology* 20:359-65.

64. _____. 1968. A functional analysis of sensory units innervating epiglottis and larynx. *Experimental Neurology* 20:366-83.

65. Code, J. F., and J. F. Schlegel. 1986. Motor action of the esophagus and its sphincters. In *Handbook of physiology: Alimentary canal*, edited by C. F. Code, 1821-839. Washington, DC: American Physiological Society.

66. Miller, A. J. 1987. Swallowing: Neurophysiologic control of the esophageal phase. *Dysphagia* 2:72-82.

---

67. Diamant, N. E. 1982. Normal esophageal physiology. In *Disease of the esophagus*, edited by S. Cohen and R. D. Soloway, 1-34. New York: Churchill Livingstone.

68. Miller, A. J. 1982. Deglutition. *Physiology Review* 62:129-84.

69. _____. 1972. Significance of sensory inflow to the swallowing reflex. *Brain Research* 43:147-59.

70. Doty, R. W., 1951. Influence of stimulus pattern on reflex deglutition. *American Journal of Physiology* 166:142-58.

71. Ardran, G. M., P. F. Benson, N. R. Butler, H. L. Ellis, and T. McKendrick. 1965. Congenital dysphagia resulting from dysfunction of the pharyngeal musculature. *Developmental Medicine and Child Neurology* 7:157-66.

72. Illingworth, R. S. 1969. Sucking and swallowing difficulties in infancy: Diagnostic problem of dysphagia. *Archives of Diseases in Childhood* 44:655-65.

73. Tuchman, D. N. 1988. Dysfunctional swallowing in the pediatric patient: Clinical considerations. *Dysphagia* 2:203-8.

74. Ardran, G. M., and F. H. Kemp. 1970. Some important factors in the assessment of oropharyngeal function. *Developmental Medicine and Child Neurology* 12:158-66.

75. Martin, G. R., C. Rudolph, C. Hillemeier, and M. B. Heyman. 1986. Dysphagia lusorum in children. *American Journal of Diseases in Children* 140:815-16.

76. Pressman, H., and S. H. Morrison. 1988. Dysphagia in the pediatric AIDS population. *Dysphagia* 2:166-69.

77. Pipes, P., and V. Holm. 1973. Weight control of children with Prader-Willi syndrome. *Journal of the American Dietetic Association* 62:520.

78. Donner, M. W. 1985. Radiologic evaluation of swallowing. *American Review of Respiratory Diseases* 131:S20-S23.

79. Logemann, J. A. 1986. Treatment for aspiration related to dysphagia: An overview. *Dysphagia* 1:34-38.

80. Logemann, J. A. 1983. *Evaluation and treatment of swallowing disorders*. Boston: College Press Publication.

81. Oestreich, A. E., and J. S. Dunbar. 1984. Pharyngonasal reflux: Spectrum and significance in early childhood. *American Journal of Roentgenol* 141:923-25.

82. Widdicombe, J. 1988. Nasal and pharyngeal reflexes. In *Respiratory function of the upper airway*, vol. 35, edited by O. P. Mathew and G. Sant' Ambrogio, 233-58. New York: Marcell Dekker, Inc.

83. Gerhardt, T., and E. Bancalari. 1984. Apnea of prematurity: Lung function and regulation of breathing. *Pediatrics* 74:58-62.

84. Berger, A. J, R. A. Mitchell, and J. W. Severinghaus. 1977. Regulation of respiration. *New England Journal of Medicine* 297:92-97.

85. Sant'Ambrogio, G., and O. P. Mathew. 1986. Laryngeal receptors and their reflex responses. *Clinics in Chest Medicine* 7:211-22.

86. Spyer, K. M., and M. P. Gilbey. 1988. Cardiorespiratory interactions in heart-rate control. *Annals of New York Academy of Sciences* 533:350-51.

87. Mathew, O. P., and F. B. Sant'Ambrogio. 1988. Laryngeal reflexes. In *Respiratory function of the upper airway*, edited by O. P. Mathew and G. Sant'Ambrogio, 259-302. New York: Marcel Dekker, Inc.

88. Morris, S. E., and M. D. Klein. 1987. *Pre-feeding skills*. Tucson, AZ: Therapy Skill Builders.

89. Rodenstein, D. O., N. Perlmutter, and D. C. Stanescu. 1985. Infants are not obligatory nasal breathers. *American Review of Respiratory Diseases* 131:343-47.

90. Miller, M. J., R. J. Martin, W. A. Carlo, J. M. Fouke, K. P. Strohl, and A. A. Fanaroff. 1985. Oral breathing in newborn infants. *The Journal of Pediatrics* 107:465-69.

91. Miller, M. J., W. A. Carlo, K. P. Strohl, A. A. Fanaroff, and R. J. Martin. 1986. Effect of maturation on oral breathing in sleeping premature infants. *The Journal of Pediatrics* 109:515-19.

92. Wilson, S. L., B. T. Thach, R. T. Brouillette, and Y. K. Abu-Osba. 1980. Upper airway patency in the human infant: Influence of airway pressure and posture. *Journal of Applied Physiology* 48:500-504.

93. Miller, M. J., R. J. Martin, W. A. Carlo, and A. A. Fanaroff. 1987. Oral breathing in response to nasal trauma in term infants. *The Journal of Pediatrics* 79:899-901.

94. Thach, B. R., and A. Menon. 1985. Pulmonary protective mechanisms in human infants. *American Review of Respiratory Diseases* 131:S55-S58.

95. Widdicombe, J. G., and M. Tatar. 1988. Upper airway reflex control. *Annals of the New York Academy of Sciences* 533:252-61.

96. Mellins, R. B. 1985. Pulmonary protective mechanisms. *American Review of Respiratory Diseases* 131:S62.

97. Mortola, J. P., and J. T. Fisher. 1988. Upper airway reflexes in newborns. In *Respiratory function of the upper airway*, vol. 35, edited by O. P. Mathew and G. Sant'Ambrogio, 303-57. New York: Marcell Dekker, Inc.

98. Bartlett, D. 1985. Ventilatory and protective mechanisms of the infant larynx. *American Review of Respiratory Diseases* 131:S49-S50.

99. Menon, A., G. Schefft, and B. T. Thach. 1985. Apnea associated with regurgitation in infants. *The Journal of Pediatrics* 106:625-29.

100. Pickens, D. L., G. Schefft, and B. T. Thach. 1986. Prolonged apnea associated with upper airway (UAW) protective reflexes in apnea of prematurity (AP). *Pediatric Research* 20:437A.

101. Thach, B. T., A. M. Davies, and J. S. Koenig. 1988. Pathophysiology of sudden upper airway obstruction in sleeping infants and its relevance for SIDS. *Annals of the New York Academy of Sciences* 533:314-28.

102. Pickens, D. L., G. L. Schefft, and B. T. Thach. Prolonged apnea in infants with respiratory syncytial virus (RSV) infection is similar to apnea of prematurity and laryngeal chemoreflex (LC) apnea. *Pediatric Research* 21:504A.

103. Leith, D. E. 1985. The development of cough. *American Review of Respiratory Diseases* 131:S39-S42.

104. Boyle, J. T., D. N. Tuchman, S. M. Altschuler, T. E. Hixon, A. I. Pack, and S. Cohen. 1985. Mechanisms for the association of gastroesophageal reflux and bronchospasm. *American Review of Respiratory Diseases* 131:S16-S20.

105. Olson, L. G., J. M. Fouke, P. L. Hoekje, and K. P. Strohl. 1988. A Biomechanical view of upper airway function. In *Respiratory function of the upper airway*, vol. 35, edited by O. P. Mathew and G. Sant'Ambrogio, 359-89. New York: Marcell Dekker, Inc.

106. Widdcombe, J. Control of airway caliber. 1985. *American Review of Respiratory Diseases* 131:S33-S35.

107. Wilson, S. L., B. T. Thach, R. T. Brouillette, and Y. K. Abu-Osba. 1980. Upper airway patency in the human infant: Influence of airway pressure and posture. *Journal of Applied Physiology: Respiratory Environment Exercise Physiology* 48:500-504.

108. Reed, W. R., J. L. Roberts, and B. T. Thach. 1985. Factors influencing regional patency and configuration of the human infant upper airway. *Journal of Applied Physiology* 58:635-44.

109. J. L. Roberts, W. R. Reed, O. P. Mathew, A. A. Menon, and B. T. Thach. 1985. Assessment of pharyngeal airway stability in normal and micrognathic infants. *Journal of Applied Physiology* 58:290-99.

110. Thach, B. T, and A. R. Stark. 1979. Spontaneous neck flexion and airway obstruction during apneic spells in preterm infants. *The Journal of Pediatrics* 95:275-81.

111. Ardran, G. M. and F. H. Kemp. 1968. The mechanism of changes in form of the cervical airway in infancy. *Medical Radiography and Photography* 44:26-54.

112. Redding, G. J., J. P. Morray, and C. Rea. 1987. Respiratory failure in childhood. In *Pediatric intensive care*, edited by J. P. Morray. Norwalk, CT: Appleton and Lange.

113. Rosen, C. L., D. G. Glaze, and J. D. Frost. 1984. Hypoxemia associated with feeding in the preterm infant and full-term neonate. *American Journal of Diseases of Childhood* 138:623-28.

114. Guilleminault, C., and S. Coons. 1984. Apnea and bradycardia during feeding in infants weighing 2000 gm. *The Journal of Pediatrics* 104:932-35.

115. Mathew, O. P. 1988. Respiratory control during nipple feeding in preterm infants. *Pediatric Pulmonology* 5:220-24.

116. Mathew, O. P., M. L. Clark, and M. L. Pronske. 1985. Apnea, bradycardia, and cyanosis during oral feeding in term neonates (letter). *The Journal of Pediatrics* 106:857.

117. Paludetto, R., S. S. Robertson, and R. J. Martin. 1986. Interaction between non-nutritive sucking and respiration in preterm infants. *Biology of the Neonate* 49:198-203.

118. Dreier, T., P. H. Wolff, E. E. Cross, and W. D. Cochran. 1979. Patterns of breath intervals during non-nutritive sucking in full-term and "at risk" preterm infants with normal neurologic examinations. *Early Human Development* 3:187-99.

119. Gryboski, J. D. 1969. Suck and swallow in the premature infant. *Pediatrics* 43:96-102.

120. Pierantoni, H. R., L. L. Wright, J. F. Bosma, and K. Bessard. 1986. The development of respiratory control during oral feeding in premature infants. *Pediatric Research* (abstract) 20:382A.

121. Johnson, P., and D. M. Salisbury. 1975. Breathing and sucking during feeding in the newborn. *Ciba Foundation Symposiums* 33:119-35.

122. Weber, F., M. W. Woolridge, and J. D. Baum. 1986. An ultrasonographic study of the organization of sucking and swallowing by newborn infants. *Developmental Medicine and Child Neurology* 28:19-24.

123. Selley, W. G., R. E. Ellis, F. C. Flack, H. Curtis, and M. Callon. 1986. Ultrasonographic study of sucking and swallowing by newborn infants (letter). *Developmental Medicine and Child Neurology* 28:821-23.

124. Mathew, O. P., Clark, M. L., and M. H. Pronske. 1985. Breathing pattern of neonates during non-nutritive sucking. *Pediatric Pulmonology* 1:204-6.

125. Negus, V. E., and T. P. Kilner. 1942. Discussion on injuries of nose and throat. *Proceedings of the Royal Medical Society* 35:315-18.

126. Peiper, A. 1963. *Cerebral function in infancy and childhood.* New York: Consultants Bureau.

127. Gould, A. 1991. Cardiopulmonary evaluation of the infant, toddler, child and adolescent. *Pediatric Physical Therapy* 3:9-13.

128. Guyton, A. C. 1991. *Textbook of medical physiology.* Philadelphia: W. B. Saunders Co.

2 *Diagnostic Tests and Procedures*

As we established in chapter 1, infant feeding is a complicated process involving multiple structural and physiological systems. When an infant presents with feeding difficulties, an ever expanding array of technological aids can be used to evaluate functions related to the feeding process. Results of such evaluation can assist in the diagnosis of feeding problems, clarify the need for intervention, and/or measure the response to treatment. Results of these tests and monitoring procedures are most useful when thoughtfully combined with the results of clinical feeding evaluation and feeding history.

The infant feeding specialist must have a basic understanding of common tests and monitoring procedures used with babies who have feeding problems, regardless of the professional practice setting. By understanding the strengths and limitations of procedures that have been completed, along with the implications of the results, specialists can integrate data from these tests into the clinical feeding evaluation. This will lead to a better understanding of the infant's feeding problems and development of more effective treatment strategies. In addition, during the clinical feeding evaluation such knowledge will allow the infant feeding specialist to consider whether additional information from specialized tests and procedures would aid in diagnosis or treatment of the feeding problem.

Selection of tests and monitoring devices must be done with care. Key to this process is the delineation of the particular features of the infant's symptomatology that are of special interest. Often there are several tests that measure closely related functions, or various aspects of the same function. Therefore, determining the specific questions that need to be answered is crucial to selecting the appropriate test.

Chapter 2 will provide the feeding specialist with a basic understanding of the purposes of the various tests, procedures, and equipment most frequently employed with infants with complex feeding disorders. In addition to a description of each test and procedure, there will be a review of its strengths and limitations. This will serve as background information for discussion of the clinical feeding evaluation of infants and the formulation of treatment.

Monitoring Physiologic Functions

Equipment used to monitor the infant's physiologic status primarily looks at the infant's ability to maintain homeostasis in the face of changing sleep states or level of activity. Heart rate, respiratory rate, and oxygen saturation are parameters that are commonly measured. The various devices that will be described can be used separately or in combination during treatment or clinical feeding evaluation.

Cardiorespiratory Monitor

The cardiorespiratory monitor or CR monitor (see figure 2-1) gives a numerical and visual display of heartbeat and respiration. The infant is connected to the monitor by a series of leads, or wires, that adhere to the chest, connecting to the monitor via a cable. The numerical readout provides information on the number of heartbeats and breaths per minute. Because these values are determined by averaging activity over a given time period (for instance, 10 seconds), they cannot reflect brief changes in either parameter. By watching the oscilloscope for the wave-form tracing of heartbeat pattern or respirations, transient changes in these parameters can be observed. The monitor can be programmed for specific upper and lower limits of heart and respiratory rate and will alarm if the infant goes beyond these limits. A summary of the strengths and limitations of the cardiorespiratory monitor is in table 2-1. See pages 139-143 for further information on using the CR monitor during feeding assessment.

Strengths
The CR monitor gives a quick approximation of the infant's status. The wave-form tracing is useful to detect the presence of short drops in heart rate (HR) or bradycardias that might not be long enough to trigger the monitor's alarm. These brief dips in heart rate may be inconsequential, but for some infants their detection is important in evaluating the feeding problem.

Limitations
The manner in which respiration, and to a lesser degree heart rate, are monitored is particularly sensitive to movement; therefore the numeric and

visual display are subject to movement artifact. This is an ever-present problem, as babies generally move despite illness. Thus the information received from the CR monitor, particularly in regard to respiratory rate, is not always accurate. Adjustments can be made in the sensitivity of the monitor in an effort to limit movement artifact, but this meets with varying success.

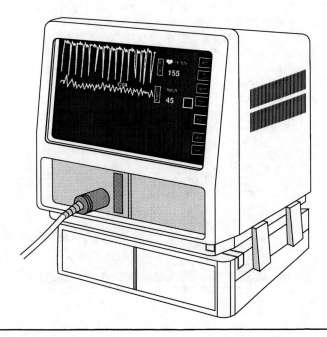

Figure 2-1 Cardiorespiratory monitor.

Table 2-1 Strengths and Limitations of the Cardiorespiratory Monitor

Cardiorespiratory Monitor—Gives numeric value and wave form tracing for heart rate and respiratory rate.

Strengths
- Gives quick approximation of status
- Alarms signal baby's distress
- HR wave form useful in observing brief changes or difficulty prior to alarm

Limitations
- Averaged values may not reflect brief changes in function
- Movement artifact can compromise accuracy

Oximetry

Oximetry monitors the oxygen saturation of capillary blood flow through an external sensor. A light probe sensor is taped around a finger, toe, hand, or foot to measure the percentage of oxygen in the capillary blood flow (see figure 2-2). Oxygen saturation is expressed as a percentage of 100. Under most circumstances, the normal infant has an oxygen saturation above 95%. Oximetry levels below 90% generally indicate some degree of hypoxia. While baseline oximetry levels may be lower for premature infants, levels below 90% are also usually undesirable in this group. For babies with other known health problems, acceptable parameters for saturation levels may be set by their physicians.

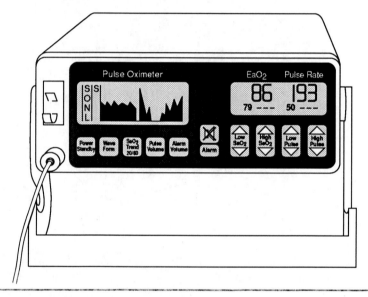

Figure 2-2 Pulse oximeter.

Oximetry can be used to determine an infant's baseline oxygen saturation, changes in the oxygen saturation in response to handling or work (such as that involved in feeding), and/or the effectiveness of oxygen therapy. While oximetry during feeding can detect changes in saturation level in response to any component of the feeding process, normal values do not necessarily indicate adequate respiratory functions during feeding. Oximetry can also be used to determine if color change (cyanosis) is secondary to a drop in oxygen saturation. Not all blue spells are the result of desaturation. On the other hand, infants can have significant desaturation without any external sign.[1] See page 143 for further information on using oximetry during clinical feeding evaluation.

Strengths

Oximetry is an easily transportable and non-invasive technique. It gives the feeding specialist ongoing, instantaneous information regarding oxygen saturation and can therefore identify the baby's response to work. Oximetry is a more reliable index of oxygen saturation than observing changes in facial color, since desaturation can occur without external cues.

The pulse oximeter probe can be left in place for extended periods without adverse effect to the skin. It can therefore provide continuous measurement over a long period of time. Thus, variability in oxygen saturations over time and during a variety of activities can be measured. Because the measurement occurs on the surface of the skin, it avoids complications that can arise from more invasive techniques.

Limitations

Although oximetry has become the most widely used method of evaluating oxygen levels, several factors limit its reliability and accuracy. Oximetry is very sensitive to movement artifact.[10] The probe is generally placed on the hand or foot; these are both body parts most babies move while feeding. Some oximeters provide a wave-form readout in addition to a numerical readout so that motion artifact can be detected. Without this type of visual display, however, the examiner cannot be confident about the accuracy of the saturation levels.

The natural pigmentation of the infant's skin can affect the oximetry reading. Since oximetry values are computed by the degree of infrared light absorption, pulse oximetry may overestimate the oxygen saturation of darkly pigmented infants.[11] External ambient light sources and infrared heating sources (such as those used with certain warmers) can also impair accuracy of oximetry readings.[12] In addition, anemia or the amount of fetal hemoglobin still present in the baby's blood can result in an inaccurate estimation of true oxygen saturation levels.[10]

Oximetry readings can vary with the type of oximeter used. Some oximeters will display numerical values that are averaged over several seconds; others display point-by-point values that may be more precise. Oxygen saturation levels can vary plus or minus 1% to 3% at 90% saturation or above.[13] This relatively small inaccuracy in saturation could reflect larger proportional differences in true blood oxygen levels, which could be significant for some babies.

When evaluating saturation levels for a particular infant, the feeding specialist needs to consider the relationship between oximetry values and partial pressures of oxygen (PaO_2) that could be obtained through an arterial blood gas. An accurate oxygen saturation level of 95% would be equal to a PaO_2 of 74.2 mm Hg; a saturation level of 90% would be equal to a PaO_2 of 57.8 mm Hg.[14] If a baby has oxygen saturation levels of 90%, considering the standard error of measurement of the oximeters, the "true" saturation may be as low as 88%. This would translate to a PaO_2 of 55 mm Hg, a value that, if sustained, could place the infant at considerable risk for respiratory compromise. Thus, oximetry values should be interpreted somewhat conservatively, especially at borderline values. The baby's clinical response (i.e., whether the baby is feeding poorly or adequately), should also strongly be considered when interpreting oximetry values. Strengths and limitations of oximetry are summarized in table 2-2.

Table 2-2 Strengths and Limitations of Oximetry

Oximetry—External sensor monitors oxygen saturation of capillary blood flow.

Strengths
- Non-invasive and transportable
- Monitors one aspect of baby's response to work
- Can help determine the significance of problems coordinating, such as swallow and breathe
- More reliable than observing color change

Limitations
- Affected by perfusion
- Affected by movement (movement artifact)
- Often done for brief period of time
- Some units may obscure brief changes because of averaging values

---

Pneumogram

Technically, a pneumogram is a hard-copy tracing of respiratory function. Clinically, it generally includes additional tracings of related functions. In its simplest form it may be a two-channel study based on chest wall excursion and heart rate. Recently, computerized technology has allowed development of multichannel equipment that can simultaneously record information on parameters such as heart rate, respiratory rate, oxygen saturation, nasal airflow, and esophageal pressures (see figure 2-3). This study is done at bedside, generally over 12 to 24 hours.

The monitoring equipment used in these studies gives exact values rather than averaged values, so subtle changes in the parameters are identified and the extent of an infant's compromise can be determined accurately. Continuous hard copy or computerized data allows careful evaluation of the relationship between the parameters, so an understanding of the sequence of events that leads to the infant's compromised status can be developed. If activity and behavioral observations are recorded during the study, the interpretation becomes even more sensitive. If feeding periods have been indicated, detailed evaluation of the infant's physiologic responses to feeding can also be completed.

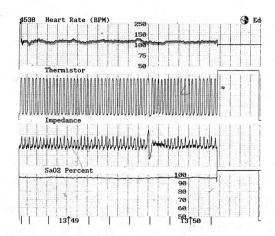

Figure 2-3 Print-out from a four-channel pneumogram. (Courtesy of N. Davis, M.D., Seattle, WA)

The pneumogram is often the first test used to evaluate an infant for idiopathic sleep apnea or obstructive apnea felt to be due to gastroesophageal reflux. The results must be interpreted by specially trained physicians. A summary of the strengths and limitations of the pneumogram is found in table 2-3.

Table 2-3 Strengths and Limitations of the Multichannel Pneumogram

---

Multichannel Pneumogram—Detailed hard copy of respiratory activity related to other parameters.

Strengths
- Identifies interrelationships between measured parameters
- Picks up data lost to visual monitoring alone
- Differentiates between various types of respiratory control problems (i.e., central versus obstructive apnea)

Limitations
- Requires specialized equipment
- Needs special training to interpret
- May have lag time for interpreting

A positive feature of the pneumogram is its ability to record data that would be lost on visual monitoring alone and to relate external events to physiologic changes in the baby. It is also useful for differentiating between central and obstructive apnea. With multichannel studies, a large amount of information can be gathered in a bedside test.

Limitations
The interpretation of the pneumogram requires specialized skill and training. As more channels are added, equipment becomes more specialized and the cost of the procedure increases.

Polysomnogram

The polysomnogram, or sleep study, is a multichannel recording of respiration, airflow, chest and diaphragm movement, oxygen and carbon dioxide levels, heart rate, and esophageal pressures. This data is correlated with information on sleep state, which is collected by EEG recordings. Babies are generally monitored for the length of two complete sleep cycles, including the awake period that precedes sleep. This test is used by physicians to evaluate problems in central ventilatory control, such as idiopathic sleep apnea. It is not a test employed by feeding specialists, nor is it necessarily related to feeding. Many babies, however, who have a disorder of central ventilatory control first manifest these difficulties during feeding.

For example, a baby may present with a history of blue spells during feeding. On clinical feeding evaluation, the baby is noted to have normal control of the suck/swallow/breathe process. As the baby becomes drowsy during feeding, however, the ventilatory pattern changes and cyanosis develops. The polysomnogram could be useful in evaluation of this type of problem as it looks at the baby's physiologic parameters during all states of consciousness. As the sophistication of the bedside multichannel pneumogram increases, many problems previously evaluated by the polysomnogram will no longer require evaluation with this more complicated test. Strengths and weaknesses are summarized in table 2-4.

Strengths
Since this test measures the greatest number of variables, it has the best potential to interpret the interrelationship between these variables. It is able to differentiate between central and obstructive apnea and apnea secondary to seizures. Since pressure transducers are placed in the esophagus, the sleep study can differentiate between whether the obstructive apnea is due to gastroesophageal reflux or to airway collapse. In addition, a feeding can be included in the test period, providing data about many physiologic functions during feeding.

Limitations

This test requires a specialized sleep lab and is therefore not widely available. It is expensive and requires specialized expertise and equipment to interpret.

Table 2-4 Strengths and Limitations of the Polysomnogram

Polysomnogram—Multichannel recording of respiration, airflow, chest and diaphragm movement, oxygen and carbon dioxide levels, heart rate, sleep state (EEG and EOG), esophageal pressure. Mostly done during sleep—baby goes through two sleep cycles.

Strengths

- Most sensitive to interpreting relationship between variables
- Strongest study for evaluating problems of respiratory control
- Can be done awake during feed

Limitations

- Requires specialized sleep laboratory
- Expensive and requires special expertise to interpret

Radiologic Procedures

The radiologic studies described here are used to evaluate gastroesophageal reflux (GER), structural abnormalities, and/or swallowing function. The rationale behind evaluating structural integrity and swallowing as they relate to feeding is relatively clear. The relationship between GER and feeding performance, however, may be less clear. Gastroesophageal reflux is the return of gastric contents, either milk alone or mixed with stomach acid, into the esophagus. It can have considerable impact on the infant's feeding behavior. Symptomology resulting from GER can include: worsening of respiratory disease; apnea and/or bradycardia; failure to thrive; and esophageal irritation leading to irritability or refusal to eat. A more detailed discussion of GER and its interactions with feeding is found in chapter 6.

Technetium Scan

During a technetium scan (also referred to as gastroesophageal scintigraphy or a milk scan) a small amount of radionuclide isotope (200u Ci technetium labeled sulfur colloid) is added to the feeding, radioactively labeling the

---

food. The baby is fed in the usual manner via bottle or breast, swaddled, and positioned supine under the camera. A gamma camera images the infant, recording the location of the "labeled" material. Images are made every 30 seconds over a one-hour period after the feeding, looking for the presence of material in the esophagus (see figure 2-4).

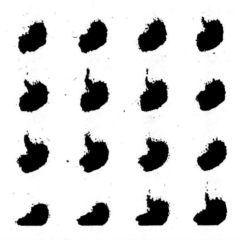

Figure 2-4 Images from a technetium scan.

The number of reflux episodes and the height of refluxed material in the esophagus is calculated and compared with standards. Gastric emptying can be computed by measuring the percentage of food remaining within the stomach after one hour. If food stays in the stomach longer than average there is a greater chance for reflux. Strengths and weaknesses of the technetium scan in comparison to other radiologic tests can be found in table 2-5.

Strengths
The technetium scan provides information regarding several important parameters of GER. It will measure both acid and alkaline reflux—anything that comes up out of the stomach—so it is unlikely to miss reflux events should they occur. It is able to measure the height of the reflux in the esophagus. Airway protective responses or aspiration are more likely if the reflux is frequently to the level of the pharynx. The contribution of delayed gastric emptying to the reflux problem can be determined and treated if necessary. Despite ingestion of the radioactive tracer, this substance is not absorbed and total radiation exposure is low relative to other radiologic procedures. Additionally, the exposure does not change regardless of how long images are taken.

Table 2-5 Strengths and Limitations of the Technetium Scan

Technetium Scan—Radionuclide isotope given with feeding and imaged each 30 seconds for 1 hour after feeding.

Strengths

- Measures both acid and alkaline reflux
- Evaluates gastric emptying
- Evaluates height of reflux
- Relatively low radiation exposure

Limitations

- May be oversensitive
- GER measured for a short time period
- Not continuous, so can't know how long each episode lasts

Limitations

The technetium scan has been criticized for being overly sensitive to reflux and having a high false positive rate. Two factors may contribute to this view: supine positioning may exacerbate reflux activity, and normative values for infants of various ages are not available. While "standards" are used to interpret this study, all infants spit up or reflux to some degree and it is not clear at what point this becomes a pathologic process.

Reflux is measured only for a short period of time—one hour after eating. The technetium scan may therefore miss episodes of GER that occur after this time. One may assume, however, that if significant GER is observed within the hour after eating, then some reflux events will occur as long as food is in the stomach. Lastly, the technetium scan does not take a continuous reading. Therefore, the length of the reflux episodes is unknown.

Barium Swallow

The barium swallow, also known as the esophagram or upper GI, is primarily used to evaluate structure and function of the esophagus and stomach. Structural anomalies, such as tracheoesophageal fistulas, or dysfunction in esophageal motility, are often diagnosed by barium swallow. During this procedure, barium is placed in the esophagus either by oral feeding or via nasogastric tube. The infant is positioned supine on a board with the head restrained in midline and the arms lifted over the head and restrained alongside the ears. The board can be rotated along the body axis so that barium flows into all the crevasses of the esophagus and structures may be observed from all angles (see figure 2-5, page 74).

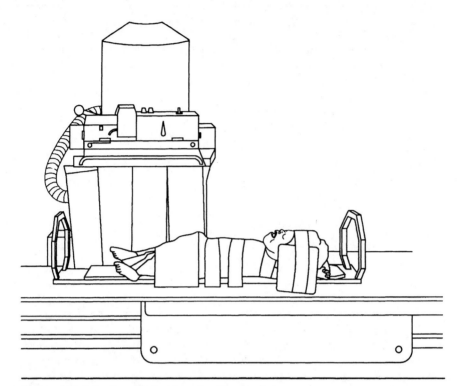

Figure 2-5 Infant positioned for a barium swallow.

The images are viewed via a fluoroscope camera so real-time events can be observed; however, generally only still photographs are taken for later review. Although swallowing can be viewed at the beginning of the study, the general area of interest during a barium swallow is the esophagus. Esophageal motility can be evaluated as the barium flows into the stomach. Once the barium enters the stomach, the radiologist can observe for the presence of spontaneous reflux or attempt to elicit GER by giving pressure to the abdomen. The amount of radiation exposure to the infant is proportional to the time of exposure, which is generally brief. Strengths and limitations are summarized in table 2-6.

Strengths
The barium swallow is an excellent tool to evaluate structural abnormalities and anatomic detail, as well as esophageal motility. If gastroesophageal reflux is observed, the duration and height of the refluxed material in the esophagus can be assessed.

Limitations
The barium swallow has several limitations in evaluating swallowing and gastroesophageal reflux. Because the test is brief, some episodes of spontaneous GER are likely to be missed. As the relatively small amount of

barium used does not compare to a full feeding, reflux may not be triggered in the test conditions. If a reflux episode is seen, the frequency of such an event is still unknown.

Swallowing function observed during a standard barium swallow may not reflect typical performance, as the conditions differ markedly from the feeding situation. The position is supine and restrained, with the infant often crying and upset. Nipple holes may be extremely enlarged to encourage rapid ingestion of an adequate amount of barium for imaging. Generally only one or two swallows are observed, and without saving a real-time image, it is not possible to review the swallowing sequence in detail at a later date.

Table 2-6 Strengths and Limitations of the Barium Swallow

Barium Swallow—Barium placed in upper esophagus by NG or nipple.
  Primarily monitors function of esophagus, may attempt to measure GER.

Strengths
- Identifies structural abnormalities
- Evaluates height of GER in esophagus

Limitations
- Done in a restrained supine position
- No real-time permanent record
- Does not simulate eating process
- Poor measure of GER—too short a time period
- Limited evaluation of swallowing

Videofluoroscopic Swallowing Study

The videofluoroscopic swallowing study (VFSS), also known as the modified barium swallow, is specifically designed to evaluate the pharyngeal swallow. Similarities to the barium swallow described above include use of the same moving-action fluoroscope camera and the introduction of barium to image structures and function. In the VFSS, however, the normal feeding situation is simulated with regard to position and feeding techniques, the area of interest is the pharynx, and a video image is the permanent record of the study. The similarities and differences between the VFSS and standard barium swallow are outlined in table 2-7. The purpose of this study is not only to document whether or not aspiration is occurring, but also to show the reason for the aspiration and the point at which it

---

occurs. Table 2-8 lists the primary parameters that can be evaluated with the VFSS. Table 2-9 outlines the strengths and limitations.

Table 2-7 Comparison of the Standard Barium Swallow and VFSS

Similarities:
- Same type of camera is used
- Barium is introduced by mouth

Differences:
- Positioning
- Method of introducing barium
- Anatomic area of interest
- Type of permanent record

For evaluating infants, the fluoroscope table is tilted vertically and a feeder seat is placed on the ledge in a semireclined position (see figure 2-6). Positioning can be customized by adding cloth rolls to stabilize the head, shoulders, and trunk. The images are enhanced if the fluoroscope is used with magnification. The fluoroscope is connected to a standard VHS video-recorder so that the study can be recorded for later review, possibly in slow-motion or stop-action formats for more detailed analysis. If a frame counter is connected to the videorecorder, frame-by-frame analysis is possible.

Liquid barium is mixed with formula, breast milk, or pureed foods, and barium paste can be spread on crackers, allowing evaluation of all food textures. If desired, liquids can be thickened with commercial thickeners or rice cereal, or the temperature can be modified. The infant is typically fed by bottle or spoon, but in some cases small amounts of barium are introduced by syringe; this is followed by sucking on a pacifier.

Table 2-8 Primary Parameters Evaluated by VFSS

- Initiation of swallow (timing and oral control)
- Duration of pharyngeal swallow
- Adequacy of pharyngeal swallow to clear bolus
- Presence and amount of aspiration
- Timing of aspiration within the swallowing cycle
- Protective reactions in response to aspiration
- Soft palate control during swallowing
- Response to treatment techniques

DIAGNOSTIC TESTS AND PROCEDURES

Table 2-9 Strengths and Limitations of the Videofluoroscopic Swallowing Study (VFSS)

Videofluoroscopic Swallowing Study—Evaluates status and safety of pharyngeal swallow. Barium given by mouth in small amounts and in normal feeding position.

Strengths
- Permanent real-time record
- Simulates eating experience
- Ability to try various textures
- Ability to evaluate treatment techniques
- Good detail of swallowing function secondary to magnification

Limitations
- Does not identify GER or esophageal structural problems well
- Small sample of feeding

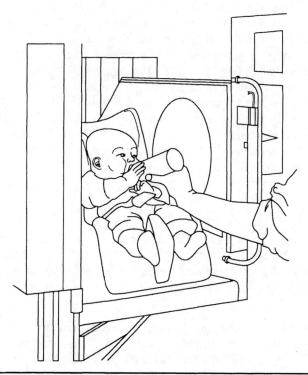

Figure 2-6 Infant positioned for a videofluoroscopic swallowing study (VFSS).

The medical personnel involved in the VFSS varies among settings. The specific combination of occupational or speech therapists with radiologists or radiology technicians will depend on the expertise, needs, and history of the facility. Regardless of the background of the personnel involved, the professionals should have expertise in infant oral-motor control, physiology of the suck/swallow/breathe process, and the influence of motor abnormalities on positioning and oral control, as well as skill in interpreting the video images of swallowing. Allowing parents to observe or assist with this procedure is often useful in enhancing their comprehension of the infant's feeding problems. This understanding may then facilitate acceptance of changes in the feeding regime, particularly if non-oral feeding is recommended.

Emergency backup equipment in the form of cardiorespiratory monitoring, oximetry, or suctioning equipment is highly recommended. It may be desirable to have a nurse or respiratory therapist present if the infant under study has a history of apneic or bradycardic events or has a tracheostomy. For personnel routinely involved in VFSS, monitoring of radiation exposure should occur according to standard hospital procedures.

The protocol used during the administration of the VFSS should be flexible enough to address each baby's individual needs. Generally, the study will begin with the bolus type, amount, and texture that is easiest or most typical for the baby. Modifications can then be made to the infant's position, feeding techniques, and the texture or temperature of the food. Changes should be an outgrowth of the information gathered during the imaging, as well as include all variations the child is expected to use during feeding. For example, microaspiration on thin liquids might lead to a trial with thick liquids. If the baby is free of aspiration using thick liquids and is beginning spoon feeding, semisolids by spoon should be observed. In some cases, a small sample of swallowing behaviors can be observed from the beginning of the feeding, the infant can be fed most of the meal, and a sampling of swallowing behaviors can be observed at the end of the meal. This procedure is useful to assess the influence of fatigue on the infant's swallowing abilities.

Although numerous feeding variations and conditions can be examined during the VFSS, careful selection is necessary to limit the amount of time taken for the study, since radiation exposure is proportionate to the duration of imaging. Logemann provides a further description of VFSS procedures in adults.[2]

Relationship between clinical feeding evaluation and VFSS: There are a number of benefits to completing a clinical feeding evaluation prior to the VFSS. First, it allows the therapist to establish a baseline of the infant's feeding behaviors to compare with the infant's performance during the swallowing study. Frequently, the feeding behavior observed on X-ray is not representative of the typical feeding behaviors. Infants can perform better or worse than their baseline. Paradoxically, there are some infants who have significant feeding disorders but who can swallow barium without difficulty. Knowing the infant's baseline performance allows the therapist to determine the significance of the feeding behavior observed during the swallowing study, thus aiding in interpretation of the study.

Performing a clinical feeding evaluation prior to a VFSS also allows the therapist to determine the types of foods and textures to observe during the swallowing study, the order in which they should be presented, and the optimal positioning of the infant during the study (or the need for adaptive equipment). A number of questions or hypotheses to be tested during the VFSS are then formulated; not just, "What is the function of the pharyngeal swallow?" but "Does swallowing function change with alterations in head position, texture, or temperature?" In this way the therapist is able to formulate and test treatment strategies and evaluate the effect of treatment on X-ray to confirm the result. Thus the VFSS is a useful tool for the evaluation of treatment effectiveness as well as for delineating the basic swallowing function.

Completing a clinical feeding evaluation before the VFSS will also confirm the need for the swallowing study. While the VFSS is an extremely useful clinical tool, the radiation exposure to the infant should not be taken lightly. When a clinical feeding evaluation of infants is performed by a skilled clinician, it may determine that feeding problems are not due to swallowing dysfunction and the VFSS is not necessary. Signs of swallowing dysfunction that might be identified during a clinical feeding evaluation and that indicate the need for a VFSS include overt signs, such as coughing or choking during swallowing or noisy, wet respirations. More subtle signs include a history of unexplained respiratory infection or illness or difficulty managing oral secretions. These clinical signs of swallowing dysfunction are discussed in detail in chapter 5.

It is important to remember that aspiration can be silent—that is, there is no outward indication during the swallow that material is being aspirated. Logemann reports that 40% of adult patients who had aspiration during VFSS were not identified as aspirating during the bedside examination.[3] While this is not a rationale for routine use of VFSS with all infants who have feeding dysfunction, it should alert clinicians to pay particular attention to the medical history, parent descriptions of feeding, and subtle indicators of potential swallowing dysfunction when determining the need for in-depth evaluation of swallowing function.

Strengths

The greatest strength of the VFSS is its ability to provide a detailed analysis of the pharyngeal swallow. It attempts to elicit the infant's typical behaviors by closely simulating the normal eating process in terms of presentation of food and position. There is the flexibility to try various textures, temperatures, and positions, allowing observation of the full range of the infant's feeding abilities. In addition, treatment techniques can be attempted during the study and their effectiveness observed. Since the swallowing study is recorded on videotape, it can be reviewed whenever desired, including in slow-motion or stop-action modes.

Limitations

The generalizability of the feeding sample observed during a VFSS has been questioned, since it is a relatively brief sampling of feeding behavior. In addition, the unusual viscosity of barium may alter the baby's swallowing response. Comparing the performance during the swallowing study to the baseline performance during clinical feeding evaluation can enhance interpretation of results.

The VFSS is not intended to be used to identify GER, as the objective of the study is to observe the pharyngeal area. It does not identify structural abnormalities well, nor does it assess esophageal function.

pH Probe

The pH probe is another diagnostic procedure used to evaluate gastroesophageal reflux. A sensor is inserted through the nose to an area just above the lower esophageal sphincter (LES) to continuously measure the acidity of the esophagus. The probe generally remains in place for 24 hours and is present for all the baby's activities during that period of time. Some pH probes are now small enough that they allow the baby to move freely with minimal restriction (see figure 2-7). The procedure generally requires at least a 24-hour hospital stay. A record is kept at the bedside to record the infant's activities throughout the day for later correlation with changes in pH.

Readings of pH are recorded for computer analysis at the conclusion of the study. Data is recorded on the total number of episodes of pH <4.0, total time with pH <4.0, number of episodes greater than 5 minutes, and longest episode of pH <4.0. Typically, episodes of pH <4.0 must last longer than 10 seconds to be recorded. This data is compiled into a reflux score, which is compared to normative data to confirm the presence of reflux. Many gastroenterologists and surgeons consider this test to be the "gold standard" for evaluation of GER.[4] Others, however, dispute this claim.[5]

The pH probe can also be run concurrently with a pneumogram so that correlations between changes in pH and heart and respiratory rates can be made. In this way, the association between acid reflux and respiratory symptoms can be confirmed. Because acid reflux events are recorded, the risk for the development of esophagitis can be assessed and the need for endoscopic evaluation of the esophagus or medications determined. Table 2-10 lists the strengths and limitations of the pH probe.

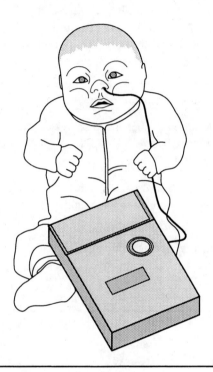

Figure 2-7 Infant being tested with a pH probe.

Strengths
A strength of the pH probe is that measurement occurs over a 24-hour period and during all of the infant's activities. Thus, it is unlikely to miss any acid reflux events should they occur. The relationship between position changes, feedings, or respiratory symptoms can be assessed when the data is compared to the bedside record. In addition, this procedure can be used concurrently with other tests for a more detailed analysis of the relationship of acid reflux to other variables. Data is obtained regarding the length and frequency of acid reflux and the ability of the esophagus to clear the reflux. A computerized score is obtained for comparison with normative data.

Limitations

Since the pH probe measures only acid reflux (pH 4.0), it would not pick up more alkaline reflux events, such as those that occur following a feeding when the gastric contents are primarily formula. Such reflux events, however, may be of vital importance for the infant who tends to aspirate or have apneic events following feeding. In addition, the pH probe will not record how high up the esophagus the refluxed material travels, since it monitors only an area approximately 3 cm above the LES. Newer models with multiple sensors may eliminate this weakness. Finally, acid reflux events must last longer than 10 seconds to be counted; therefore, the pH probe has the potential to miss many short reflux events that could lead to vagal stimulation or aspiration.

Table 2-10 Strengths and Limitations of the pH Probe

PH Probe—Sensor inserted through the nose to an area above the LES to continuously measure acidity.

Strengths

- Measures continuously over 24-hour period
- Measures length and frequency of acid reflux

Limitations

- Does not measure alkaline reflux (formula)
- May not record how high reflux travels up esophagus
- Must last more than 10 seconds to be counted

Pediatric Endoscopy

Endoscopy is the process of using a rigid or flexible tube to directly observe structures within the body for diagnosis, to obtain tissue via biopsy or aspiration, or for treatment such as the removal of a foreign body.[6] The procedure has been used for over 100 years. Reducing the size of the endoscopes for pediatric use, as well as improving the clarity of the visual images, did not occur until the early 1980s.[7,8] Advances in fiberoptics permitted the development of flexible endoscopes that can be used even with extremely small infants. Endoscopy can be used for a wide variety of purposes. This section reviews the most common forms of endoscopy used with infants who have feeding and swallowing disorders. These include the esophagoscopy, esophageal manometry, laryngoscopy, and bronchoscopy.

Esophagoscopy/Esophageal Manometry

Esophagoscopy is a procedure used by gastroenterologists or surgeons for a number of purposes: to directly observe the esophagus to view the effects of acid reflux; to obtain tissue samples through biopsy; or to identify structural abnormalities such as congenital webs, postoperative stenosis, or tumors. It can be used therapeutically for foreign body removal. A rigid endoscope is used for most procedures; however, a fiberoptic endoscope is useful for examination of the more distal gastrointestinal tract. Esophagoscopy is usually reserved for unclear diagnostic problems or to help determine the need for extensive antireflux procedures.

Esophageal manometry is used to measure the pressure in the upper and lower esophageal sphincters to assess the competence of these sphincters. An incompetent lower esophageal sphincter (LES) has a pressure less than 5 mm Hg and a length less than 1.5 cm. Often an incompetent lower esophageal sphincter is the cause of gastroesophageal reflux. Esophageal manometry is also used to evaluate the LES after a Nissen fundoplication is done for the treatment of gastroesophageal reflux.

Bronchoscopy/Laryngoscopy

Endoscopic evaluation of the upper airways (laryngoscopy) and lower airways (bronchoscopy) is used to identify abnormalities of airway size or structure, and to evaluate patency and airway dynamics. Congenital anomalies, stenosis, external compression from vascular rings or masses, or structural integrity problems such as tracheolaryngealmalacia may compromise airway patency and dynamics. Both rigid and flexible bronchoscopes are available for use even with extremely small infants, although there is some controversy regarding which type should be used.[9] Rigid endoscopy is usually performed under general anesthesia, whereas flexible endoscopy can be done at bedside. Airway size may be a determining factor regarding which type of endoscope is used. Generally, flexible endoscopes can be passed farther into the airways than can rigid bronchoscopes.

The specific indications for bronchoscopy are the evaluation of persistent stridor, lung biopsy for recurrent pneumonia, persistent wheezing that is unresponsive to bronchodilators, foreign body aspiration, or difficult intubations. Other indications may include the evaluation of an abnormal cry, hoarseness, vocal cord paralysis, upper-airway obstruction, or tracheoesophageal fistula, especially the H-type fistula.[8,9]

References

1. Garg, M., S. I. Kurzner, D. B. Bautista, and T. G. Keens. 1988. Clinically unsuspected hypoxia during sleep and feeding in infants with bronchopulmonary dysplasia. *Pediatrics.* 81:635-42.

2. Logemann, J. 1983. *Evaluation and treatment of swallowing disorders.* Boston: College-Hill Press.

3. Logemann, J. A. 1986. Treatment for aspiration related to dysphagia: An overview. *Dysphagia* 1:34-38.

4. Da Dalt, L., S. Mazzoleni, G. Montini, F. Donzelli, and F. Zacchello. 1989. Diagnostic accuracy of pH monitoring in gastroesophageal reflux. *Archive of Disease in Childhood.* 64:1421-26.

5. Orenstein, S. R., and D. M. Orenstein. 1988. Gastroesophageal reflux and respiratory disease in children. *The Journal of Pediatrics.* 112:847-58.

6. Lively, C. 1980. Pediatric endoscopy. Resident's Teaching File. Children's Hospital and Medical Center, Seattle, WA.

7. Gans, S. L., and G. Berci. 1971. Advances in endoscopy of infants and children. *Journal of Pediatric Surgery* 6:199-233.

8. Wood, R. E., and J. M. Sherman. 1980. Pediatric flexible bronchoscopy. *Annals of Otology Rhinology and Laryngology* 89:414-16.

9. Wood, R. E., and D. Postma. 1988. Endoscopy of the airway in infants and children. *The Journal of Pediatrics.* 112:1-6.

10. Hay, W. W. 1987. The uses, benefits, and limitations of pulse oximetry in neonatal medicine: Consensus on key issues. *Journal of Perinatology* 7:347-49.

11. Emery, J. R. 1987. Skin pigmentation as an influence on the accuracy of pulse oximetry. *Journal of Perinatology* 7:329-30.

12. Hay, W. W. 1987. Physiology of oxygenation and its relation to pulse oximetry in neonates. *Journal of Perinatology* 7:309-19.

13. Kopotic, R. J., F. L. Mannino, C. D. Colley, and N. Horning. 1987. Display variability, false alarms, probe cautions and recorder use in neonatal pulse oximetry. *Journal of Perinatology* 7:340-42.

14. Murray, J. F. 1986. *The normal lung: The basis for diagnosis and treatment of pulmonary disease.* Philadelphia: W. B. Saunders Co.

3 Clinical Feeding Evaluation

Although many medical tests and procedures are available to assess feeding-related functions in infants, observation of feeding should play a major role in the problem-solving process when feeding dysfunction is present. Nothing substitutes for a set of trained eyes, ears, and hands experiencing a baby's feeding problems when trying to identify the underlying causes of dysfunction and develop appropriate treatment strategies. For that reason, observation is the key component of the clinical feeding evaluation of infants (CFEI) presented in this chapter.

The feeding specialist must have a thorough understanding of normal function in the many systems that interact to culminate in infant feeding for this critical observation to be effective. In addition, a systematic method of organizing these observations is needed to insure thorough collection of data. Background information covering relevant anatomy, physiology, neural control, and maturation, as well as the impact of various medical problems on the feeding process, can be found in other chapters.

This chapter presents an overview of the process utilized during the clinical feeding evaluation of infants, describes the use of the feeding history in preparing for observation of function, and then focuses on specific observations that are made, as well as the interpretation of these observations. The following seven broad categories provide a structure for organizing observations related to infant feeding:

1. Behavior and State
2. Motoric Control
3. Response to Tactile Input
4. Oral-Motor Control
5. Sucking, Swallowing, and Breathing
6. Physiologic Control
7. General Observations

A sample form for recording specific observations during the clinical feeding evaluation of infants is found on page 154. Referring to this form while reviewing each section of the text may assist the reader in applying this material to the clinical setting.

A number of evaluations and checklists are available to assess feeding functions in the pediatric population.[1-3] The complex process of feeding by sucking, however, is generally addressed minimally. Since the focus of this text is infant feeding, the primary oral feeding method addressed in the clinical feeding evaluation of infants will be sucking, either on breast or bottle. Although many of the concepts of evaluation and treatment that are presented may be applicable to children of varying ages and abilities, spoon feeding and cup drinking will be addressed minimally.

Although a feeding difficulty may be the presenting problem and the focus of evaluation for a specific infant, the "whole" infant must be considered during the evaluation. The baby's medical status, neurologic status, neuromotor function, behavioral profile, and general developmental abilities will be important contributors to feeding function or dysfunction and may also need comprehensive evaluation. This book will not go into detail on the evaluation of these parameters but will present some basic evaluation and treatment strategies in these areas as they specifically relate to infant feeding.

The Evaluation Process

A five-step process is used in the clinical feeding evaluation of infants to guide the observation process and formulation of treatment strategies.

1. Gathering information and planning the feeding observation:
Background information on medical and social history as well as the nature of the feeding problem should be collected from chart review and/or discussions with physicians or nurses involved in the child's care. The parent or caregiver should be interviewed to determine specific concerns regarding feeding, current feeding methods, and observations that have been made during feeding. Parent feeding history will be discussed in detail in the next section of this chapter.

The information that has been gathered should be compiled to plan the feeding evaluation. Equipment that might be needed during the evaluation should be selected and gathered. For example, feeding tools (such as nipples, pacifiers, or special devices) and food of various types or textures should be readied. The need for equipment to monitor physiologic status is determined. The sequence of observation for various skills may also be planned.

2. Feeding observation:

General observations: Baseline physiologic status is noted. Posture, movement, and developmental skill should be observed briefly if these characteristics are not known to the feeding specialist.

Naturalistic observation: The typical feeding situation should be observed. This includes using the normal bottle and nipple, or breast, at a natural feeding time. In many cases it is most effective if a primary caretaker can be observed feeding the infant. If this is not possible, the feeding specialist should try to duplicate characteristics of the child's standard feeding situation but should clarify whether the feeding was typical and that problematic behaviors were actually observed.

Elicited observations: The feeding session can then be modified to elicit behaviors or to observe feeding skills that have not occurred spontaneously. The interplay of naturalistic observation and elicited responses will vary for each child, depending on the type of feeding problems. To observe some feeding behaviors, additional feedings may need to be observed. For example, if the baby has been reported to have breath-holding spells when very agitated or hungry, but was calm during the feeding evaluation and did not demonstrate this behavior, additional observations with the infant in a different state may be needed.

3. Treatment exploration:

Based on the information that has been gathered and the observations of feeding, hypotheses are developed to explain the problems that have been observed. These hypotheses can be explored by altering aspects of the feeding such as the food texture, feeding tools, position, and/or feeding techniques, and monitoring changes in performance. This process may help to clarify the underlying basis of the feeding problem, as well as suggest strategies for treatment.

For example, if a baby demonstrates an abnormal rhythm of sucking, swallowing, and breathing, external pacing or techniques to slow the rate of fluid flow might be tried. If slowing the fluid flow improves the feeding pattern, one component of the infant's problems might be poor oral control of the bolus prior to swallow. The contribution of fluid thickness and bolus size can then be explored, and various methods of reducing fluid flow may be considered as part of the treatment plan. Morris and Klein describe this process as moving between a global overview of the problem and a sequential analysis.[1] An evaluation system that incorporates both of these components tends to be efficient and effective.

4. Synthesizing information:

The information gathered during the feeding evaluation must then be synthesized into a cohesive and rational plan. It should allow the therapist to answer the following questions, which are key to developing appropriate feeding strategies.

- What is the child's level of function? In particular, how adequately and/or safely can the child's nutritional needs be met through oral feeding?

- What factors interfere with feeding function? Do developmental factors or abnormal function affect one or more of the performance areas?

- How well does the child's feeding performance "match" the caregiver concerns or expectations?

- Is additional information necessary? Must other tests or consultations be undertaken to provide adequate information to develop a treatment/management plan?

- Are there treatment techniques available that appear to improve oral feeding function?

5. *Communicating results:*

With multiple health professionals and family members involved in the evaluation process, care must be taken to effectively communicate results and suggestions for further testing or treatment techniques. Although multidisciplinary meetings are ideal, they are not always possible. Written documentation is necessary, but verbal communication is encouraged. Communicating in person or by phone allows immediate feedback to and from parents or team members, making the overall problem solving faster and potentially more effective.

Precautions and Safety Issues

All clinical feeding evaluations should be carried out in a manner that addresses the safety of both the infant and the examiner. Since feeding in some infants is accompanied by significant choking, apnea, and possibly bradycardia or cardiac arrest, the baby's safety requires that appropriate monitoring and standby assistance be available if there is any indication these conditions might exist. Precautions would include using a cardiorespiratory monitor, and having suction and oxygen equipment readily available, along with personnel trained to use this equipment and to respond to a cardiac arrest.

Since the CFEI requires the feeding specialist to place fingers in the baby's mouth, coming in contact with saliva, body substance isolation techniques should be used for the examiner's and the baby's protection. Hospital procedure gloves are the most commonly recommended means of body substance isolation.[38] They should fit snugly to better feel the structures and movement of the mouth and to insure that the baby does not pull the tip of the glove into the mouth during sucking, possibly obstructing the airway. Latex gloves may meet these criteria most effectively. While the gloves do not need to be sterile, a new pair should be used for each patient.

For the infant's comfort, fingernails should be short and the finger inserted into the mouth with the pad opposing the palate. In this position the fingernail will not poke into the palate, possibly causing a gag response. As procedure gloves may have an unpleasant taste, washing gloved hands (completely removing the soap) prior to placing them in the infant's mouth may make them more palatable. Also, if the gloved finger is wet prior to insertion into the mouth, it may slide in more easily.

Feeding History

Some information that is included in the feeding history may be available in the medical record. However, feeding-related information in the infant's chart is only one part of a complete medical history. Feeding problems may not be covered in depth, and the observations may be vague or general. For example, the record may state "the child coughs and chokes" but give no indication of how often, when during the feeding, or what happens after the coughing. Therefore, it is important to sit down with the parent or primary caretaker to take a specific feeding history.

A feeding history done in conjunction with a clinical feeding evaluation asks detailed questions about feeding behaviors and focuses on clarifying the timing of events. It not only provides a clear base of information but also assists in outlining the direction of the evaluation. General ideas regarding the source of the feeding problem may be formulated to help focus the path of the evaluation. Hypotheses that need to be tested can be developed and the feeding specialist can be prepared to have certain equipment available in order to try specific modifications. It is crucial, however, that the feeding specialist not decide what the problem is prior to actually observing the infant. Although parent history may point clearly to a particular problem, deciding this is the problem before watching a feeding may close the feeding specialist's eyes, ears, and hands to other important information during the evaluation process.

Taking the feeding history may be the first encounter the feeding specialist has with the parents or caregivers, and it will address what is often an emotionally charged area. Since this interview may set the tone for all future interactions with the caregivers, including how well they will comply with treatment techniques, rapport building is extremely important. As questions regarding their infant's feeding may sound threatening, information needs to be gathered in a supportive manner. The loss of self-confidence and control the parents may be feeling when their baby's feeding is not successful needs to be acknowledged.

Mothering and feeding are intimately linked. A mother's confidence and capability in her role as a mother may feel threatened when the baby has feeding difficulties. Many factors play a part in how deeply an infant's feeding difficulties will affect a mother's feeling about her own mothering skills. These may include the number of children she has mothered, her overall level of self-confidence, the presence of adequate support systems, or the type of problem her baby has.

Following are examples of ways to acknowledge the parent's loss of control and minimize feelings of inadequacy while taking a feeding history.

- "I'll be asking a lot of questions related to your baby's feeding. I know many parents don't routinely observe these things. I'm not expecting that you will have noticed all these things either, but if you have observed some of them it may help us discover what the feeding problem is."

- "I know it's hard when a baby is having trouble feeding. We all expect babies to be able to feed when they are born. If your baby is having trouble feeding, you might assume that it is your fault, and that you are doing something wrong. Feeding for a baby is a very complicated process, and at times things go wrong even if we are trying our best. If we work together to discover what the problem is, we can find a way to make the feeding better."

- "I know none of your other children had feeding problems. You may be frustrated that the techniques that worked for your other children did not work for this baby. This baby may have difficulties that your other children did not have. Your experience as a mother has probably enabled you to handle the baby's difficulties longer than an inexperienced mother. Together we most likely will be able to find ways of dealing with this feeding difficulty."

Taking a Structured Feeding History

The feeding history is a structured interview with questions divided into six broad categories. A complete interview form is shown on pages 150-153 to assist in structuring the interview. A brief description of each category follows.

Parent description of the problem: Parents or caregivers are initially asked for a description of the problem. This allows them to be in control of the first part of the interview and acknowledges the importance of their views regarding the infant's feeding. It also provides the examiner with information on their perception of the magnitude of the feeding problem.

State/behavior: General questions are asked about the baby's typical state and behavior. This helps determine if these characteristics might interfere with feeding and provides information on the baby's response to feeding.

Schedule: Information on the feeding schedule helps determine basic nutritional intake and the amount of time spent feeding the baby each day. It may provide clues to the parents' perception of the adequacy of their baby's diet.

Method of feeding: This information allows the feeding specialist to provide a "typical" feeding during the clinical feeding evaluation, or helps determine whether the baby's behavior during the evaluation differed from the usual behavior.

Feeding problems observed by parent: Parental feeding observations alert the feeding specialist to specific problems to look for during the actual observation of feeding. They provide information on the parents' perceptions of any relationships between events during the feeding.

Other factors: These questions provide input on factors that may seem unrelated to feeding but may potentially play a role in the feeding problems (for example, a history of frequent upper-respiratory infections).

Interpretation of Feeding History

Table 3-1, page 92, describes clusters of symptoms that may be reported during the feeding history. Although it is unlikely that one symptom in a cluster will be diagnostic of a particular problem, a group of symptoms may suggest a potential problem area or point to the need for further evaluation. This area should then receive careful attention during the feeding observation process. Also note that many of the symptoms may be associated with several problem areas, so interpretation of any one symptom needs to be in the context of other findings.

Table 3-1 Interpretation of Feeding History

Cluster of Symptoms:	Suggests need for:
• parent description of swallowing problem • gulping sounds • noisy breathing only with feeding • takes pacifier well, won't take bottle • excessive drooling; need for oral suctioning • history of respiratory illness: pneumonia, asthma, etc.	Careful assessment of swallow
• sleepy baby • poor cues re: when to feed • difficulty with feeding transitions • agitated, cries a lot, sleeps poorly • difficulty initiating sucking • poor rhythm	Careful assessment of state/behavior
• parent describes sucking problem • history of frequent changes of nipple • history of enlarging nipple hole • difficulty initiating sucking	Careful assessment of oral-motor control
• frequent spitting up, vomiting • agitated, excessive crying • sleeps poorly • draws knees to chest with crying	Consider presence of GER
• sleepy baby • falls asleep prior to taking full feed • sweating • many colds • chronic nasal congestion • sucking becomes disorganized in middle of feeding • slow sucking rhythm • feeding lasts longer than 30 min.	Careful assessment of endurance
• likes spoon better than sucking • chronic nasal congestion • uneven sucking rhythm • forgetting to breathe • coughing, choking	Careful assessment of coordination of sucking, swallowing, and breathing

Table 1-3 *(continued)*

• excessive gagging	Careful assessment of tactile responses
• very particular about nipple shape	
• problems with transitions, especially to spoon	
• history of tube feeding	
• color change has been noted	Assessment of physiologic parameters
• baby forgets to breathe	
• medical history of apnea and/or bradycardia with feed	
• sweating	
• baby is fed too often	Careful assessment of parent knowledge regarding infant feeding needs
• baby not fed frequently enough	
• baby is not given adequate amount of formula, though parent perceives it as adequate	
• inappropriate feeding position	

Behavior and State

By observing an infant's behavior, information can be gathered on how well the infant is able to deal with the environment and adapt its behavior to changing environmental demands. The environment may include internal input from the baby's own body; the sights, sounds, and smells of the general environment surrounding the infant; and/or specific movement or activities imposed on the infant. Behaviors can range from social engagement, to self-regulatory, to stress or avoidance behaviors. Interwoven with a baby's behaviors are the various states of alertness or attention within the infant's repertoire. These states are communicated via behaviors that can range from sleep to active interaction to passive inattention to crying.

Through observations of the baby's behaviors and state, the feeding specialist can determine how well the baby is handling a situation—specifically the feeding process. Behaviors of stability and adaptation will be observed when feeding is going well. If avoidance or stress behaviors are observed, a dysfunction in some component of the feeding process can be presumed.

Als[4] has provided a model for understanding the role of state and behavioral cues in determining the stability and organization of a particular infant, and literature in this area continues to expand. An infant's response to the environment and the quality of its interactions can be manifest through behaviors in any of four hierarchical systems: the autonomic or physiologic system, the motoric system, state system, or the attentional system. The baby with state stability and attentional regulation is described as demonstrating: clear, robust sleep states; rhythmical, robust crying; effective self-quieting; reliable consolability; and, when awake, robust, focused, shiny-eyed alertness and/or animated facial expressions such as frowning, cheek softening, mouth pursing to an ooh-face, cooing, and attentional smiling.[4]

This section discusses behaviors as they relate to state and attentional changes. Physiologic and motoric behaviors that relate to feeding performance will be included in the broader sections on physiologic and motor control.

States of Alertness

As described above, an infant's state is a constellation of behaviors that signals a level of alertness or consciousness. It can also signal how available the baby is for interaction or for functional skills such as feeding. Brazelton provides a descriptive and clinically useful list of states of alertness.[5] These are summarized below and will be referred to by number in subsequent sections.

State 1—Deep sleep: The baby is asleep and has a regular respiratory pattern. The eyes are closed, with no eye movements. There is no spontaneous activity, though jerks or startles may be seen. Responses to external stimuli are delayed.

State 2—Light sleep: The eyes are closed, though rapid eye movements may be noted beneath closed lids, and occasionally eyes may open briefly. There is low-level motor activity present, with movements quite random. Respirations are frequently irregular and sucking movements may be seen.

State 3—Drowsy or semi-dozing: The eyes are open but dull and heavy-lidded or closed with eyelids fluttering. The infant may look dazed and "unavailable." The activity level is variable, though movements are generally smooth with mild startles. Frequently state changes can be seen with stimulation.

State 4—Quiet alert: The infant is strongly focused on a stimulus (often auditory or visual). There is a bright, almost glazed look, though the focus of attention can change easily after a brief delay. Motor activity is minimal.

State 5—Active alert: There is considerable motor activity, including thrusting of the extremities. The baby often responds to stimuli with more movement. Brief "fussy" periods may be noted.

State 6—Crying: The infant is crying intensely. It is difficult to break through the crying with any stimulus.

There is not one optimal state for feeding every baby. It is important to remember that there is a wide range of variability within babies and among babies regarding which state is optimal for feeding. Many babies feed adequately in state 3, 4, or 5 and occasionally may feed while in state 2. Some babies feed best only when very awake and alert; other babies have better feedings when they are drowsy or in light sleep.

Expectations regarding the states of alertness a baby demonstrates and the baby's ability to transition between states are related to age. Premature infants will spend minimal time in states 4 and 5. Their states may seem disorganized and lack clarity when compared to a full-term baby. Full-term babies should have clear differentiation between states, although they may spend only a small amount of time in states 4 and 5. An older baby will spend more time awake and alert and will have clearer and more predictable changes of state.

How to Evaluate

When assessing state and behavior as they relate to feeding, it is important to consider whether the baby has a repertoire of behaviors and states that allows the baby to be successful at the functional skill of feeding. State and behavior should be observed throughout the CFEI, during the feeding history as well as during the direct observation of feeding. The therapist should note the presence of stress signals and observe whether these are a factor during feeding or nonfeeding times. The parents' response to the baby's stress signals and the amount of intervention or support they supply to the baby should be noted. Below is a list of questions that will guide the therapist's observation of state and behavior as they relate to feeding. These observations can be recorded on the CFEI observation form.

Range of states: What is the baby's state before the feed? in the middle? at the end? Does the baby's state provide a foundation for functional feeding?

State stability: How stable or fragile is the state? How much change in the environment can the baby tolerate and maintain an adequate, steady state for feeding? How much help is necessary from the examiner to maintain an appropriate state for feeding?

Stress signals: Does the baby show any of the state-related stress signals listed in table 3-2? How frequently are these stress cues observed and what are their antecedents? Do they occur mainly during feeding or nonfeeding times? Following the demonstration of stress signals, does the baby make any attempt at self-regulation?

Table 3-2 State-Related Stress Cues

- diffuse sleep or awake states with whimpering sounds, facial twitches, and discharge smiling
- eye floating; roving eye movements
- strained fussing or crying; silent crying
- staring
- frequent active averting
- panicked or worried alertness; hyperalertness
- glassy-eyed, strained alertness; lidded, drowsy alertness
- rapid state oscillations; frequent buildup to arousal
- irritability and prolonged diffuse arousal
- crying
- frenzy and inconsolability
- sleeplessness and restlessness

Adapted from Als[4]

Interpretation

The basic question that must be addressed is whether the baby's state or state control is interfering with the ability to feed. If it appears that it is interfering, the examiner must first determine the optimal feeding state(s) for that particular baby. Then it must be determined whether the baby can achieve an appropriate state, either independently or with intervention. Even a baby who is able to maintain a calm alert state may show subtle behavioral cues of gaze aversion or rapid shifts in muscle tone that indicate some aspect of the feeding process is stressful. The feeding specialist must determine which techniques are useful in changing and/or maintaining the appropriate state for feeding (see chapter 5).

An infant's distribution of states, as well as ability to move smoothly between states, is dependent on a number of variables. These include the age or maturity of the infant, neurologic integrity, and the baby's general well-being. Physiologic variables such as hunger or a point in the sleep-wake cycle can also influence an infant's state control.[5] At times, these factors may impact state in ways that the feeder is not able to modify. In

---

other words, in some cases it may not be possible to bring the baby to a functional state for feeding. For example, a baby who is in the deep sleep portion of the sleep cycle may not be able to be aroused adequately for optimal feeding, though the baby may feed well at another time. Or, a baby who feeds best in a drowsy state may become so hungry that frantic crying is initiated. The baby may not be able to be calmed adequately to reach an optimal state for oral feeding, though careful timing of the next feeding may lead to successful feeding. Babies who are in pain or discomfort for any reason may utilize sleep or crying states as a way to cope with that discomfort, thus interfering with feeding.

If factors are present that might interfere with appropriate state control for feeding, such as immaturity or neurologic impairment, the infant may have a prolonged need for state-related intervention. This can also be seen in babies with ongoing medical problems such as bronchopulmonary dysplasia or congenital heart disease. The stress of the medical condition may be an overriding factor impacting the infant's state and behavior. While state-related interventions may assist in the feeding process, there may be times when only improvement in the underlying medical condition will alleviate the state control difficulties interfering with feeding.

Motoric Control

Several areas of motoric control that do not specifically include oral-motor skills are important when evaluating infant feeding. These include overall neuromotor control, development of specific motor skills, motoric behaviors, and the infant's feeding position. Normal functioning and/or integrity of these areas supports the feeding process. Abnormal functioning in any of these areas may limit the success of feeding. Observation of a baby's motoric control can occur during any portion of the CFEI or at a separate time. Observations of motoric control can be recorded on the CFEI form.

General Neuromotor Control

Evaluation
General neuromotor control includes elements of muscle tone, primitive reflex activity, and the development of antigravity postural control. Whether or not a formal evaluation of neuromotor control is completed, at least a brief assessment of the infant's overall neuromotor control should be done before beginning a feeding evaluation. This background information is important, as problems in oral-motor control or in feeding posture/position may be related to a larger picture of abnormal neuromotor control.

Formal evaluation of neuromotor control can be done using a variety of formats. Some examples of evaluation tools are: the Movement Assessment of Infants (MAI),[6] the INFANIB,[7] and the Dubowitz Neurological Assessment of the Preterm and Full-Term Infant.[8] Informal assessment can occur when the feeding specialist changes or wraps the baby prior to feeding or through a brief screening before beginning the feeding observation. During formal or informal assessment of neuromotor control the following specific questions should be considered:

Tone: What is the overall muscle tone at rest? How does overall muscle tone change with activity? What is the quality of the baby's movement?

Primitive reflexes: To what degree does primitive reflex activity influence posture and movement? (Not simply, Are the reflexes present or absent?)

Posture: How are tone and reflexes reflected in resting postures or during active movement? How well does the baby move against gravity?

Interpretation

Since the baby's neuromotor control provides a background of support for the feeding process, when feeding difficulties arise the feeding specialist must consider whether the baby's tone, posture, and/or reflexes are interfering with feeding. For effective feeding, muscle tone must be balanced. Tone should be high enough to allow movement but not so high that it interferes with smoothly coordinated movement. Abnormal muscle tone or posture may also interfere with appropriate positioning during feeding or may contribute to oral-motor control problems.

Although abnormalities in neuromotor control can be a sign of neurologic dysfunction, they can have other causes in the premature or medically fragile infant. Neuromotor abnormalities may be a reflection of (1) immaturity, as in the variable motor patterns noted at each gestational age; (2) the effects of the extrauterine environment on the immature fetus, such as shoulder retraction or hip abduction in a weak infant positioned without support; or (3) habitual postural responses developed secondary to medical interventions, for example, the hyperextended head and neck posture often seen in chronically intubated infants. It is the feeding specialist's role to differentiate between acquired abnormal postural patterns and neurologically based tone and postural abnormalities.

Various handling activities (as discussed in chapter 5 under Tone, Posture, and Position) may be used prior to (or possibly during) the feeding, to modify neuromotor problems in a way that improves the feeding. Some of these techniques may be utilized during the evaluation process to determine their effectiveness. For example, the feeding specialist might work to reduce extensor tone, elongate the neck, and/or bring the shoulders into a less elevated, retracted position. In addition, the feeding position may be modified to modulate tone while the baby is eating. When faced with significant neurologically based abnormalities (for example, a baby with significant sequelae from severe birth asphyxia), handling activities may modify the position or neuromotor control but still not enable the infant to cross the threshold and become a functional oral feeder.

Development of Specific Motor Skills

Evaluation
Although it is not necessary to know the specific developmental level of the baby in order to complete the feeding evaluation, it is important to know if the infant's skills approximate age expectations or are significantly delayed. Specific developmental levels can be evaluated using a variety of standardized tools such as the Bayley Scales of Infant Development,[9] the Gesell Developmental Scales,[10] or the Peabody Scales of Development.[11] Formal developmental testing does not need to accompany the CFEI, but a brief screening of the infant's developmental skills will round out the evaluation process.

Interpretation
Knowing the level of an infant's motor and interactive development allows the feeding specialist to consider feeding skills in the context of overall development. It can be determined if feeding performance is "developmentally appropriate," not just "age appropriate," aiding in the establishment of realistic expectations. For example, the choice of position to feed the baby will be influenced by the overall level of gross motor control. Likewise, decisions to introduce various food textures or skills such as cup drinking may be influenced by the infant's overall level of development rather than age.

Motoric Behaviors

Evaluation
These are motoric responses to the environment that can indicate how stressful the baby finds the environment and how well the baby is able to adapt to stressors. Als describes the baby who is motorically stable as demonstrating smooth, well-modulated posture, well-regulated tone, and synchronous, smooth movements with efficient motor strategies at the appropriate developmental level.[4] Motoric strategies a newborn may use for self-regulation in the face of environmental stress include hand clasping, foot clasping, finger folding, hand-to-mouth maneuvers, grasping, suck searching and sucking, and hand holding.

Unlike neuromotor control and developmental level, which may be evaluated both before and during the feeding observation, motoric behaviors are primarily evaluated during the feeding, as they indicate the baby's perception of stress with feeding. Important motoric behaviors that may be seen in response to stress are listed in table 3-3. When these motoric behaviors are observed, the examiner must try to identify the specific source of the stress as well as observe the infant's attempts to cope with the source of stress.

Table 3-3 Motoric Stress Cues

- Motoric flaccidity:
  Trunk, extremities and face (gape face)
- Motoric hypertonicity:
  Hyperextensions of the legs—sitting on air, leg bracing
  Hyperextensions of the arms and hands—saluting, airplaning, finger splays
  Truncal hyperextensions—arching, opisthotnus
  Hyperflexions—fetal tuck, fisting
- Facial grimacing
- Frantic, diffuse activity
- Frequent twitching

Adapted from Als[4]

Interpretation
Motoric stress signals are often difficult to differentiate from neuromotor abnormalities. In fact, the type of motoric stress behaviors an infant demonstrates is usually related to the infant's overall neuromotor control. For example, a baby with disorganized movement patterns may respond with frantic, diffuse activity and squirming, whereas the baby with neurologically increased tone may respond to stress by arching.

Initially the feeding specialist must try to determine whether motoric behaviors such as tonal variations and movement disorganization are the result of neuromotor impairment or responses to stress. Without making this distinction, treatment may be ineffective. For example, if a baby is arching, presumably due to neurologically based increased extensor tone, handling and movement activities may be initiated to decrease extension and increase flexor control. If the extension is actually due to excessively rapid liquid flow from the bottle, this baby's problem will not have been solved. Continuing to feed a baby in a manner that is stressful, over time, may inadvertently increase feeding problems.

If it is determined that stress factors are responsible for abnormal motor behaviors, the *timing* of motoric stress signals provides important clues about the source of stress. For instance, a baby who becomes frantic just after swallowing is giving cues that swallowing may be dysfunctional. The baby who stiffens when the bottle is placed in the mouth, on the other hand,

---

CLINICAL FEEDING EVALUATION

may perceive the tactile components of the feeding process as stressful. Since the ultimate goal is to eliminate or modify the source of stress (not just to modify the motor behavior), we must be able to identify this underlying problem. It is therefore critical to be aware of what is happening during the feeding at the time of the stress cue, as the same motoric behavior may have different causes in different children and at different times.

Feeding Position

Evaluation

One way the three aspects of motor control described above influence feeding is in how they come together in the feeding position. Poor positioning may compromise an infant's ability to feed effectively, but improvements in positioning may assist the feeding process. The posture or position assumed during feeding can be a reflection of the infant's overall motoric integrity, the infant's response to the environment, or the knowledge of the feeder. Although normally feeding babies are relatively adaptable and can feed in a variety of positions and alignments, babies with even slight feeding problems may need, or benefit from, very specific positions for optimal feeding.

Proper alignment of the head, neck, trunk, and extremities is important to feeding performance. In the optimal position for infant feeding (see figure 3-1, page 102), the head and neck assume a neutral to slightly flexed position and are given stable support. Overall body posture reflects slight flexion. The trunk is neutrally aligned and well supported in a semireclined position, with orientation of the head and extremities about the midline. Prior to four months, some degree of shoulder elevation is normally present. After that, the shoulders should assume a typically depressed position during feeding. The hips should be flexed, but 90° of hip flexion is not necessary in the infant feeding position.

The head and neck have a key role in the feeding position, as there is a strong interaction between head and neck position and feeding function. Bosma has proposed a neurological link between the maintenance of the patency of the pharyngeal airway and the development of head and neck posture[12] (see chapter 1, page 44). He suggests that craniocervical posture begins with stabilization of the pharyngeal airway in the baby. The airway remains key in postural mechanisms throughout life. In development, once the maintenance of the pharyngeal airway is achieved, it begins the process of craniocervical postural control. Likewise the control and competence of head and neck posture is important for a competent pharyngeal swallow. Thus, using proper positioning during a feeding session not only will affect respiratory mechanisms, oral-motor control, and swallowing control, but it may also assist in the development of early head and neck postural responses.

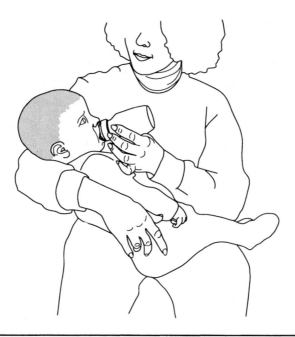

Figure 3-1 Proper feeding position, showing alignment of head, neck, and trunk.

During the CFEI the infant's feeding position should be assessed in comparison to the "optimal" position described above. In addition to observing alignment of the infant's body, paying particular attention to the head and neck, the observer must note the degree of support the feeder provides to the baby. It must be determined whether the amount of support matches the baby's intrinsic postural control. For example, the newborn will require firm support throughout the head, neck, and trunk, whereas the four-month-old, who has gained some postural control of the head and trunk, will require less support. The overall position that is used (e.g., baby in the crook of the arm, en face, fully reclined) should be recorded, as it may impact the infant's alignment and the potential for interaction between the baby and feeder.

Interpretation
If the feeding position is felt to be less than optimal and potentially interfering with feeding, the underlying problems need to be identified in order to structure an appropriate intervention plan. Factors that may play a role include the following.

Abnormal muscle tone: Tone may be either too high, too low, or not well modulated. For example, with increased tone, marked neck and back extension may be seen. With low tone, excessive neck flexion, chin tucking, and truncal collapse may be noted.

Inappropriate developmental expectations: Although the baby may be fed in a position appropriate for its chronological age, this may be developmentally inappropriate if motor delays are present. For example, a baby who is fed in an upright seated position before achieving adequate head and trunk control may have the head turned to the side and neck extended during feeding, possibly compromising oral-control of the bolus.

Environmental stressors: If the baby is uncomfortable for any reason either from internal or external stimuli, the baby's motoric stress responses may compromise the feeding position. For example, arching or flailing movements may be observed during feeding in response to inability to coordinate swallowing and breathing.

Feeder's body mechanics: The feeder may not be providing adequate support for the infant during feeding. This may be due to the feeder's lack of knowledge about feeding infants or the feeder's body type. If the feeder is not comfortably positioned, it will also be reflected in his or her body mechanics while handling the baby. Common problems are: a parent who supports the baby's neck, rather than head, and allows the baby's head to tip over the parent's arm in an extended position (see figure 3-2); holding the infant in a very reclined position; and tucking the infant's arm under the feeder's arm, leading to shoulder retraction and poor midline orientation.

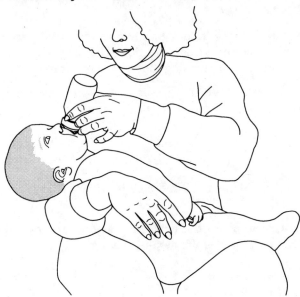

Figure 3-2 An example of poor feeding position, with excessive neck and trunk extension.

Summary of Interpretation of Motoric Control

The evaluation of an infant's motoric control requires skill and attention to detail. The interplay between the baby's inherent central nervous system integrity and the baby's response to the environment may be manifest in similar behaviors. Yet if these behaviors have very different underlying causes, the treatments may be different, if not conflicting, as illustrated in the following example. Sorting through the multiple possibilities of why a motoric behavior is observed is the art of evaluation and a key to effective treatment. Example:

The feeding specialist observes that a baby arches during feeding. Possible interpretations of this response include:

- There is neurologically abnormal extensor tone, which suggests the need for handling to modify the tone and/or changes in the feeding position.

- The child may have gas or some other GI discomfort and arch only at the end of the feeding. More frequent burping throughout the feeding may be needed.

- The flow of liquid may be too fast, and the baby is pulling away to protect itself. This may be seen more frequently at the beginning of the feeding when the baby's sucking is strongest. A change of nipple may be indicated.

- The baby has respiratory problems and is trying to maintain the airway in the most open position. The baby may need nebulizer treatments prior to feeding to improve respiratory status.

- The baby is not hungry. Feeding needs to be postponed to a later time.

- The baby is orally aversive to the touch of the nipple or the taste of the formula. Treatment for oral normalization needs to be instituted.

- The baby is used to being fed lying down with the bottle propped. Gradual introduction of more appropriate feeding positions needs to occur.

Successful intervention for this problem depends on correct identification of the underlying causes of the motor behavior.

Response to Tactile Input

The mouth is the infant's oral sensorium and first "handle on the world." Infants, even preterm infants, come into the world with a relatively sophisticated tactile system that affords them survival as well as discriminatory skills. Tactually elicited reflexes and responses that are present at birth allow the infant to seek out and obtain nutrition safely. The ability to accept touch to the cheeks, lips, gums, and tongue is therefore a prerequisite for feeding, and thus the infant's survival. Newborns can communicate preferences or likes and dislikes via tactile responses, with wide variability seen in infant preferences. Normal infants get pleasure from oral tactile experiences, seeking them out for purposes other than nutrition, and show adaptability to tactile input in the oral area. For example, during the first few months of life, babies can adapt to various shapes of nipples and pacifiers.

This section will look at two aspects of tactile responses in infants—oral reflexes and behavioral responses to tactile input.

Oral Reflexes

The oral reflexes develop quite early in utero. The swallowing reflex has been observed in the fetus at 12 to 14 weeks[43] and the gag reflex at 18 weeks.[14] These oral reflexes are defined as programmed responses to a specific sensory input, generally a tactile stimulus, and they become modified or integrated into functional activity with increased maturity. The expression of oral reflexes at any age can be quite varied, depending on a number of factors, such as state or hunger. Eliciting specific oral reflexes during the clinical feeding evaluation may provide information on the baby's neurologic maturity or integrity as well as on the quality of its response to tactile input. The interplay of the reflexes with the child's functional feeding skills, however, is generally more important than the presence or absence of specific reflexes.[15]

Oral reflexes fall into two categories: adaptive and protective. The adaptive oral reflexes, which include the rooting reflex and the sucking reflex, assist in the acquisition of food. Other adaptive oral reflexes, such as the palmomental reflex, have less functional importance in the feeding process and therefore are not included in the CFEI.

The protective oral reflexes are designed to protect the airway during feeding and to expel foreign material should it enter the airway. These include the gag reflex and the cough reflex. Observations of the adaptive and protective oral reflexes can be recorded on the CFEI form.

Adaptive Oral Reflexes

Evaluation and Interpretation

Rooting reflex: The purpose of the rooting reflex is to help the baby locate the food source. A touch or stroke to the baby's lips or cheeks causes the baby to turn its head toward the stimulus and open the mouth. In newborns, the presence of this response is quite variable and is based on factors such as state and satiation.

When the reflex is absent or diminished, it is usually of little functional significance to feeding, as the feeder can place the nipple in the baby's mouth, particularly during bottle-feeding. During breast-feeding, however, the ability to root and open the mouth is an important part of effective latch-on. If the reflex is absent or diminished, it may signal poor tactile receptivity or neural integration, either of which could be problematic in other aspects of feeding.

Excessive rooting may indicate hypersensitivity or lack of inhibition and can interfere with initiation of sucking. Eliciting the rooting reflex may assist in evaluating jaw movement (using it to observe mouth opening) and neck movement (using it to observe head turning).

Sucking reflex: While sucking is reflexively based in the newborn, there is a gradual transition to full volitional control of sucking by four to six months of age. It is generally accepted that the purpose for the reflexive basis of sucking is to insure that the young infant obtains nourishment. The elicitation of the reflex can vary depending upon whether the stimulus is nutritive or non-nutritive, and may be inhibited by factors such as satiation or state.

Applying light touch from a nipple or finger to the lips or tongue of the very young infant will initiate the complex of movements that comprise sucking. The nipple is drawn into the mouth and rhythmic sucking begins. If the nipple is removed during active sucking, the baby will attempt to find it by flexing its head. If the sucking response is initially absent, it should be reevaluated under different conditions of hunger or alertness. In the very young infant, a consistently absent or hyporesponsive sucking reflex often indicates depressed neurologic status.

Suck-swallow response: As commonly described, the "suck-swallow reflex" may be a misnomer. In the young infant, reflexively based nutritive sucking introduces a bolus of fluid to the back of the mouth, where the reflexively based portions of swallowing are elicited. These two events happen in such rapid succession that they often appear to be a single action. At all ages and stages of infant feeding, however, sucking and swallowing are distinct responses. They are highly integrated with breathing in a rhythmic pattern that is subject to more influences than a simple reflex. This process is discussed in detail in chapter 1 and on page 122 of this chapter.

In the CFEI, therefore, sucking and swallowing are considered as separate but related functions, rather than combined in a "sucking-swallow reflex." It is particularly important to assess sucking and swallowing separately when there may be swallowing dysfunction.

Protective Oral Reflexes

Evaluation and Interpretation

Cough: Two mechanisms trigger reflexive coughing. The first is foreign material that actually enters the upper airway. This stimulates the laryngeal receptors, which then trigger a cough to expel the foreign material and protect the airway. Stimulation to bronchial receptors by excessive secretions will also trigger coughing, with the purpose of clearing the lower airways of foreign material or mucus that interferes with gas exchange. This cough is referred to as a "deeper" cough, though in practice it may be difficult to distinguish between the two coughs auditorily. The type of cough usually can be inferred only from the circumstances surrounding its elicitation. Coughing may also be noted as part of a strong gag response.

Although it may not be possible to elicit a cough during the CFEI, there are two reasons that it is important to observe for spontaneous coughing. First, the presence of the protective laryngeal cough is prerequisite for safe infant feeding. Second, excessive coughing from laryngeal triggers suggests that some dysfunction in the suck/swallow/breathe triad is allowing aspiration or penetration of food or secretions to occur. Information about coughing can be gathered from the primary feeder. If information regarding an infant's ability to cough and protect the airway is needed in a baby who is non-orally fed, a cough may be observed during a strong gag response, as when an NG tube is placed, or during oral suctioning.

All infants cough and splutter periodically during feeding. It is important, however, to note the baby's physiologic response to the cough, how quickly the baby recovers, and how frequently the coughing occurs. When an infant coughs, noting the events surrounding it can help determine if it was triggered by laryngeal or bronchial receptors. Material that enters the airway and triggers a cough can be descending (as in swallowing) or ascending (as in GE reflux). Coughing seen during sucking generally indicates substances are entering the airway as they descend. If coughing is seen frequently when the bottle is out of the baby's mouth and/or when the baby's position is changed, substances may be entering the airway as they ascend from GE reflux.

Although the presence of a cough is imperative for safe feeding, observing that a cough is present does not necessarily indicate that the infant is a safe feeder. Many infants with swallowing dysfunction are observed to cough at some times, but do not cough routinely when they aspirate foods during swallowing. This is called silent aspiration. In some infants the cough is present but not effective in clearing the airway, so aspirated material enters the lungs. Even if a coughing response is noted, if the infant demonstrates other evidence of aspiration or swallowing dysfunction, a full evaluation of the swallowing mechanism with a videofluoroscopic swallowing study (see chapter 2) should be completed if oral feeding is considered.

Gag: The purpose of the gag reflex is to protect the baby from ingesting items that are too large to be handled by the esophagus and/or digestive system (and thus could become lodged in the pharynx and block the airway). It is elicited by touch-pressure to receptors located on the tongue or pharyngeal wall, causing a reverse peristaltic movement in the pharynx and at times a cough. The site for elicitation of the gag reflex changes with increasing age. In the newborn it is elicited in the mid-tongue area. As the baby matures, the site gradually moves back to the pharyngeal wall or posterior portion of the tongue.

Eliciting a gag response is uncomfortable for an infant and therefore can interfere with observations of the baby's normal feeding function. In evaluating feeding function in babies who are apparently normal neurologically, it is generally not necessary to elicit a gag response. Reasons for eliciting the gag response include observing palatal movement and function, establishing a comprehensive baseline of neurologic function, or monitoring change in the neurologic assessment. Instances of spontaneous gagging during feeding should *always* be noted, along with indications of what triggers those responses. A gag reflex that is too easily stimulated indicates hyperesponsivity, which can interfere with feeding. If the gag is not present, the baby may be neurologically depressed.

Many clinicians suggest that it is not safe to feed babies who show minimal or no gag reflex. It should be emphasized that the purpose of the gag is to protect the digestive system from large objects and, hence, protect the airway from blockage. The infant diet, however, is liquid and does not contain firm solid boluses that could become trapped in the pharynx. As coughing is the mechanism that provides protection to the airway from aspiration of liquids, the presence and effectiveness of the cough, not the gag, should be the primary consideration in decisions regarding the safety of infant feeding. An absent or diminished gag, however, may indicate decreased responsivity of the pharyngeal receptors. In this case it is possible that diminished responses might also be found in other pharyngeal receptors, such as those that trigger the swallow. Therefore, in some infants an absent or diminished gag may be a clue to inadequate triggering of swallow. While an absent or diminished gag reflex does not mean that oral feeding should be excluded, it does suggest that the feeding specialist should proceed with caution if oral feeding is pursued.

Behavioral Responses to Tactile Input

To be a successful feeder, the baby must have appropriate registration and perception of tactile input as well as appropriate adaptive responses. The baby must adapt to the tactile components of the tools used in feeding, such as the bottle, breast, spoon, or cup. The baby must also perceive the presence and characteristics of food in the mouth in order to make the correct motoric responses.

Evaluation
Observation of the baby's behavior provides the feeding specialist with information about the baby's ability to register and respond to tactile stimuli. Evaluation can occur in two ways: (1) by observing spontaneous behavioral responses to the tactile aspects of typical feeding maneuvers, and (2) by structured sensory examination, presenting graded tactile input to determine the behavioral threshold for acceptance or rejection. In most cases the baby's responses during feeding will provide sufficient information regarding the infant's ability to handle tactile input. Casual acceptance of the tactile experiences accompanying feeding generally indicates that there is no problem in this area.

A structured sensory examination will be needed with some babies to clearly delineate difficulties with the tactile components of the feeding process. This is accomplished by presenting graded sensory input. Grading must occur in two areas: (1) the area on the face or mouth that will be stimulated first, and (2) the type of tactile input that will be used. Tactile input should be presented progressively from the easiest to tolerate (least threatening) to the most difficult to tolerate.

Area of the face: Stimuli should first be presented distal to the mouth, then moving progressively closer to it. Begin with the cheeks and move toward the lips, gums, and tongue. When the threshold for the elicitation of a negative or aversive response is very low, stimulation to the arms or head may need to precede stimulation to the face and mouth. When applying stimulation inside the mouth, the point at which the gag reflex is stimulated and the magnitude of the gag should be noted to determine if this level of sensitivity is commensurate with the baby's developmental level.

Type of tactile input: This should be graded from firm and smooth (firm pressure from fingers or a toy) to soft and smooth (e.g., stuffed animal or soft finger touch) to prickly or unusual (e.g., rubber hedgehog toy). For a child who is taking some solid food, tolerance of food textures should also be evaluated in a similar graded manner. Move from smooth/pureed to chunky (junior foods, cottage cheese) to crunchy (crackers).

The infant's behavioral responses should be observed as the feeding specialist presents tactile stimuli (whether in the spontaneous feeding situation or during structured assessment of tactile functions) and recorded on the CFEI form. Some babies may view tactile stimulation as stressful, so the behaviors reflecting this stress may be observed in motoric, state, or physiologic stress signals (described in other portions of this chapter). In particular, behaviors that may be observed are gagging, grimacing, arching, turning away, crying, and/or vomiting. Other cues may be much more subtle such as eye avoidance, sneezing, yawning, or slight shifts in muscle tone.

Interpretation
A baby with normal registration and response to tactile stimulation will acknowledge the tactile input, show reasonable tolerance to it, and perhaps exhibit some responses indicating pleasure. A baby's response to tactile input could vary with the baby's developmental level. For example, a baby who is in a period of stranger anxiety will be less accepting of tactile input provided by a stranger than by the parent. All babies have times when they demonstrate stress-related behaviors to tactile input. This may be noted more frequently if they are exploring a new texture and/or letting an object move further into the mouth than appropriate for the maturity of their gag. Therefore, seeing some stress-related behaviors does not in itself indicate a tactile problem. The feeding specialist needs to consider the degree of the response, the persistence of the response, and whether or not it is interfering with feeding performance.

A wide range of behaviors can be observed that are indicative of dysfunction in tactile processing, and these behaviors tend to form a continuum of function containing several broad categories: hyporesponsive, hyperresponsive, aversive, and absent (see figure 3-3).

Absent Responses: When tactile responses are severely diminished or absent, a significant sensory impairment should be suspected and oral feeding may not be possible. This level of dysfunction, however, is typically associated with other oral-motor impairment, such as in the cranial nerve dysfunction of Moebius syndrome, facial palsies, or significant neurologic compromise.

Hyposensitive Responses: In this case, a large amount of stimulation is required to elicit a response, the responses are slow, or they are only partially complete. In an infant with this type of decreased sensory awareness, the quality of oral-motor control and feeding may suffer, though functional feeding is generally possible. Inadequate lip closure and/or trouble forming and handling the bolus may be observed. Swallowing difficulty may also be seen, either due to difficulty with bolus formation and/or due to poor triggering of a swallow related to decreased pharyngeal sensitivity.

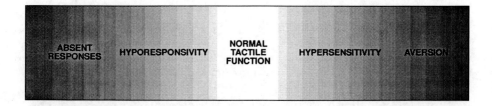

Figure 3-3 Continuum of tactile responses.

Hypersensitive Responses: A hypersensitive response is one that is heightened or exaggerated out of proportion to the magnitude of the stimuli. For example, gagging when the tip of the tongue is touched would be a hypersensitive response in a newborn, as even at that early age the gag reflex is typically elicited halfway back on the tongue. Other examples are infants who turn their heads away when the lips are touched with a bottle and those who push toys away when oral exploration is encouraged. Many babies who have a low threshold for oral-tactile stimuli and demonstrate hypersensitive responses may nonetheless be willing to engage in some oral-tactile activity within their limited range.

Aversive Responses: While similar to hypersensitive responses, aversive responses are stronger, more negative, and generally include a behavioral component. A baby with aversive responses may cry, grimace, wiggle, arch away, or keep the mouth closed when asked to feed. If the feeder persists, the baby may begin to gag and if that sign is not heeded, vomit. These responses may also be observed merely on the visual presentation of the spoon or bottle.

Both hypersensitive and aversive responses can be part of a global tactile processing problem or localized to the face and mouth or more specifically to a certain part of the mouth, most frequently the tongue. The aversive and hypersensitive responses may be to touch only or may include response to tastes, temperatures, textures, or smells.

While hypersensitive responses may interfere with feeding, aversive responses often preclude oral feeding.

Factors Contributing to Abnormal Tactile Responses

A number of factors may contribute to the development of hypersensitive and aversive response to tactile stimulation. These include (1) immaturity or chronic illness, (2) unpleasant oral-tactile experiences, (3) delayed introduction of oral feeding, and (4) neurologic impairment.

Many infants born prematurely with immature central nervous systems are not equipped to deal with the intensity and multitude of stimuli present in the extrauterine environment, particularly the neonatal intensive care unit. Premature infants have difficulty registering and processing sensory information. They often are overly sensitive to stimuli and unable to buffer or filter sensory input due to lack of inhibitory controls.[4] Chronically ill infants may be at the mercy of their physiologic status, with all their resources harnessed toward simple survival. In this state, the slightest increase in sensory stimuli may prove to be overwhelming. When immaturity, lowered threshold to stimuli, and lack of regulatory filtering mechanisms are present, an infant may respond to stimuli either by tuning out or developing hypersensitive, and then aversive, responses.

Sick babies also undergo many negative and traumatic oral/facial experiences during the course of medical treatment. Many have been intubated repeatedly or for long periods of time. They have had their faces taped and retaped to hold endotracheal tubes and feeding tubes. They have been suctioned frequently through the endotracheal tube or directly into the mouth. If the endotracheal tube has been in the mouth, they may have been unable to engage in simple hand-to-mouth behavior or sucking on a pacifier. These babies often experience a period of relative oral deprivation combined with aversive oral stimuli. They learn a pattern of defensive behavior to stimulation in and around the oral area. This learned response tends to persist well beyond the end of the medical interventions and is often reflected in their hypersensitive and aversive responses when oral feeding is introduced. To such a baby, normal attempts at oral feeding may be interpreted as noxious and further reinforce hypersensitive or aversive responses.

For the medically compromised infant, the introduction of oral feeding may also be delayed. Not only is the introduction of bottle or breast often delayed, but the progression toward solids or cup drinking also lags. Illingworth and Lister, in a classic article, discuss the role of the critical or sensitive period for the acquisition of oral feeding skills.[16] This period is the time when the infant is most ready to learn a particular skill if the appropriate stimuli are applied. If this critical or sensitive period is missed, learning the skill at a later time will be more difficult, if not impossible.

Many infants with complex feeding disorders have not been fed by mouth for long periods of time, and the onset of oral feeding has been significantly delayed. Having missed the critical period, their response to the sensory components of feeding and their acquisition of oral skills are impaired.

In conjunction with the factors discussed above, or independent of them, an infant may also have impaired neurologic function. In this case any aspect of sensory processing may be deficient. Sensory registration and/or responses may be inadequate. Such dysfunction can result in hypersensitive or aversive behavior to tactile stimulation, though it can also lead to hyposensitive responses.

Oral-Motor Control

The clinical feeding evaluation of infants assesses oral-motor control as it relates to sucking, since this is the infant's primary method of obtaining nourishment. Although developmental changes in sucking are likely,[1] they are poorly understood. Therefore, this portion of the CFEI focuses on how the individual structures perform mechanically to produce functional sucking. These structures—tongue, jaw, lips/cheeks, and palate—work together to create compression and suction, which brings fluid into the mouth to nourish the infant. Chapter 1 provides a detailed description of the sucking process and characteristics of sucking.

To evaluate the functional contribution of each structure to the feeding process, the characteristics of the resting position as well as the components of movement need to be considered. In evaluating movement, it is important to go beyond observing these structures and to actually feel them working together. This is best done by using the examiner's gloved finger in the baby's mouth and eliciting sucking. Older babies may not suck readily on a finger, so the function of the various structures may need to be inferred from observation of nutritive sucking and/or non-nutritive sucking on a pacifier, knowing that there is a greater chance of inaccurate observation. Although using the finger or a pacifier to evaluate sucking provides information on the mechanics of the suck, it does not provide information on the function of sucking seen during oral feeding, since that involves the coordination of sucking with swallowing and breathing.

In describing the characteristics of position and movement for each oral-motor structure, certain words will be emphasized. These correspond to observations that are included on the CFEI form.

Tongue

The tongue serves multiple functions in the mechanics of sucking. These are related to the creation of negative pressure, bolus formation, and propulsion. They include the following:

- In breast-feeding, the tongue is active in bringing the nipple into the mouth, shaping it, and stabilizing its position. On the bottle, it is not needed to draw the nipple into the mouth, but it does help to stabilize the position of the nipple.

- The tongue helps to seal the oral cavity. Anteriorly, in conjunction with the lower lip, it seals against the nipple. Posteriorly, it seals against the soft palate, until the palate is lifted for swallowing.

- By changing configuration, the tongue is the primary means of increasing volume of the oral cavity to create negative pressure and suction.

- The tongue provides a compression force against the nipple to express liquid from the nipple.

- By forming a "central groove," the tongue channels liquid toward the pharynx.

- It assists in forming the bolus and holding it in the oral cavity in preparation for triggering the swallow.

Evaluation

Characteristics of position: As the baby opens its mouth to receive the nipple or finger, the resting position of the tongue should be observed. A normally functioning tongue will appear *soft*, though with a well-defined shape that is relatively *thin* and *flat*, with a moderately *rounded tip*. There should be evidence of a slight *central groove* in the anterior-posterior direction (see figure 3-4). The tongue should lie in the *bottom of the mouth* between the lower gum ridges. It does not protrude over the lips and is not seen when the mouth is closed. In newborns, the relative size of the tongue in relationship to the oral cavity makes it appear that the tongue fills the oral cavity. It may cover the gums, touching the inside of the lower lip. With increasing age, the tongue moves back in the mouth. It also becomes more mobile, so a greater variety of positions is observed.

Several deviations of tongue position can be observed. *Tongue-tip elevation* brings the tip of the tongue in opposition to the upper gum ridge or the palate behind the alveolar ridge. When this occurs, the tongue tip may also be excessively pointed or rounded. An elevated tongue tip is often held in place fairly strongly, making it difficult to insert a finger or nipple. The tongue can appear humped (in an anterior-posterior direction) or *bunched* (compressed in a lateral direction). Neither position allows the formation of a central groove. A *retracted* tongue is held posteriorly in the mouth, with the tongue tip well behind the alveolar ridges. The tongue tip may be elevated in addition to being retracted, or the back of the tongue may be bunched. A retracted and bunched tongue position can be seen when the jaw is normally proportioned and is often seen in association with micrognathia. In this case, the tongue may appear even more retracted than it actually is relative to the small jaw.

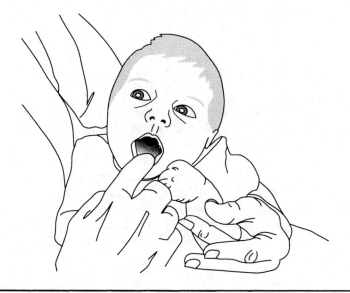

Figure 3-4 Central grooving of the tongue.

Abnormalities of the tone of the tongue can relate to position. Bunched, retracted, or humped tongues tend to accompany high muscle tone; resistance is felt when the tongue is touched. If tone is low, little shaping or resistance is felt when palpating the body of the tongue. The lower-tone tongue may protrude. When the tongue is *protruded,* the tip rests forward, on the lips or over the lower gum ridge. A protruded tongue may seem excessively soft and wide. When *asymmetry* is present, the tongue may deviate at rest or with spontaneous movement to either side. There also might be asymmetry of tone, with one side more bunched or flat.

Characteristics of movement: When sucking is elicited by placing a finger inside the baby's mouth, the normally functioning tongue will become *cupped* around the finger, forming a distinct central groove. Tongue movements on the finger will be in either an *in-and-out* direction (with a stronger movement in the "in" direction) or an *up-and-down* direction. All movements will be of *small excursion* and should have a *rhythmic* quality. The tongue will compress the finger during sucking, but the pressure should vary with the tongue's rhythmic movements.[17-19]

A tongue thrust, one type of deviation in tongue movement, results in an in-and-out pattern of movement with a strong protrusion or push "out." It is often associated with other findings of increased tone. A *flat* tongue, or one that does not cup around the finger to create a central groove, may be seen in some babies. When the tongue is flat, the feeding specialist's finger is not well stabilized. The finger may tend to slide to the side of the tongue or depress into the tongue without meeting resistance. *Clonus* may be felt in the tongue either before sucking begins or during sucking pauses. *Fasciculations* can also be observed. Tongue movements may also *lack rhythm.*

Interpretation

Tongue-tip elevation and retraction and a tongue in a bunched or humped position are all possible indications of increased oral tone. A tongue with these characteristics may not be able to move flexibly to create appropriate or adequate intra-oral negative pressure. Tongue-tip elevation and retraction can also be a reflection of the infant's effort to maintain stability in the head, neck, or mouth area through postural fixation ("fixing") and can be an indication of lower postural tone. A strongly elevated tongue tip can block adequate nipple placement and at times can be a primary cause of feeding difficulties. The following case example will demonstrate this problem.

Case example:

Jason was a 3-week-old former 36-week premature infant who had a relatively benign neonatal course. He had been home from the hospital for about 1 week and was not eating well. He seemed hungry but would cry excessively shortly after he began sucking on the bottle. He was taking very little formula. He showed several signs of increased tone throughout the body and in the oral area—increased trunk/neck extension, tightly pursed lips, limited mouth opening, and strong tongue-tip elevation. Observation of parents feeding him revealed that they slid the bottle into his semiclosed mouth while he began strong sucking movements. Although he sucked vigorously no bubbles returned into the bottle. Due to the poor mouth opening and strong tongue-tip elevation, the parents were sliding the bottle into his mouth with the nipple *under* the tongue. Jason then made unproductive sucking movements, became frustrated, and cried. With treatment activities to improve mouth opening, reduce tongue-tip elevation, and facilitate correct nipple position, feeding immediately improved.

During sucking the tongue forms a central groove along the median raphe, which creates a channel for the liquid to travel from the anterior to the posterior portion of the mouth. When a tongue is retracted, bunched, or humped, or has extremely low tone, it may lack the ability to form an adequate central groove, leading to poor control of the liquid. The ability of the tongue to form and hold the bolus in the posterior portion of the mouth is a crucial component in the correct timing of the initiation of swallowing. If this function is impaired, liquid may spill prematurely into the vallecular or piriform sinuses, timing of the swallow may be poorly coordinated, and aspiration is possible.

A retracted tongue is either pulled into (indicating high tone) or falls into (indicating low tone) the posterior portion of the oral cavity. If the tongue is quite retracted, and perhaps bunched, with the tip fairly far back in the mouth, there may be inadequate contact between the tongue and nipple. This can interfere with the development of adequate negative pressure. When hypotonia or generalized weakness is present, the tongue is unable to resist the force of gravity and may passively fall to the back of the mouth. If the tongue is markedly retracted, particularly in conjunction with a small or recessed jaw, the tongue may at times obstruct the pharyngeal airway, potentially causing apnea and bradycardia. The baby may appear to have obstructed breathing, which suddenly clears as the position of the tongue changes. The potential for obstruction from a retracted tongue is greater when structural abnormalities like the Pierre-Robin malformation are present.

Asymmetries of tongue position or movement generally reflect some type of neurologic impairment. If asymmetries in tongue movement or position are observed, cranial nerve dysfunction should be considered. Fasciculations can also be an indication of an underlying nervous system problem.

Tongue protrusion at rest is frequently associated with overall hypotonia in the infant. The tongue shape may lack definition with the tip quite rounded. The infant with a hypotonic, protruded tongue may have difficulty shaping or stabilizing the nipple during sucking or in forming an adequate central groove. Tongue protrusion may also interfere with lip seal during sucking.

A tongue thrust, which implies a forceful outward component, needs to be differentiated from simple tongue protrusion. Observation of the tongue at rest and during active sucking is necessary. Tongue thrust during active sucking is generally associated with increased tone, particularly increased extensor tone and possibly CNS abnormality. The tongue is generally firm, often with a pointed tip. Since the tongue is moving in an in-and-out direction rather than an up-and-down direction, it will not be able to create adequate negative pressure. If liquid is obtained, it is done primarily by nipple compression. Tongue thrusting may also hinder proper anterior-posterior movement of the bolus for swallowing. Part of the bolus may move forward, leading to fluid loss at the lips.

When smooth, rhythmic movements of the tongue are not present, incoordination of sucking, swallowing, and breathing may result. Although abnormal rhythmic movement of the tongue may be due to central nervous system factors, dysfunction in swallowing or breathing can also lead to abnormal tongue movement and rhythm. This is discussed in more detail in chapter 1, and page 122 of this chapter.

Jaw

The role of the jaw in the mechanics of sucking is twofold:

- It provides a stable platform for movements of the tongue, lips, and cheeks.
- Slight downward movement of the jaw during sucking assists in expanding the size of the sealed oral cavity to create negative pressure or suction.

Evaluation

Characteristics of position: At rest the normal infant has a *neutral* jaw position, with the upper jaw and lower jaw loosely opposed so that the lips touch. Both gum ridges are in direct opposition in the anterior-posterior and lateral planes. Deviations that may be noted include a *recessed* jaw, where the lower gum ridge is posterior to the upper gum ridge, or the jaw may be depressed, with the mouth typically *open*. *Asymmetries* or lateral deviations can also be seen.

Characteristics of movement: Normal jaw movement is *smooth*, in *small excursions*, with a *rhythmic* quality. Jaw instability can be reflected in *large excursions* that indicate poorly graded movement. Although the range of movement may be wide or excessive, the movement itself may be quite rhythmic. Abnormal *jaw thrusts* are forceful, downward movements whereby the jaw appears to jut forward. These may also be in a large excursion, but they may demonstrate more force and less rhythm than the pattern of poorly graded large excursions. Jaw thrusts are frequently associated with overall increased extensor tone. Infants may also demonstrate inadequate mouth opening. *Lack of range* of jaw movement represents a problem of passive range of movement. If passive range is present, but active opening is limited, initiation of feeding may be difficult. *Clenching* or tonic biting is a problem of active movement that limits mouth opening. Phasic or intermittent *biting* may also be seen. *Clonus* and *tremors* can also be seen in the jaw.

Interpretation

Deviations in resting position may reflect muscle-tone abnormalities. The baby with low muscle tone often has a resting posture with the mouth loosely opened. On the other hand, an open mouth in conjunction with strong neck extension may be related to increased muscle tone, particularly increased extensor tone. With the mouth and jaw open, regardless of whether the cause is increased or decreased tone, the ability to adequately seal the lips will be impaired.

Asymmetries of the jaw may reflect asymmetric muscle tone or strength, but they may also be secondary to structural defects, torticollis, or deformation from in utero positioning. Another structural problem is the small, recessed jaw (micrognathia), discussed in detail in chapter 6. It can be associated with a retracted tongue position and difficulty maintaining an adequate airway, or can lead to poor contact with the nipple, causing inadequate sucking. Even a mildly recessed jaw, which many normally functioning infants have immediately after birth from in utero positioning, can interfere significantly with breast-feeding, where direct opposition of the gum ridges is necessary for adequate compression of the areola and milk ducts.

Abnormal movement patterns of the jaw, such as clenching and thrusting, generally reflect increased muscle tone. Jaw thrusting is often accompanied by tongue thrusting. Biting may be secondary to increased tone but may also reflect the infant's attempt to hold the nipple in place when tongue movements are not functional. Poor mouth opening due to lack of range of movement or clenching can interfere with nipple placement and the initiation of feeding, as well as limiting jaw excursion necessary for developing adequate negative pressure.

The position in which the infant is fed may also impact jaw function. If the infant's neck is positioned in extension or hyperextension, jaw stability is generally compromised, which leads to large jaw excursions during feeding. Increased jaw excursion may interfere with lip seal and result in fluid loss. Increased jaw excursion may also result in ineffective tongue movement and inadequate suction, leading to greater work to obtain a given volume of formula. When feeding is inefficient, the infant expends a large amount of energy for a minimal amount of nutrition.

Lips and Cheeks

During sucking the functions of the lips and cheeks include the following:

- On the breast, the lips help locate the nipple and bring it into the mouth. This is not necessary on the bottle, as the nipple is placed in the baby's open mouth.

- The lips stabilize the nipple position within the mouth.

- The lips assist in forming the anterior seal around the nipple.

- The cheeks provide stability to maintain the shape of the mouth. In young infants, the fat pads provide the majority of the positional stability. As the infant grows, the fat pads diminish and the cheek muscles provide more active stability.[34]

- The cheeks provide lateral boundaries for food on the tongue, aiding in bolus formation.

Evaluation

The descriptors of position and movement of the cheeks and lips are similar; therefore they will be described together. The *fat pads* (or sucking pads) of the cheeks should be visible through 6 to 8 months of age, giving the child a puffy-looking cheek.[1] Even the premature baby who is starting to feed should have some evidence of a fat pad, though it may not be as substantial as in the full-term baby. As the fat pads disappear, the baby has increased muscle control for stability of cheeks. The cheeks should appear *soft*, though well defined, with evidence of tone and activity during sucking.

The lips should also appear *soft* at rest. During sucking they should loosely *shape to the nipple*, and the examiner should notice slight *pressure at the corners*. The amount of pressure or lateral lip seal will increase as the baby matures. The lips tend to seal more firmly during the intake phase of sucking and loosen somewhat during refilling of the nipple. This occurs so quickly during active sucking that it may go unnoticed.

Deviant patterns are most noticeable in the lips. These include very tight lips that are pulled back in a *retracted* manner. This is certainly a characteristic of the older baby with cerebral palsy, but in infants tight lips more typically are noted to be *pursed*. This can be observed as the finger or nipple is being inserted. The lips can also be *loose* or floppy and not shape to the nipple.

Interpretation

Problems noted with the lips and cheeks can lead to a number of feeding difficulties. Lips that are quite loose, actively and passively, may be associated with generalized hypotonia. With poor lip seal, the amount of suction the infant can generate will be impaired. Thus, the baby's feeding efficiency will diminish. When lips are loose, floppy, and not sealing well around the nipple, the tongue may protrude to assist. If there is a poor seal, periodic breaks in suction (smacking sounds) may be noted during sucking. Liquid may also leak from the corners of the mouth or center of the lower lips.

Tightly pursed lips may make nipple insertion difficult. Although lip pursing may not contribute markedly to bottle-feeding difficulties, it can impair both latch-on and active sucking during breast-feeding. This pattern and the underlying increased tone it may represent can potentially interfere with more mature feeding skills and should be followed closely.

Cheek function can be compromised by tone that is either too high or too low. If the cheeks have low tone and are unstable, some of the negative intra-oral pressure that is generated may pull the cheeks into the oral cavity, compromising suction on the nipple and decreasing feeding efficiency. If the inherent stability of the fat pads is diminished and the baby does not develop muscular cheek stability, it may be harder to maintain lip stability and adequate seal on the nipple.

Palate

Both the hard and the soft palate (the velum) are important structures to consider when evaluating the mechanics of sucking and feeding. They serve both purely structural or positional functions as well as being a part of the dynamic action of sucking. Their roles include the following:

- The hard palate assists with positioning and stability of the nipple within the mouth.
- The hard palate works with the tongue to compress the nipple.
- The soft palate works with the tongue to create the posterior seal of the oral cavity.
- The soft palate elevates during the swallow, allowing passage of the bolus and occluding the nasal cavity to prevent nasal reflux.

Evaluation

During physical inspection of the baby's mouth, the feeding specialist should look at the shape of the hard palate. The hard palate should be *intact* and smoothly contoured, and it should roughly approximate the shape of the tongue. *Abnormally shaped* hard palates may be narrow, grooved, high arched, or quite flat. *Clefts*, or openings, in the hard palate may also be seen (see chapter 6). There could be asymmetry or grooves of the alveolar ridge.

The soft palate should be observed for structural integrity, though submucous clefts cannot be visualized. Soft palate movement is difficult to appreciate, even during sucking on the finger. By eliciting a gag reflex while the mouth is open, palatal movement may be observed, but this will not reflect the quality of velar closure during the feeding process. Formula routinely escaping through the infant's nose during feeding or emesis may indicate *abnormal soft palate movement*. A snorty or stuffy sound to the baby's breathing may also be an indication of a velar problem. Further evaluation of soft palate function is possible with a videofluoroscopic swallowing study (VFSS), discussed fully in chapter 2.

Interpretation

In utero and after birth, the shape of the hard palate is contoured by the continual pressure of the tongue as it rests against the palate with the mouth closed. In babies who have been orally intubated for prolonged periods, the pressure and contact on the palate are abnormal. The tongue cannot contact the palate to assist in this shaping, and the palate is in constant contact with the endotracheal tube. In addition to having the endotracheal tube pressing against the palate, orally intubated babies frequently have their mouths open, further limiting tongue contact with the palate. These infants therefore often develop very narrow, high-arched palates. While such babies often have feeding problems, the specific role of abnormal palatal shape is not clear. A narrow or highly arched palate can also be observed in the absence of intubation and may be due to excessive tongue thrusting, congenital malformation, or perhaps a family trait.

Clefts of the hard or soft palate may be present and interfere with the generation of negative pressure during sucking. Small submucous clefts and problems with complete palatal closure may allow intermittent suction, though feeding will be inefficient. Clicking noises, representing these breaks in suction, may be heard. Additional details on clefts are found in chapter 6.

Sucking, Swallowing, and Breathing

The mouth is often considered the "organ of feeding." Thus, the traditional assumption has been that problems with feeding stem from problems in using the mouth. Since infants feed by sucking, the sucking process is often implicated as the source of problems. Many of the feeding problems seen in infancy, however, have their basis in difficulties that do not arise in the mouth.

Although the infant's primary method of feeding is by sucking on the bottle or breast, sucking is only one of three components in the process of ingesting nourishment by nipple. Swallowing and breathing are also intimately related in the nipple-feeding process, forming the suck/swallow/breathe triad of functions. In assessing the infant with feeding difficulties we must therefore carefully evaluate the integrity of sucking, swallowing, and breathing individually, as well as consider the coordination or organization of these components in the feeding process.

Rhythmicity is the hallmark of normal infant sucking. Dysfunctional feeding is often characterized by inefficient, discoordinated, and dysrhythmic feeding behaviors. Rhythmicity is an important component of many bodily functions, including heart rate and respiration. Few other bodily functions, however, require such intricate timing as the coordination of sucking, swallowing, and breathing. These three events occur with remarkable speed and repetition in infancy.

Structurally, however, feeding and breathing share a common space. The pharynx is the crossroad between these two functions, serving as a conduit for air going to and from the lungs and for food going to the esophagus. It is this dual role that underlies the problems seen in suck/swallow/breathe incoordination. A dysfunction or immaturity in any of these three systems will have a profound effect on the other two systems and thus on the baby's feeding ability. Therefore, evaluation of suck/swallow/breathe coordination must take into account problems observed in each of the three major systems, as well as the infant's level of maturity. This section reviews evaluation and interpretation procedures for each of these three subsystems separately and then for the process of coordinating sucking, swallowing, and breathing. Observations can be recorded on the CFEI form.

Sucking

Sucking is the final product integrating the motor activity of the individual oral structures in infant feeding. A detailed description of the sucking process and characteristics of sucking can be found in chapter 1, and development of sucking in the premature infant covered in chapter 6. In the preceding sections, the role of individual structures in this process has been described, but the overall characteristics of sucking must also be evaluated.

Evaluation

The infant's suck should be evaluated during both non-nutritive and nutritive sucking. Non-nutritive sucking is evaluated first so that it can be considered in isolation from the added functions of bolus formation, swallowing, and respiratory coordination. Whether sucking is evaluated nutritively or non-nutritively, the hungry baby should be able to *initiate* sucking spontaneously with minimal encouragement.

Non-nutritive suck (NNS): Ideally this is evaluated by allowing the baby to suck on the examiner's finger. If this is not possible, some information can be gained by observing sucking on a pacifier or nipple. A primary consideration is *strength* of suck. This includes the force of the tongue *compression* on the examiner's finger and the negative pressure, or *suction*, which is generated. The relative contribution of these two forces should be determined.

The degree of negative pressure is determined by the amount of resistance the infant gives when the examiner attempts to remove the finger or nipple from the baby's mouth. There may be a slight smacking or clicking noise when suction is broken to remove the finger.

Compression is the force of the tongue on the finger during sucking. Neither of these forces should be confused with biting, a strong clenching of the jaws around the nipple to maintain its position. Frequent clicking noises indicate that there are *breaks in suction* intermittently throughout the sucking process.

Sucking should feel well *coordinated,* with the structures working together in a smooth and effective manner. There should be *rhythm* to the sucking, with bursts of six to ten sucks between short pauses. The sucking rate is approximately two sucks per second.

Nutritive sucking (NS): When liquid flows through the nipple, other characteristics of sucking can be evaluated. During bottle-feeding, the return of bubbles into the bottle reflects the flow of fluid through the nipple. The *strength* of nutritive sucking will be reflected by the baby's resistance on the nipple as well as the number of bubbles returning into the bottle. When sucking is strong and well *coordinated,* there will be an active and steady return of bubbles into the bottle, indicating efficient sucking. If the suck is weak, the flow of bubbles will be reduced; sucking is inefficient and little fluid is ingested. When there are few bubbles returning to the bottle, but there are other indications that the suck is strong, the nipple hole may be blocked. An extremely strong suck may collapse the nipple, also reducing the flow of bubbles. The infant generating *suction* will give some resistance as the nipple is withdrawn from the mouth. If the infant primarily generates *compression*, the bottle will be withdrawn easily, unless the infant bites the nipple.

Loss of liquid out of the mouth during nutritive sucking should be noted. Although slight fluid loss is not a concern, continual fluid loss should be noted. As in non-nutritive sucking, clicking or smacking noises generally represent *breaks in suction* and should be recorded. The rate of sucking is approximately one suck per second. While this varies among infants, for any baby it should always be slower than the rate of NNS. Nutritive sucking should also be *rhythmic*. This rhythmicity is a primary indicator of the coordination between sucking, swallowing, and breathing and is covered in detail below.

Interpretation
A baby's suck must be strong enough to obtain nutrition without undue effort. A weak suck may reflect generalized weakness or the infant's compromised medical status. Although a strong suck is desirable, a suck that is too strong can lead to problems. It can collapse a nipple, particularly a soft nipple, leading to air swallowing and/or frustration due to poor liquid flow. If a strong suck is paired with a fast-flow nipple, food may be ingested too rapidly and air swallowing may occur. Either of these can contribute to greater emesis.

Case example:

Jeffery was a 3-month-old term infant referred for evaluation of persistent vomiting and slow weight gain, but not truly failure to thrive. All studies for gastroesophageal reflux proved negative, so he was referred for a CFEI. Observing his feeding, the feeding specialist noted that he had an extremely strong, robust, and very fast rate of sucking, with some air swallowing. He took four ounces of formula in less than five minutes. Shortly after feeding, during burping, he had a large emesis. It appeared that his rapid rate of formula ingestion, combined with slight air swallowing, was leading to emesis. He was provided with a slower-flow nipple, and his mother was taught techniques to slow the rate of his sucking. His emesis improved significantly, and weight began to increase.

When evaluating NS and NNS, if the tongue is providing firm pressure on the finger or nipple, yet the baby's feeding is inefficient, there may be inadequate negative pressure. The baby may be able to create a compression force to squeeze fluid from the nipple but is not able to create suction to draw fluid from the nipple. Bottle-feeding efficiency will be particularly compromised. This situation may reflect a problem in tongue control. Possibly the tongue does not groove well or does not move adequately. Insufficient negative pressure may also result from inadequate seal of the oral cavity, as the creation of negative pressure requires a sealed cavity. In this case, tongue movement could be normal, but integrity and function of the palate (hard and soft) and lips should be assessed. In particular, clefts of the hard or soft palate may be present, or velopharyngeal closure may be inadequate.

Poorly coordinated or inefficient sucking often reflects inadequate motoric control of one or more oral structures (as described in the sections above) or difficulty in coordinating and integrating oral movements. Loss of liquid may also reflect problems with control of specific oral structures, such as poor lip seal, thrusting tongue movements, or poor bolus formation by the tongue and cheeks.

Assuming the infant is in an optimal state for feeding, inability to initiate sucking can result from excessive rooting when the nipple is presented. The baby may begin to root wildly back and forth and be unable to inhibit the rooting reflex to latch on to the nipple. Some babies may also orient to the nipple with wide jaw extension and be unable to smoothly close the mouth.

Abnormal non-nutritive sucking rhythms may reflect poor neurologic integrity or generalized motor control problems. When normal sucking rhythms are noted during non-nutritive sucking yet there are abnormal sucking rhythms with nutritive sucking, other aspects of the suck/swallow/breathe triad probably are involved, as discussed in detail below.

Swallowing

The most comprehensive evaluation of swallowing function is done with the videofluoroscopic swallowing study or VFSS (see chapter 2). External observation of swallowing function during the clinical feeding evaluation, however, can provide useful information. In particular, these observations, along with the medical and feeding history, can help determine the need for a VFSS. Specific clinical indications for a VFSS are listed in table 3-4 and described in detail below.

Table 3-4 Clinical Indications of Swallowing Dysfunction

- Coughing or choking during swallowing
- Inability to handle own oral secretions
- Noisy, "wet" upper airway sounds after individual swallows or increasing noisiness over course of feeding
- Multiple swallows to clear a single bolus
- Apnea during swallowing
- History of frequent upper-respiratory infections or pneumonias

---

Although the VFSS is a very powerful and useful test, it is not appropriate to use with every infant presenting with a feeding problem. Careful guidelines for appropriate use must be developed, taking into consideration the radiologic risks to the infant versus the yield of information from the test. In making the decision to do a VFSS, it is important to take a comprehensive view of the infant's situation, including the feeding expectations and how information from the VFSS will be used. If it is suspected that the baby may be aspirating, but physicians and/or parents are unlikely to change oral feeding methods (for instance, oral feeding is one of the child's few pleasures, or the child's prognosis is poor), doing a VFSS to confirm the aspiration may not be appropriate.

Evaluation and Interpretation

Coughing and choking: Coughing and choking during feeding may be an indication of a primary swallowing problem leading to aspiration. They can also be the result of incoordination of sucking, swallowing, and breathing. For a full discussion of coughing and choking see pages 107 and 138.

Handling of secretions: An important clinical sign of swallowing dysfunction is the inability to handle oral secretions. If an infant requires frequent oral suctioning, there may be some impairment of spontaneous swallowing. The frequency of suctioning is often related to the

---

degree of swallowing dysfunction; the more suctioning that is needed, the more impaired the swallowing abilities. In this case, excessive pooling of secretions in the pharynx may cause airway obstruction and can lead to oxygen desaturation and bradycardia. Although drooling can also be a sign of swallowing dysfunction, it may instead reflect poor oral-motor control or sensation with a normal swallowing mechanism. Inability to handle secretions is generally the result of poor triggering of swallowing. It may lead to aspiration before or after the swallow, as secretions spontaneously slide down the hypopharynx and into the open airway.

Specific cranial nerve involvement is one possible cause of an inability to handle secretions. Overall depressed central nervous system function, like that seen in birth asphyxia, is another possible cause. Specific lesions of the brain-stem area responsible for the motoric or sensory control of swallowing can also be a cause.

Oral feeding is generally not safe for a baby who cannot handle secretions. In this case, the role of a VFSS needs to be carefully considered. For the infant with marked difficulty handling oral secretions, the VFSS will probably only confirm that the baby has significant swallowing dysfunction, either including aspiration or putting the baby at high risk for aspiration. In doing the study, the infant will have radiation exposure and the likelihood of aspirating barium, yet it is unlikely that any techniques would be identified that could improve swallowing enough to make it safe for oral feeding. While the VFSS could provide a baseline from which to measure change, it is suggested that the VFSS be delayed until the infant is handling secretions fairly completely. At this point it is more likely that the information from the VFSS will be useful in decisions relating to the initiation of oral feeding.

Multiple swallows: The examiner should assess whether the baby is able to clear a bolus with a single swallow or requires more than one swallow for the same bolus. Multiple swallows suggest that the bolus may not be organized adequately in the oral area, the swallow may not be triggered appropriately, and/or pharyngeal peristalsis may be insufficient to clear the bolus in one swallow. Careful evaluation of oral-motor control may delineate the difficulty. If oral control appears adequate, a VFSS will be helpful to clarify which factor is resulting in multiple swallows and to assess possible interventions.

Noisy breathing: The presence of wet- or congested-sounding breathing should be noted during the evaluation. By listening to the respirations carefully, it is often possible to determine if these sounds are coming from the nasal cavity, oropharynx, or pharynx. The location of the sounds suggests potential types of swallowing dysfunction. It is also important to consider the timing of these sounds. They may be present prior to feeding, develop or change during feeding, and/or become more pronounced after feeding.

If noisy breathing is present before the feeding begins and remains relatively unchanged with the feeding, then the cause is more likely respiratory than swallowing. If the noise appears to arise in the nose and worsens during the feeding, insufficient velar elevation leading to nasal reflux should be considered and confirmed through a VFSS.

If the baby's breathing becomes noisier as the feeding progresses and appears to originate in the pharynx, there may be inadequate pharyngeal peristalsis, leading to pooling or poor clearance of liquid in the pharynx.[22] Infants with residual food in the pharynx following the swallow often present with extremely noisy, wet-sounding breathing that is worse following feeding. They are literally breathing through material (formula or secretions) in the hypopharynx. Aspiration can occur as the material is inhaled or passively falls into the open airway after the swallow occurs. VFSS should be used to confirm this suspicion.

Frequent respiratory infections: In some cases there is little or no evidence of swallowing dysfunction during the clinical feeding evaluation, but the baby has a history of frequent, unexplained respiratory illness and infection, including pneumonia. This suggests the presence of aspiration. Oral feeding and sucking patterns are often normal. Coughing may or may not be present, but is not excessive. When aspiration is confirmed with VFSS (frequently microaspiration), the infant is described as having silent aspiration.

Because the feeding patterns of these infants appear normal, evaluation of this problem may be lengthy and circuitous. The initial focus may be on the respiratory symptoms; asthma or cystic fibrosis may be considered. Interestingly, some babies with asthma do have a component of silent aspiration, either ascending from gastroesophageal reflux or descending during swallowing.[23]

Treatment for silent aspiration depends on the point at which the aspiration occurs in the swallowing cycle. Many times, silent aspirators respond well to therapeutic intervention and go on to have a decrease in respiratory symptoms once their swallowing problems have been addressed. Other times, positioning, dietary manipulations, and oral-motor therapy do not improve the silent aspiration sufficiently, so that non-oral feeding methods are required for some or all of the infant's intake.

Gulping: A "glunk" or clicking sound may be present with all or some of the swallows. This sound generally indicates air swallowing, which may lead to excessive spitting. In some cases the air swallowing may trigger a vagally mediated apnea and/or bradycardia as the large food-and-air bolus stimulates the pharyngeal stretch receptors.

Although this observation helps to identify air swallowing clinically, the VFSS is not able to assess air swallowing. If therapeutic techniques to decrease air swallowing and gulping decrease apnea, bradycardia, and/or emesis, no further evaluation is necessary. If apnea or bradycardia persist after the air swallowing is reduced, then further evaluation of swallowing function may be indicated. If no swallowing dysfunction is found, evaluation of respiratory function may be useful.

Quality of Respiration

To evaluate the respiratory system in relation to feeding, basic physiologic parameters as well as the quality of respiration must be considered. Our respiratory system is a complicated, interactive system that is able to adapt to the body's physiologic needs as those needs change with activity or stress. In order to match oxygen requirements to the task at hand, changes occur in the rate and depth of breathing, effort involved in breathing, heart rate, and shape of the airway.

For infants, feeding is aerobic exercise and therefore physiologic work. By its nature, work taxes the respiratory system, so there must be some degree of respiratory reserve to meet the increased demands. A variety of changes must be made to allow the infant to cope with the increased work load without compromise.

During infant feeding, breathing and swallowing must be smoothly integrated. The exquisite timing of these two functions allows feeding to appear effortless and remain free of choking or aspiration. (Detailed discussion of the interaction of these two functions is found in chapter 1). When the quality of respiratory function is diminished, the coordination of the suck/swallow/breathe triad will be compromised, potentially leading to feeding difficulties. The interdependency of these three systems can be seen in changes that occur in infant feeding during the common cold. When the baby's nose is congested, there will be difficulty breathing during eating; the baby may then be unwilling to eat, and intake declines.

Evaluation and Interpretation
Several parameters need to be considered when evaluating the quality of respiratory function during feeding. These include: (1) respiratory effort, (2) changes in respiratory pattern, and (3) the sound of the respirations.

Respiratory effort: The infant's "work of breathing" or *respiratory effort* needs to be evaluated both before and during the feeding. Increased respiratory effort, or respiratory distress, can be noted in subtle ways such as nasal flaring or grunting on exhalation. More obvious signs of increased work of breathing include retractions, wherein certain areas of the chest are drawn in by the increased strength of inhalation.

Retractions may occur at a variety of locations: between the ribs (intercostal), above the clavicles (supraclavicular), below the rib margins (subcostal), in the notch at the base of the neck (suprasternal), or at the distal sternal margin (xyphoid).

There is a continuum of severity for retractions. Respiratory distress is greater when the amount of retraction is large and there are many sites involved. At the extreme end of this continuum is a "paradoxical" pattern of breathing. In this pattern, when the infant forcefully contracts the diaphragm in an attempt to move air, the abdomen protrudes. Simultaneously the chest wall and sternum are drawn inward due to the high negative pressure generated within the thorax. This produces a "see-saw" pattern of chest and abdominal movement during breathing and suggests impending respiratory failure.[39]

An obvious by-product of increased respiratory effort is fatigue. In normally feeding young infants this fatigue is reflected in their falling asleep shortly after feeding. If the work of breathing is already increased prior to feeding, frequently the infant will not take an adequate volume before fatiguing and ending the feeding.

For some infants, respiratory effort is high at baseline and throughout the feeding. For others there may be distinct points when changes in respiratory effort occur. These should be noted. The timing and magnitude of increased respiratory effort will affect the infant's potential to be a totally oral feeder. If the infant's respiratory effort and work of breathing is high at all times, so the infant has little respiratory reserve for other activity, the degree of effort the baby should expend in feeding must be considered. In this case, the feeding specialist and other members of the medical team must determine if the work of feeding will compromise the infant's already fragile system.

Changes in respiratory pattern: The frequency and duration of inspiration, expiration, and pauses between respirations can vary. Some variations, however, are abnormal and imply dysfunction in central regulation of breathing.

Apnea. This is the cessation of respiratory airflow of any duration.[20] Short apneas of less than 15 seconds can be normal at all ages. Although short pauses in respiration are technically known as apnea, referring to them as respiratory pauses differentiates them from longer apneic pauses that are abnormal. Apnea becomes pathologic when the respiratory pause is longer than 20 seconds or is associated with cyanosis, abrupt pallor, hypotonia, or bradycardia (see figure 3-5).

Apnea can be central, obstructive, or mixed. In central apnea there is no respiratory effort. The diaphragm does not move, as it is not receiving signals from the central respiratory center in the brain stem. In obstructive apnea, there is respiratory effort but no air exchange. The diaphragm continues to move, but airflow is blocked, usually due to upper airway obstruction. This obstruction may be caused by collapse of the airway secondary to tracheomalacia or laryngospasm. Gastroesophageal reflux (GER) can also lead to obstructive apnea. Refluxed material can directly block the airway, impeding airflow, though more typically refluxed material stimulates sensory receptors, triggering a vagally mediated laryngospasm.

Mixed apnea is a combination of central and obstructive apnea. The infant may initially have a central apneic event. As the baby attempts to initiate respiration, there may be no airflow secondary to obstruction of some sort.

During feeding, a baby can have both central and obstructive apneic events. Central mechanisms are primarily responsible if a baby holds its breath for an extended period during nutritive suck-swallow bursts (see page 134 for further information on this abnormal pattern of suck, swallow, breathe coordination). Obstructive apnea can also occur during feeding when the airway is blocked by the bolus itself, if there is structural collapse of the airway, or if a vagally mediated broncho- or laryngospasm occurs. In either case, the baby may recover spontaneously and without compromise, or the apnea may lead to oxygen desaturation and possibly bradycardia.

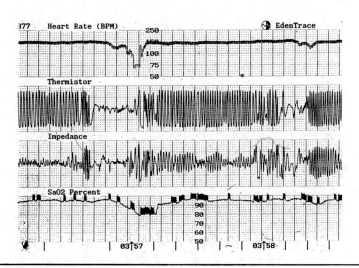

Figure 3-5 An episode of central apnea recorded on a multichannel pneumogram. (Courtesy of N. Davis, M.D., Seattle, WA)

Periodic breathing. This is a breathing pattern in which there are three or more pauses in respiration of greater than 3 seconds duration, with less than 20 seconds of respiration between the pauses.[20] For example, a baby may take five short breaths followed by a 10-second pause, repeating this pattern several times (see figure 3-6). This type of breathing pattern can be normal in some instances, particularly in premature babies. Excessive or prolonged periods of periodic breathing are not normal and can lead to oxygen desaturation.

The presence of periodic breathing suggests that the infant has difficulty with central control of respiratory rhythms. Since sucking, swallowing, and breathing during feeding require exquisite coordination, dysrhythmic breathing could lead to decreased coordination of these three key functions. If immaturity of the central rhythm-generating mechanisms is leading to periodic breathing, such immaturity might also directly lead to dysrhythmic coordination of sucking, swallowing, and breathing.

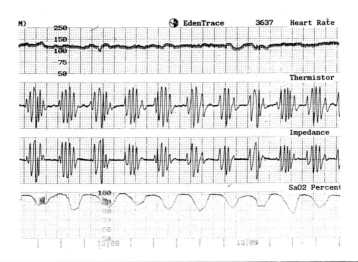

Figure 3-6 Periodic breathing recorded on a multichannel pneumogram. (Courtesy of N. Davis, M.D., Seattle, WA)

Sound of respirations: In the normally functioning infant, respirations are smooth and quiet. Little sound is heard on inspiration or exhalation. Audible sounds during any part of the breathing cycle indicate a problem with the patency of the upper or lower airways. Any process that alters the shape of the airway will create "noise." What this noise sounds like and when it occurs are important features to observe when evaluating the quality of respirations for feeding.

Stridor. Stridor is a harsh, raspy respiratory noise heard predominantly on inspiration and caused by narrowing or obstruction of the airway. Softer expiratory noises may also be heard. There are many causes of stridor, but some of the more common include: tracheo- or laryngomalacia, vocal cord paralysis, extrinsic compression of the trachea (such as a vascular ring), or subglottic hemangioma.[21] In tracheo- or laryngomalacia, the airway collapses to a slitlike opening, resulting in air turbulence, which produces stridor. There is substantial respiratory effort on inspiration, and the baby may show signs of respiratory distress.

When a baby has stridor, the work of breathing may be so increased during feeding that the baby fatigues prior to taking adequate nutrition. An infant with stridor may also have difficulty coordinating swallowing and breathing and/or have oxygen desaturation during feeding.

Wheezing. In contrast to stridor, wheezing is a forced, high-pitched noise that occurs primarily on exhalation, although inspiratory components may be present. It is due to constriction of the smaller airways, which makes it difficult for the baby to push air out. The baby uses increased force for exhalation, and the length of the exhalation may be increased. Inflammation and bronchoconstriction result in wheezing and can be due to a variety of factors, including asthma or reactive airway disease.

Microaspiration during feeding, which is frequently silent aspiration, can lead to reactive airway disease, which then results in wheezing. If the baby's respiratory sounds are quiet before feeding but become increasingly noisy over the course of or at the end of feeding, with increasing wheezing, microaspiration should be considered.

Coordination of Sucking, Swallowing, and Breathing

The smooth integration of sucking, swallowing, and breathing during nutritive feeding allows the infant to feed efficiently and effectively. If a problem is present in any one component, feeding may be compromised. In addition, the central mechanisms that coordinate these three functions into a smooth, rhythmic package must be intact. Because rhythmicity is the hallmark of normal sucking, evaluating rhythm during nutritive sucking is the primary means of assessing the coordination of sucking, swallowing, and breathing.

As described in detail in chapters 1 and 6, the infant has maturational changes in sucking patterns over time[24] as well as changes in sucking pattern over the course of the feeding.[25-27] Differences in sucking and breathing rhythm have been observed between nutritive and non-nutritive sucking.[28-30] These developmental changes as well as the functional components of the suck/swallow/breathe triad need to be considered during the CFEI.

Evaluation and Interpretation

Evaluation is always done during nutritive sucking. The primary method of evaluating the coordination of sucking, swallowing, and breathing is by carefully *listening* to the infant during feeding. The feeding specialist should determine the ratio of sucks to breaths. Swallows may be heard, but they are usually inferred by the sucking sequence and flow of the liquid. Recently, Vice et al. have described a potentially useful method for assessing the relationship of swallowing to sucking and breathing through cervical auscultation.[41]

Normal rhythmic pattern: Mature nutritive sucking is organized into a series of sucking bursts and pauses. During sucking bursts, respirations are interspersed with sucking and swallowing. During pauses only respirations are observed. Figure 3-7a shows the normal sucking burst-and-pause pattern. The beginning of a feeding in both term and preterm infants is characterized by long, continuous sucking bursts with few pauses. Toward the end of the feeding, sucking bursts are shorter, with more frequent and somewhat longer pauses.[26,31]

The ratio of sucks to swallows changes over the course of a feeding and with increasing maturation.[30] Newborns, whether they are breast- or bottle-fed, generally have a 1:1 ratio between sucking and swallowing, with a breath associated with each swallow. As the feeding progresses, this ratio changes to 2:1 or 3:1. Older infants will more frequently have two to three sucks prior to each swallow, and there will be one or more breaths between swallows. When the swallow occurs, it suppresses breathing at some point in the respiratory cycle. That is, infants are not able to swallow and breathe simultaneously, as had once been thought.[32] Chapter 1 provides more detailed information on the normal coordination of sucking/swallowing and breathing.

Prolonged sucking (feeding-induced apnea): In this abnormal sucking pattern (figure 3-7b), the baby has lengthy sucking bursts without interspersing breaths appropriately. There may be no respiration for at least 5 sucks and upward to 20 sucks, which could last from 5 to 25 seconds. The infant is not able to "pace" respirations with swallowing and may be described as having pacing difficulties. The end point of this prolonged sucking may take many forms. First, sucking may cease independently after numerous sucks, with the infant then compensating with rapid, panting respirations. This can cause the baby to become fatigued and have difficulty taking adequate volume. Second, sucking may cease only as the infant sputters and coughs in a poorly timed effort to breathe, putting the infant at increased risk for aspiration. Lastly, often the sucking burst terminates when the baby becomes cyanotic and/or bradycardic from this feeding-induced apnea. Interestingly, some infants continue to make sucking motions for several seconds before taking a breath even when the nipple is removed from the mouth.

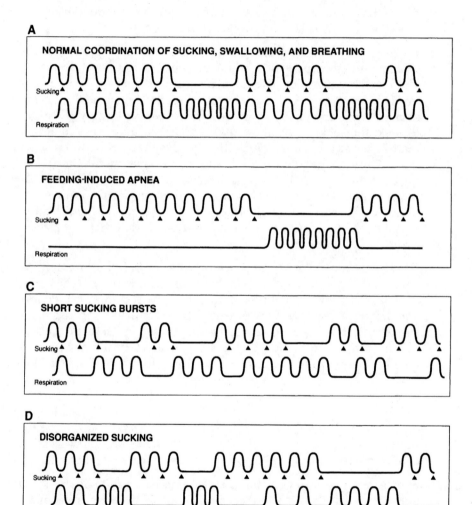

Figure 3-7 Normal coordination of sucking, swallowing, and breathing compared to abnormal patterns. Each ▲ represents a swallow.

Babies who demonstrate this pattern of prolonged sucking may have strong, rapid sucking activity. The prolonged sucking pattern occurs most frequently at the beginning of a feeding, when the baby is in the most eager phase of eating. As sucking and swallowing slow toward the middle or end of the feeding, and intermittent sucking predominates, the baby may return to a normal respiratory pattern during sucking. This type of feeding-induced apnea is observed in full-term and preterm infants, but it is seen more frequently in premature infants, especially between 34 and 38 weeks gestation.[26]

When this prolonged sucking pattern is noted, it appears that the swallowing accompanying feeding may "over-suppress" respiration. The mechanism responsible for this pattern is unclear, but it might involve a central process such as a laryngeal chemoreceptor mechanism[27,31] and/or a physical mechanism. If a baby is hungry and eager to suck, the sucking/swallowing rate and flow may be so high that there is physically not adequate time for respirations between swallows. Since this pattern is typically seen in premature infants, inadequate maturation of the central brain-stem processes that regulate coordination of sucking, swallowing, and breathing could be involved. If feeding-induced apnea persists for 10 to 30 seconds, it can lead to oxygen desaturation. It is this oxygen desaturation that can lead to cyanosis and bradycardia.[27]

The significance of prolonged sucking patterns in full-term infants is unclear. Perhaps these infants still have some immaturity of the brain-stem mechanisms regulating the integration of sucking, swallowing, and breathing rhythms. On the other hand, this may be an early and subtle indicator of specific neurological dysfunction. The experience at our center has been varied. On follow-up, several term infants who had no other problems in the newborn period besides prolonged sucking have gone on to have neurologic and developmental problems such as seizures, cerebral palsy, and developmental delay. On the other hand, a number of infants appear to be developing normally. Perhaps this type of early feeding difficulty in a full-term infant is a red flag for future neurological or developmental difficulties. Careful observation of development during the first year of life is indicated for these infants.

Short sucking bursts: In this abnormal feeding pattern, the infant takes only one to three sucks before pausing (figure 3-7c). There is an appropriate suck/swallow/breathe ratio, but the pauses are too frequent and too long, particularly early in the feeding. Efficiency and intake can be compromised. This pattern of short sucking bursts is generally related to either swallowing or respiratory difficulties.

If the swallow is delayed, is not complete, or is poorly triggered due to inadequate bolus formation, this pattern may represent the baby's attempt to prevent further liquid from entering the mouth until the previous bolus has exited the oral cavity. There may also be poor oral-motor control interfering with effective bolus formation and impeding the speed of the swallowing reflex. If this is the case, the infant may be purposefully slowing down the sucking process to allow for better oral preparation prior to swallowing. In either case, the shortened sucking burst can be an adaptive mechanism by the infant to limit sequential boluses.

If the baby has respiratory distress, a high respiratory rate (for example, more than 75-80 breaths/minute while feeding), works excessively to breathe during feeding (as observed in sternal or clavicular retractions), and/or has poor respiratory reserve, the baby may be pausing after only a few suck/swallows to rest and to "catch its breath" or to organize the swallow/breathe sequence. In this case, the infant is adapting to limited respiratory function by "self-pacing." This compensation should be supported until the underlying respiratory problem can be improved. Full intake, however, may not be achieved by nipple-feeding.

Disorganized sucking: This is a very disorganized and uneven sucking pattern (figure 3-7d). The duration of bursts and pauses may vary considerably. Even if burst and pause times remain somewhat consistent, there is an uneven pattern of breathing and swallowing within the sucking burst. Frequent coughing or choking is often observed. This pattern may be a result of general disorganization of state and behavior, neurologic deficit, mild respiratory difficulties, or an incompatible nipple-flow rate.

Differences in sucking rhythm between nutritive and non-nutritive sucking: The observation of differences in coordination, rhythm, and/ or strength between nutritive sucking (NS) and non-nutritive sucking (NNS) is important. If the NNS pattern is more appropriate, it can indicate that although oral abilities may be adequate, something about the presence of liquid is causing problems for the baby.

Several factors can lead to a difference between NS and NNS. This observation can be an indication of swallowing dysfunction. The infant may alter the strength or rhythm of sucking to limit the amount of fluid taken in. Another possibility is that the coordination of breathing with frequent swallowing is too difficult for the baby, so NS is less vigorous than NNS. Respiratory distress or other respiratory dysfunction can account for this. Tactile problems can also be considered, as the sensation of liquid entering the oral area is quite different from the nipple alone. Experiential or behavioral difficulties must be considered in older babies. For example, a baby who was pushed or forced to nipple despite many difficulties may later refuse to feed but still enjoy NNS.

Coughing/choking: Since coughing is the primary protective response that keeps fluids from entering the airway, the presence of a cough during the feeding process typically indicates that some fluid has entered or nearly entered the larynx. All babies sometimes have food that "goes the wrong way" and stimulates coughing or sputtering. Frequent, hard coughing or choking during feedings or coughing associated with physiologic change is indicative of a problem outside the normal spectrum of infant sputtering.

Frequent coughing during the suck/swallow/breathe process often reflects ongoing aspiration. Aspiration may also be occurring more often than the coughing is heard, as in silent aspiration. It is important to note the frequency and timing of the coughing or choking during the feeding, and whether it is associated with changes in color, heart rate, or respiratory rate. Coughing or choking while feeding, accompanied by changes in other physiologic parameters most likely reflects swallowing problems.

Coughing and choking between feedings or toward the end of feeding, when the stomach is full, or may be triggered by GE reflux ascending to the laryngeal area. Coughing associated with changing the baby's position could also be triggered by GE reflux and/or reflux of food that remains in the esophagus due to poor motility. When esophageal motility is impaired, liquid can back up during periods of continuous sucking. If it then reaches the level of the larynx, coughing may occur. This should be considered in infants who have had surgical repair of tracheal esophageal fistula, when esophageal motility is often impaired (see chapter 6).

It is important to differentiate between coughing because of a swallowing problem and coughing due to an acute or chronic respiratory disease. If the infant has an active respiratory illness, aspiration may not be the trigger for the coughing. In some infants, drinking milk products can cause increased mucus production and secretions in the lungs. These may then trigger bronchial coughing.

Physiologic Control

As stated previously, feeding is a baby's work. The infant has physiologic and autonomic responses to that work in the same way that adults respond to any form of exercise. To fully evaluate the feeding process in infants with difficulties, their physiologic response to this work must be considered. Parameters such as heart rate, respiratory rate, and oxygen saturation, as well as autonomic and visceral indicators of stress, therefore, should be addressed. Both clinical observations and sophisticated technical equipment (reviewed in chapter 2) help in evaluation of these parameters. For babies whose presenting feeding problems are frequent coughing or choking, cyanosis, apnea, and/or bradycardia, it is suggested that a cardiorespiratory monitor, and possibly an oximeter, be used to assist in monitoring the infant's physiologic responses during the CFEI.

Healthy, normally feeding infants will remain physiologically stable throughout the feeding process. Respiration and heart rate may increase somewhat, though respirations will remain smooth and changes in heart rate will never be dramatic. Their color will remain pink and stable, and they will show stability in their viscera.[4]

In order to accurately interpret changes in physiologic responses during feeding, it is crucial to be aware of the baby's behavior, as well as the specifics of the feeding situation, at the time the physiologic changes occur. This is particularly true if the physiologic changes are sudden, such as an abrupt color change or bradycardia. For example, a baby may be feeding well and maintaining physiologic stability, but when lifted to burp becomes cyanotic and bradycardic. This would suggest that there is something about position change that is the trigger for the cyanosis and bradycardia, as opposed to a sucking or swallowing difficulty. The feeding specialist must become sensitive to these relationships in order to provide the most thorough interpretation of the results of the CFEI. (Information on physiologic control can be recorded on the CFEI form.)

Heart Rate

Evaluation

An *initial* or baseline prefeeding heart rate (HR) and *postfeeding* HR should be established. HR should be monitored throughout the feeding with notations of *highest* values, *lowest* values, abrupt changes, and events related to any of the HR observations. HR is most easily followed using a cardiac-respiratory monitor, which allows observation of the wave-form pattern, provides an averaged numeric value, and sounds an alarm if the baby goes beyond the preset upper and lower limits.

If a CR monitor is not available, it is possible to take the pulse before and after the feeding, though it is more difficult to obtain information on the HR during a feeding in this way. Dips in HR will not be noticed. Brief episodes of bradycardia with self-recovery may not be recognized, and more significant bradycardic episodes will be noted only as the baby has become more compromised and demonstrates cyanosis or change in level of consciousness.

Interpretation

Baseline HR values, when the baby is awake and quiet, need to be considered in relation to "normal" values. For the full-term neonate, HR typically falls between 120 and 140 beats per minute (BPM), though rates from 70 to 170 BPM can be acceptable under certain conditions.[35,40] While there may be wide variability in normal heart rates among infants, there is generally less variability within one infant. Therefore, it is important to determine the appropriate baseline rate for a particular infant before interpreting changes in HR. Heart rate tends to be lower during sleep and higher with activity. During work, such as feeding, it is common to see the HR increase 10 BPM over the baseline value.

In premature infants, resting HR is generally higher than the values given for term neonates, with heart rates of 160 to 180 BPM not uncommon. Baseline HR declines with age, though average values do not change substantially during the first year.[40] By 3 years of age, a child's normal HR falls between 70 and 150 BPM.[36]

If the baseline HR is elevated (tachycardia), or the HR shows a dramatic increase with feeding, or it remains high for a prolonged period after the feeding, the work of feeding may be excessive for that baby. The increased heart rate, however, must be considered in terms of other variables. If the infant is gaining weight and having no other signs of significant physiologic stress, feeding may be quite reasonable and the tachycardia of no functional significance. If the infant is not gaining weight well, fatiguing quickly, and/or having difficulty completing feedings, increased HR may suggest that the baby is working too hard to feed effectively. The infant may in fact be burning more calories during feeding than it is taking in. Additional support to the cardiorespiratory system (medication, supplemental oxygen, etc.) or nutritional support through supplemental non-oral feeding may be needed.

Bradycardia, a drop in heart rate to below 90 or 100 BPM, when observed with feeding, is a significant and possibly life-threatening event. Feeding must be modified to eliminate this response, or oral feeding may need to be discontinued. Several mechanisms can trigger a bradycardic event. It may result from either central or obstructive apnea. Aspiration, structural anomalies that intermittently occlude the airway, or vagally mediated laryngospasm can cause obstructive apnea that would lead to bradycardia. A prolonged sucking pattern (see page 134), or feeding-induced apnea, can also lead to bradycardic episodes. Apnea itself does not cause bradycardia, but it leads to decreased oxygen saturation. Arterial chemoreceptors then respond to reduced oxygen levels in the blood by slowing the heart rate. Bradycardia can also be triggered directly through stimulation of the laryngeal and pharyngeal chemo- and baro- (stretch/pressure) receptors, as described in chapter 1.

By observing the wave-form pattern on the CR monitor, transient dips in HR may be noted. Such events may be missed if the examiner is primarily relying on numeric values or alarms for feedback on HR. These dips are generally caused by mechanisms similar to a true bradycardic event. Such an event is typically not dangerous. If it is seen occasionally it may be a slight "lurch" in the system or may reflect immaturities that the baby adjusts to and outgrows. Multiple transient drops in HR during feeding, however, are more noteworthy; they may compromise feeding and require further investigation.

Respiratory Rate

Evaluation
An *initial* prefeeding respiratory rate (RR) should be established when the infant is awake, alert, and calm. Throughout the feeding it is important to document changes in RR: what the *highest* and *lowest* values are, trends over the period of the feeding, what the *post-feeding* RR is, and how soon after feeding it returns to baseline. Apneic pauses impact RR and must be noted. They are addressed in detail on page 130 with other qualitative aspects of respiration.

The RR can be followed using a cardiac-respiratory (CR) monitor. However, this method has several limitations (also see chapter 2). First, the numeric reading is an averaged value, so it will obscure information regarding brief to moderate respiratory pauses or short bursts of rapid, "panting" respirations that occur during sucking pauses. Each of these relatively transient findings can have an impact on feeding. In addition, because of the method by which data on respiratory rate is generally collected on the CR monitor, it is particularly susceptible to movement artifact. Therefore, if the infant is wiggling or being rocked or patted, values may be inaccurate. An alternate means of assessing RR is to count respirations for 15- to 30-second periods before, during, and after the feeding and multiplying this number by four or two to derive the breaths per minute. During the feeding, it is best to measure RR during a pause in sucking.

Interpretation
To interpret an infant's respiratory rate in relation to feeding, the baseline rate must first be compared to normal values. While rates of 30 to 60 breaths per minute (BPM) are considered typical for full-term newborns,[35,36] the infant's state of alertness during the measurements of RR must be considered. In a study directly observing respiratory rate in a large sample of infants 0 to 6 months of age, Morley et al. found significant differences in RR when infants were awake and content, as compared to crying or sleeping.[37] Respiratory rate was highest when infants were awake and lowest during sleep. Interestingly, the RR for sleeping babies was roughly

between 30 and 60 BPM. When awake the mean RR was 58 BPM, with a range of 30 to 80 BPM. The RR of older infants was not significantly different from that of younger infants across this age span.

In regard to feeding, the most important finding is a high respiratory rate, or tachypnea. If one considers that an infant might take 40 to 60 nutritive sucks per minute, and that each suck is accompanied by a swallow and breath, nutritive sucking will limit the RR to 40 to 50 breaths per minute. This is a slight reduction from the typical mean value described above (58 BPM) and agrees with observations of Mathew and Shivpuri that RR decreases during the continuous phase of sucking.[27,31] Recovery of RR occurs during intermittent sucking when there are more frequent and longer pauses, with RR at baseline values by the end of the feeding.

If, however, the resting RR is 70 BPM, the infant obviously needs more frequent breaths to maintain homeostasis. A reduction to 40 BPM during continuous nutritive sucking is a significant change and may compromise the infant's status or make it difficult for the infant to cope with the respiratory demands of feeding. If the infant is not able to adequately meet its own respiratory needs during feeding, the baby is at risk for oxygen desaturation as well as fatigue. In addition, when the RR is very high there is an increased risk of discoordination between sucking, swallowing, and breathing. The infant's gasping for a much needed, though poorly timed, breath could lead to aspiration.

An important issue is: At what point is the respiratory rate too high for safe, effective feeding? There is not a clear answer to this question. Instead, RR needs to be considered in the context of the infant's overall health. The healthy baby with a baseline RR of 70 to 75 BPM while awake may be able to compensate for the reductions in ventilation imposed by feeding. However, the infant with any evidence of respiratory dysfunction (for example, a baby recovering from infant respiratory distress syndrome, or with bronchopulmonary dysplasia, or a baby with congenital heart disease) with a RR of 70 to 75 BPM may not have the respiratory reserve to cope with these same reductions in ventilation imposed by feeding. Such an infant may become compromised during feeding, may be inefficient, and/ or may be unsafe for oral feeding. For infants with any evidence of respiratory compromise, a conservative guideline might be that RR should not be over 65 to 70 BPM at rest to initiate feeding. In making such judgments, it is crucial to measure RR in a consistent state. These values are for the awake, content infant and may be lower for a sleeping infant.

In infants with some degree of respiratory compromise, the overall RR may actually increase during feeding, in an attempt to compensate for the significantly reduced ventilation during sucking. This may particularly be observed during the sucking pauses as the infant attempts to recover from the dip in RR during continuous sucking. While increases of up to 10 BPM are generally clinically acceptable, greater increases indicate that feeding is putting undue stress on the infant. Feeding should probably be terminated if RR goes above 80 BPM. In some cases, even small increases in RR move the infant into the area where ventilatory needs cannot be met during oral feeding. Infants whose RR increases during feeding should be monitored after feeding to determine how long it takes them to return to baseline values. A prolonged recovery is another indication of the stress feeding places upon the infant, as well as the "cost" to the infant.

Oxygen Saturation

Evaluation
Oxygen saturation is the amount of oxygen present in the blood and available for exchange at the tissue level. A pulse oximeter with external sensor is generally used to measure oxygen saturation in capillary blood flow. Oxygen saturation is expressed as a percentage of 100.

Pulse oximetry readings can be influenced by a variety of factors and therefore should not necessarily be regarded as absolute values. Oximetry readings are quite susceptible to movement artifact. Since most babies move while feeding, this may significantly affect the accuracy of the oximetry results. The presence of anemia, ambient light sources, skin perfusion, and the infant's natural skin pigmentation can all cause pulse oximetry values to vary.[42] In addition, a pulse oximeter's accuracy can vary +/- 1-2% at 90% oxygen saturation or above. This small change in pulse oximetry saturation, however, can reflect relatively large differences in blood oxygen levels.[42] These differences between saturation levels and true blood oxygen levels could be significant for some infants. Interpretation of pulse oximetry readings during feeding must take these factors into consideration. Chapter 2 provides additional information on the strengths and limitations of oximetry.

Interpretation
The normal infant has oxygen saturation above 95% in most conditions. For preterm babies, oxygen saturation above 90% is generally considered acceptable. Saturations below 90% indicate some degree of hypoxia. For some infants, oxygen saturation below 90% will be considered acceptable based on the infant's particular disease process. This is particularly true for babies with congenital heart disease who cannot maintain higher oxygen saturations due to the mixing of oxygenated and unoxygenated blood.

Desaturation may be an isolated event and seen without significant observable changes. Color change is not a reliable means of assessing oxygen saturation, since infants can have significant desaturation without external changes in color, HR, or RR.[33] Infants tend to have a cyclic oscillation of oxygen saturation during feeding. In the beginning, during the continuous sucking phase, oxygen saturation will dip slightly and then return to baseline during the intermittent sucking phase. However, some infants, particularly premature infants, may not recover adequately and may continue to have oxygen desaturation throughout the feeding.[27,33]

Providing supplemental oxygen is one method of improving oxygen saturation. If this is effective, immediate changes in oxygen saturation values should be observed. Not all conditions, however, will respond to the provision of supplemental oxygen. With certain types of congenital heart disease or very severe bronchopulmonary dysplasia, supplemental oxygen may not bring saturations into the normal range.

Color

Evaluation
During the CFEI, the easiest way to assess color is by observing the face and neck, paying particular attention to the color around the mouth (*circumoral*) and around the eyes (*circumorbital*). Observe the infant's color *initially* at rest to establish a baseline, then monitor *changes* in color during the feeding. It is again important to notice if color changes are related to specific events, suggesting mechanisms that may trigger these changes. Although the basic pigmentation of the baby's skin will influence how easily the examiner can perceive these differences in facial color, all babies manifest changes in color from physiologic sources regardless of their ethnicity.

Interpretation
Normally there is a *pink* blush to the skin. *Pale,* whitish skin suggests either poor oxygen saturation or poor perfusion. Typically the degree of concern would be mild if a pale color is noted, but this can be associated with poor endurance. The infant may be a *dusky/gray* color, leading to greater concern regarding cardiorespiratory function. *Circumoral* or *orbital cyanosis* is noted when tissues around the infant's mouth or eyes become gray or blue. Mildly dusky color and circumoral or orbital cyanosis may develop slowly over the course of a feeding, suggesting a slow, steady decline in oxygen saturation. A sudden change in color suggests that there has been an acute event, such as a period of apnea or sudden drop in oxygen saturation. If an infant's color becomes *blue/purple,* there has been an acute compromise and immediate medical support is required. If a baby turns *red* or *ruddy* during the feeding, it may be accompanied by straining, grunting, or crying. This does not indicate cardiorespiratory problems, but rather it is reflective of the increased effort the infant uses during these activities. The stress of these activities, however, can influence feeding.

Autonomic Stress Signals

Evaluation and Interpretation

Autonomic stress signals, or stress cues, are similar to those previously discussed in relation to state and motoric behavior; they are indications that the infant perceives something in the environment as stressful. In this case, however, they are physiologic responses, and thus their importance as indicators of stress may be overlooked. The stress cues in this domain that have been identified by Als[4] are listed in table 3-5. When a number of signs are observed during feeding, it suggests that the infant is experiencing major stress. Their presence may also provide important information on an infant's feeding or swallowing performances, so these stress responses have been discussed in detail throughout this chapter.

Table 3-5 Autonomic Stress Cues

Autonomic Signs of Moderate Stress

- Sighing
- Yawning
- Sneezing
- Sweating (diaphoresis)
- Hiccupping
- Tremoring
- Startling
- Gasping
- Straining

Autonomic Signs of Major Stress (when seen with feeding)

- Coughing
- Spitting up
- Gagging/Choking
- Color change
- Respiratory pauses
- Irregular respirations

Adapted from Als[4]

Endurance

Poor intake and poor weight gain are generally the results of decreased endurance. Either the infant fatigues before finishing the feeding, thus getting inadequate calories, or the baby takes the required amount but has expended excessive calories in the process. Some diagnoses associated with poor endurance include: prematurity, bronchopulmonary dysplasia (BPD), congenital heart disease, diaphragmatic hernia, or structural abnormalities like tracheal stenosis or Pierre-Robin malformation. Regardless of the diagnosis or presence of respiratory compromise, decreased endurance results in poor growth. The younger and smaller the infant is, the greater the impact of limited endurance on feeding.

Eating is an infant's aerobic exercise or work. Calories are burned to produce work, so when infants are working extremely hard to breathe or feed, they will use a proportionately higher number of calories for those activities. Unless these calories are replaced, often through higher volumes of food, there will be poor weight gain. Unfortunately, babies with poor endurance often struggle to take minimum volume, so the ability to take larger volumes is questionable.

Infants with problems of endurance may have normal oral-motor control and normal coordination of the suck/swallow/breathe mechanism. Such babies will feed well but will stop early in the feeding before they have accomplished adequate intake. They will have frequent, lengthy pauses to rest and/or will feed for excessively long periods of time. Attempting to push such infants to take more usually proves pointless, as they will refuse, gag, or simply let liquid run out of the mouth. When these babies are finished, they are finished. Often babies with limited endurance are still awake after feeding but are unwilling to take more.

General Observations

After observing the feeding, the examiner should record general information about the *method of feeding* (breast or bottle) and the type of bottle and nipple used. The *length of the feeding* and *amount taken* should be recorded to determine feeding efficiency. The *reason for ending* the feeding should be described. A baby who cries and won't take more is providing a different message (something is wrong) than a baby who falls asleep when finished ("I've had enough"—even though the intake may or may not be adequate for nutrition). It should also be noted whether the baby has had any emesis (*spitting*), including *when* during the feeding, how frequently, and *how much*. In addition, any *respiratory support*, such as oxygen by nasal canula or blowby oxygen, should be noted, including the amount.

References

1. Morris, S. E., and M. D. Klein. 1987. *Pre-feeding skills*. Tucson, AZ: Therapy Skill Builders.

2. Jelm, J. 1990. *Oral-motor/feeding rating scale*. Tucson, AZ: Therapy Skill Builders.

3. Furuno, S., K. A. O'Reilly, C. M. Hosaka, T. T. Inatsuka, T. L. Allman, and B. Z. Eisloft. 1979. Hawaii Early Learning Profile (HELP), Palo Alto, CA: VORT Corporation.

4. Als, H. 1986. A synactive model of neonatal behavioral organization: Development in the premature infant and for support of infants and parents in the neonatal intensive care environment. *Physical and Occupational Therapy in Pediatrics* 6:3-53.

5. Brazelton, T. B. 1984. *Neonatal behavioral assessment scale*. Philadelphia: J. B. Lippincott Co.

6. Chandler, L. S., M. S. Andrews, and M. W. Swanson. 1980. *Movement assessment of infants: A manual*. Rolling Bay, WA.

7. Ellison, P. H., J. L. Horn, and C. A. Browning. 1985. Construction of an infant neurological international battery (INFANIB) for the assessment of neurological integrity in infancy. *Physical Therapy* 65:1326-31.

8. Dubowitz, L., and V. Dubowitz. 1981. The neurological assessment of the preterm and full-term newborn infant. In *Clinics in developmental medicine #79*. Philadelphia: J. B. Lippincott Co.

9. Bayley, N. 1969. *Bayley scales of infant development*. Berkeley, CA: The Psychological Corporation.

10. Knobloch, H., and B. Pasamanick. 1974. *Gesell and Amatruda's developmental diagnosis: The evaluation and management of normal and abnormal neuropsychologic development in infancy and early childhood*. Hagerstoum, MD: Harper and Row.

11. Folio, M. R., and R. R. Fewell. 1983. *Peabody scales of development and activity cards*. Allen, TX: DLM Teaching Resources.

12. Bosma, J. F. 1988. Functional anatomy of the upper airway during development. In *Respiratory function of the upper airway*, edited by O. P. Mathew and G. Sant'Ambrogio, 47-86. New York: Marcel Dekker, Inc.

13. Tuchman, D. 1988. Dysfunctional swallowing in the pediatric patient: Clinical considerations. *Dysphagia* 2:203-8.

14. Tucker, J. 1985. Perspective of the development of the air and food passages. *American Review of Respiratory Disease* 131:S7-S9.

15. Ingram, T. T. S. 1962. Clinical significance of the infantile feeding reflexes. *Developmental Medicine Child Neurology* 4:159-69.

16. Illingworth, R. S., and M. B. Lister. 1964. The critical or sensitive period, with special reference to certain feeding problems in infants and children. *The Journal of Pediatrics.* 65:839-48.

17. Ardran, G. M., F. H. Kemp, and J. Lind. 1958. A cineradiographic study of bottle-feeding. *British Journal of Radiology* 31:11-22.

18. Ardran, G. M., F. H. Kemp, and J. Lind. 1958. A cineradiographic study of breast-feeding. *British Journal of Radiology* 31:156-62.

19. Smith, W. L., A. E. Erenberg, A. Nowak, and E. A. Franken. 1985. Physiology of sucking in the normal term infant using real-time US. *Radiology* 156:379-81.

20. Infantile apnea and home monitoring. 1986. National Institutes of Health Consensus Development Conference Statement 6:3-4.

21. Tunnessen, W. W. 1987. Stridor—Listen carefully! *Contemporary Pediatrics,* 4:51-54.

22. Logemann, J. 1986. Treatment for aspiration related to dysphagia: An overview. *Dysphagia* 1:34-38.

23. Orenstein, S. R., and D. M. Orenstein. 1988. Gastroesophageal reflux and respiratory disease in children. *The Journal of Pediatrics.* 112:847-58.

24. Wolff, P. H. 1968. The serial organization of sucking in the young infant. *Pediatrics* 42:943-56.

25. Mathew, O. P. 1986. Regulation of breathing during oral feeding. *The Indian Journal of Pediatrics* 53:432-33.

26. Mathew, O. P. 1988. Respiratory control during nipple feeding in preterm infants. *Pediatric Pulmonology* 5:220-24.

27. Shivpuri, C. R., R. J. Martin, W. A. Carlo, and A. A. Fanaroff. 1983. Decreased ventilation in preterm infants during oral feeding. *The Journal of Pediatrics* 103:285-89.

28. Daniels, H., H. Devlieger, P. Casaer, M. Callens, and E. Eggermont. 1986. Nutritive and non-nutritive sucking in preterm infants. *Journal of Developmental Physiology* 8:117-21.

29. Lepecq, J. C., M. T. Rigoard, and P. Salzarulo. 1985. Spontaneous non-nutritive sucking in continuously fed infants. *Early Human Development* 12:279-84.

30. Weber, F., M. W. Woolridge, and J. D. Baum. 1986. An ultrasonographic study of the organization of sucking and swallowing by newborn infants. *Developmental Medicine Child Neurology* 28:19-24.

31. Mathew, O. P., M. L. Clark, M. L. Pronske, H. G. Luna-Solarzano, and M. D. Peterson. 1985. Breathing pattern and ventilation during oral feeding in term newborn infants. *The Journal of Pediatrics* 106:810-13.

32. Wilson, S. L., B. T. Thach, R. T. Brouillette, and Y. K. Abu-Osba. 1981. Coordination of breathing and swallowing in human infants. *Journal of Applied Physiology: Respiratory Environmental Exercise Physiology* 50:851-58.

33. Garg, M., S. I. Kurzner, D. B. Bautista, and T. G. Keens. 1988. Clinically unsuspected hypoxia during sleep and feeding in infants with bronchopulmonary dysplasia. *Pediatrics* 81:635-42.

34. Morris, S. E. 1982. *The normal acquisition of oral feeding skills: Implications for assessment and treatment.* Islip, NY: Theraputic Media.

35. Crane, L. D. 1986. Cardiopulmonary management of the high-risk neonate: Implications for developmental therapists. *Physical and Occupational Therapy in Pediatrics* 6:255-81.

36. Gould, A. 1991. Cardiopulmonary evaluation of the infant, toddler, child, and adolescent. *Pediatric Physical Therapy* 3:9-13.

37. Morley, C. J., A. J. Thornton, M. A. Fowler, T. J. Cole, and P. H. Hewson. 1990. Respiratory rate and severity of illness in babies under 6 months of age. *Archives of Disease in Childhood* 65:834-37.

38. Centers for Disease Control. 1987. Recommendations for prevention or HIV transmission in health-care settings. *Morbidity and Mortality Weekly Report* 36 (supplement 25).

39. Aloan, A. 1987. *Respiratory care of the newborn.* Philadelphia: J. B. Lippincott Co.

40. Chow, M. P., B. A. Durand, M. N. Feldman, and M. A. Mills. 1984. *Handbook of pediatric primary care.* New York: John Wiley and Sons.

41. Vice, F. L., J. M. Heinz, G. Giuriati, M. Hood, and J. F. Bosma. 1990. Cervical auscultation of suckle feeding in newborn infants. *Developmental Medicine and Child Neurology* 32:760-68.

42. Hays, W. W. 1987. Physiology of oxygenation and its relationship to pulse oximetry in neonates. *Journal of Perinatology* 7:309-19.

43. Inniruberto, A., and E. Tajani. 1981. Ultrasonographic study of fetal movements. *Seminars in Perinatology* 5:175-81.

Feeding History

1. **Parent description of problem**

2. **State/behavior**
    Describe your baby's disposition.

    What is baby's state/behavior throughout the day?

    What is baby's wake/sleep pattern?

    What does the baby act like when you first give the bottle/breast?

    What does the baby act like during feeding?

    How do you know the feeding is over?

    If the baby is also fed by spoon, is there a difference in behavior between spoon and bottle/breast?

3. Schedule

How you know when to feed the baby?

How often is the baby fed?

How long does the feeding take?

How much does the baby take?

4. Method of Feeding

Is baby fed by bottle or breast?

Does the baby take any spoon foods?

If there was a transition (breast to bottle, or introduction of spoon foods) how did baby adjust?

Were there any special circumstances around transition?

Type of bottle used?

Type of nipple used?

Formula used?

Spoon foods tried?

Position used?

5. **Feeding Problems Observed** by Parents. If the baby has been fed with varying methods/equipment, were the same observations made with all of the feeding methods? If any of these observations have been made by the feeder, it is important to clarify how frequently they occur and when during the feeding they occur. Frequency may be related to magnitude of the problem and the same symptom can suggest different problems depending on when in the feeding it is seen.

Does the baby:

have trouble sucking? When? How often?

have dysrhythmic or disorganized sucking? When? How often?

have trouble swallowing? When? How often?

have a "gulping" sound with swallowing? When? How often?

forget to breathe while feeding? When? How often?

have noisy breathing during feeding? When? How often?
Is this noisy breathing hard at nonfeeding times?

cough, choke, or gag? When? How often?

have any changes in color of the face or area around mouth or eyes? What color? When? How often?

sweat during feeding? When? How often?

spit up or vomit? How much? How often? During or after the feed? When during feed?

6. Other Factors
Does the baby:
take a pacifier? Does the baby like it better than bottle/breast?

have many colds?

have chronic nasal congestion?

drool a lot or need help managing secretions (i.e., require suctioning)?

have a history of respiratory illness, asthma, or pneumonia?

cry frequently and draw the legs up to the stomach, or have other behaviors suggesting abdominal discomfort? When in relationship to feeding? How often?

have a history of tube feeding? Gather details.

Clinical Feeding Evaluation of Infants

Name: _____   Date: _____

State

Initial	1	2	3	4	5	6
Midfeed	1	2	3	4	5	6
After	1	2	3	4	5	6
Functional for feeding	Yes	No				
Stable	Yes	Moderately		Minimally		No
Stress cues						

Motor Control

Tone	Hypotonic	Normal	Hypertonic
Reflexes	Appropriate		Dominant
Posture			
Developmental level			
Stress signals			
Feeding position			

Tactile

Reflexes:

Rooting	+	–	+ / –
Sucking	+	–	+ / –
Cough	+	–	+ / –
(preceding events)			
Gag	+	–	+ / –
(preceding events)			

Behaviors:

Hyporesponsive	Hypersensitive
Absent	Aversive

Oral-Motor

		Normal	Deviant
Tongue:	Position	soft thin flat round tip bottom of mouth central groove	tip elevated retracted humped bunched protruded asymmetric
	Movement	in/out up/down cups nipple rhythmic small excursions	thrust flat clonus fasciculations lacks rhythm
Jaw:	Position	neutral	recessed hangs open asymmetric
	Movement	small excursions smooth rhythmic	thrusts large excursions biting clenching clonus lacks ROM tremors
Lips/Cheeks:	Position	C: fat pad L/C: soft	L: retracted L: pursed
	Movement	L: shape to nipple L: pressure at corners	L: loose
Palate:	Position & Movement	intact	abnormal shape hard palate ? movement problem soft palate cleft

Suck, Swallow, and Breathe

Sucking:

Strength	Non-nutritive			Nutritive		
	Strong	Moderate	Weak	Strong	Moderate	Weak
Suction	Yes	No		Yes	No	
Compression	Yes	No		Yes	No	
Coordinated	Yes	No		Yes	No	
Breaks in suction	Yes	No		Yes	No	
Initiates sucking	Yes	No		Yes	No	
Loss of liquid				Yes	No	
Rhythmic	Yes	No		Yes	No	

Swallowing:

doesn't manage secretions
multiple swallows
noisy breathing (when?)
history of respiratory infection
gulping

Respiratory Quality:

Increased respiratory effort
apnea   periodic breathing
wheezing   stridor

Coordination of S/S/B: Rhythm

normal, rhythmic   feeding-induced apnea
short sucking bursts   disorganized

Difference between NS and NNS

Yes	No	
Coughing/Choking		
None	Sometimes	Frequently

Physiologic Control

	Initial	high	low	post-feeding
Heart rate				
Respiratory rate				
Oxygen saturation				
Response to O₂				
Autonomic stress signals				
Endurance				
Color	Normal			

$Response\ to\ O_2$

Color

Initial:
pink
pale
dusky/gray
circumoral-orbital cyanosis

Normal · Moderate · Low

Change to:
pale
dusky/gray
red/ruddy
blue/purple
circumoral-orbital cyanosis

General

Length of feed
(reason for ending?)
Amount taken
Bottle used (or breast)
Nipple used
Spitting
(when? how much?)
Respiratory support

4 Problem-Driven Models for the Comprehensive, Multidisciplinary Assessment of Infant Feeding

Infant feeding is a highly integrated, multisystem skill and thus may be compromised by dysfunction in one or more of the contributing systems. Figure 4-1 (see page 160) graphically depicts the interrelated nature of the infant's physiologic, motoric, and organizational abilities and parental attributes that combine for effective infant feeding. When feeding dysfunction is identified, numerous methods are available to evaluate the many components of infant feeding and its related functions, as described in the previous chapters. The feeding specialist's task is to organize a comprehensive assessment efficiently in order to determine the specific underlying cause of the infant's feeding problems. Implicitly, this process will involve a group of multidisciplinary health-care professionals working together, along with the infant's family.

This chapter presents a series of multidisciplinary "problem-driven models" that can serve as a flexible framework for systematically determining the underlying cause(s) of infant feeding problems. These models are based on the principle that if the problem is well defined, the specific causes for the problem can be more accurately determined, and the treatment will then be most effective (see figure 4-2, page 161).

Team Process

In some centers "feeding teams" have been established to carry out the comprehensive assessment and treatment process. As feeding problems may stem from a variety of systems, the availability of multiple medical and allied health specialists is optimal. Because infant feeding problems are often quite complex, a large number of clinicians may become involved in the diagnostic and treatment process. Therefore, even if no formal team is designated, an informal team often develops on a case-by-case basis. It is therefore important to understand the potential role and contribution of the various team members. These roles are summarized in table 4-1.

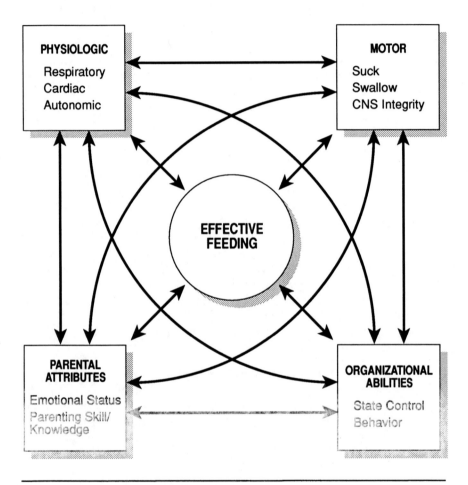

Figure 4-1 The multisystem, integrated nature of infant feeding.

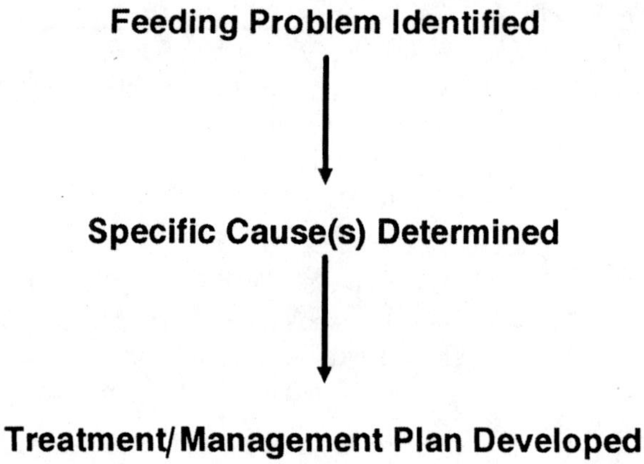

Feeding Problem Identified

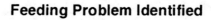

Specific Cause(s) Determined

Treatment/Management Plan Developed

Figure 4-2 Sequential activities in assessment and treatment of infant feeding problems.

Table 4-1 Potential Members of a Feeding Team and Possible Roles

Potential Team Members	Role in Assessment Process
Parents	Provide historical and current information on the feeding problem. Careful history, as well as parental report or demonstration of the feeding problem, can help to narrow the focus of the evaluation.
Occupational/Physical/ Speech Therapists	Any one may be the primary feeding specialist and carry out the feeding evaluation. Occupational and physical therapists may also evaluate general motor components and position during feeding. Speech therapists may relate oral-motor findings during feeding to speech and language.
Nutritionist	Able to determine optimal nutritional needs. Can suggest dietary modifications to achieve best caloric intake.
Social Worker	Assesses parent resources, strengths, and limitations. May help parents clarify their feelings about the baby's feeding problems and treatment.

Table 4-1 *(continued)*

Nurses	Includes hospital nurses, clinic nurses, community nurses, and clinical nurse specialists. The nurse may help initially identify the feeding problem. Nurses may also provide support for treatment/management strategies that are implemented.
Primary Physician	May initially identify the feeding problem. Often coordinates the feeding evaluation process. Could be a general pediatrician, developmental pediatrician, neonatologist, or family practice physician.
Gastroenterologist	Can provide assessment of esophageal and gastrointestinal anatomy and function, including assessment of GE reflux, GI motility, and malabsorption.
Pulmonologist	Can provide detailed evaluation of all aspects of pulmonary function and, in some cases, central respiratory control.
Otolaryngologist (Ear, Nose, and Throat)	Can identify structural abnormalities in the nose, pharynx, larynx, and trachea. Also provides surgical treatment for these problems.
Radiologist	Often involved in conducting studies of feeding-related functions using fluoroscopy, ultrasound, and nuclear medicine scans.
Neurologist	Can help identify neurologic basis of feeding problems, such as CNS damage or cranial nerve dysfunction.
Cardiologist	Assesses and plans treatment for congenital heart defects and other cardiac dysfunction.
General Surgeon	Provides surgical management of structural anomalies such as TEF and cleft palate. Performs surgery for placement of gastrostomies, central lines for parenteral nutrition.
Specialized Surgeon	Handles very specialized areas of surgical management, such as neurosurgery or cardiovascular surgery.

Physicians

In the process of assessing and managing feeding problems, physicians generally participate in the capacity of either manager or specialist.

Manager: The physician as manager is often the person initially presented with the feeding problem. He or she will frequently oversee the evaluation and treatment process. Pediatricians (both general and developmental), neonatologists, and family practitioners may function in this capacity.

Specialist: At times these physicians may initially identify a feeding problem and oversee the evaluation and treatment process. It is more likely that they would provide special diagnostic tests or procedures or specialized management in regard to the feeding problem. This group includes gastroenterologists, otolaryngologists (ear, nose, and throat), pulmonologists, neurologists, cardiologists, and surgeons (both general and specialized).

Allied Health Specialists

At times these clinicians may initially identify a feeding difficulty and bring it to the attention of a physician for comprehensive assessment. More often, however, their role is in providing pieces of assessment information that are valuable in the problem-solving process and/or in helping to implement the treatment. Allied health specialists might include occupational therapists, physical therapists, speech pathologists, nurses (including floor nurses in a hospital, clinic nurses, specialty nurses, and lactation consultants), nutritionists, and social workers.

The Infant Feeding Specialist

The professional who takes on the role of feeding specialist is generally an occupational therapist, a physical therapist, or a speech pathologist. In the comprehensive assessment of infant feeding problems, the feeding specialist is the team member who generally carries out the clinical feeding evaluation of infants (CFEI). Depending on the results of this process, the feeding specialist may also play a role in developing and carrying out the treatment plan.

The CFEI is an important element in the comprehensive assessment process. In the CFEI the feeding specialist is: (1) gathering detailed information on the feeding history and background of the feeding problems, (2) thoroughly observing the infant's feeding skills and difficulties, and (3) formulating hypotheses regarding the underlying causes for the feeding problems (see chapter 3).

Although the function or role of the CFEI in the comprehensive assessment process will vary from case to case, it is crucial that the feeding specialist not view this evaluation as an isolated element. It must be seen as part of a much larger process of assessment and problem solving. At times (e.g., when the infant's medical characteristics are well understood) the CFEI may focus fairly narrowly on understanding one function, such as oral-motor control, in order to develop a treatment plan (see case 5). At other times the CFEI may play a lead or pivotal role in determining the direction for further medical assessment and arriving at underlying medical causes for the feeding problems (see case 2). As the feeding specialist cannot initially know which role the CFEI will play in the overall problem-solving process, it is imperative to begin with a broad perspective on the potential outcomes when carrying out a CFEI.

To be effective in this role, the feeding specialist must

- have a thorough understanding of infant feeding mechanisms, including related systems that may impact feeding (see chapter 1). The feeding specialist can lend a "holistic" approach to the overall assessment process, by looking at the problem from the perspective of many systems rather than only ruling out problems in one system.

- have an adequate understanding of the tests and procedures that are related to this comprehensive problem-solving process (see chapter 2). This allows the feeding specialist to make appropriate suggestions for further evaluation of the problem and to integrate the results of various studies into the findings of the CFEI. This knowledge helps the feeding specialist fit the CFEI into the "big picture" of comprehensive assessment.

- understand the comprehensive problem-solving process in order to use the CFEI to play an important role in overall medical diagnosis and management, as well as in the development of specific feeding treatments.

- have excellent communication skills. This is crucial to working with parents and other caretakers in gathering information, and then in teaching treatment techniques. These skills are also needed to communicate results of the CFEI, hypotheses, or suggestions for further study, as well as treatment plans, with the medical team. Only through sound communication will the most efficient and effective assessment and management process be possible.

Identifying the Feeding Problem

A feeding behavior does not become a "feeding problem" until it does not meet the expected performance for that infant. For a "normal" baby without any medical diagnoses or complications, we expect that the infant will take the required amount efficiently, without color change or other physiologic compromise, and will gain weight. So, for example, if the infant takes less than is optimal; does not gain weight; has apnea or cyanosis; coughs, chokes, or gags frequently; or takes excessively long to feed, typical expectations are not met and a feeding problem exists.

The expected performance may be influenced by the infant's medical diagnosis. A 34-week premature infant may not take a complete feeding or may cough and choke and show slight color change. Although these are not typical feeding behaviors for a term baby, in this infant they may be accepted as appropriate for the gestational age. If they are persistent, oral feeding may even be postponed for a short time without concern. If these same behaviors are noted when this baby reaches 38 weeks gestation, and if other medical problems are resolved, the baby is not feeding as expected, so a feeding problem exists. Similarly, a baby with cleft lip and palate may cough or choke periodically while fed with a squeeze bottle. This can be expected as the baby and feeder become comfortable with the rhythm of this system. If the infant does not receive adequate calories, however, a feeding problem exists.

When a feeding problem exists, it must be clearly delineated so that the underlying cause or causes can be determined. The key reasons that the baby is not meeting expectations must be identified. These reasons must be stated in terms of the problem rather than in terms of a medical diagnosis. In other words, for the premature infant described above, the feeding problem is not prematurity but cyanosis with feeding, or inability to complete the feeding. For the baby with cleft lip and palate, the feeding problem is inadequate intake. Using a problem-driven model rather than a diagnosis-driven model in the comprehensive assessment of infant feeding problems is necessary because (1) many infants with feeding problems carry no medical diagnosis, and (2) when a medical diagnosis does exist it may or may not be related to the feeding problem. Focusing on the feeding problem keeps the clinician's mind open to alternate explanations which may ultimately be unrelated to the known primary diagnosis.

Basing the determination that a feeding problem exists on whether the infant meets expectations for feeding implies that it is the clinician's responsibility to be knowledgeable about the feeding expectations for infants with a variety of conditions. In addition, although many changes and much maturation take place in infancy, which can at times lead to resolution of

---

certain minor feeding problems, it is the clinician's responsibility to not underestimate the significance of a potential feeding problem by assuming that the infant will "grow out of it."

There are several reasons why it is often prudent to begin the assessment process soon after the feeding difficulties are initially identified. First, feeding difficulties that begin as fairly simple problems related to a medical diagnosis may easily become extremely complex as the infant and caregivers develop feeding patterns that may compound the initial problem. Second, seemingly simple problems like coughing with feeding can at times be related to significant conditions such as chronic aspiration. And finally, many techniques are available to assist infants with common feeding problems such as "poky" feeding, thus relieving much parental stress and anxiety.

In the problem-driven models described here, the presenting feeding problem is used to determine which model to follow during the problem-solving process. As infant feeding problems are often complex, initially several problems may be present that would trigger the use of different models. These models have been developed to determine the underlying cause(s) for the feeding problems even when the problems follow a variety of "paths." The process is usually more clearly focused when the model is selected based on the primary problem; that is, the problem that is most persistent or most compromising to the infant.

Comprehensive Assessment of Infant Feeding

The goal of any assessment of infant feeding problems is to determine the underlying cause, or constellation of causes, for the feeding dysfunction. The number of systems and people that may be involved in this process attests to the complexity that may develop. Efficiency and effectiveness in pursuing this task, therefore, requires a framework for the assessment. Such a framework must

- take into account the multisystem nature of infant feeding;

- follow a logical sequence to avoid unnecessary tests, procedures, and specialists, but without allowing critical gaps in the assessment sequence; and

- be flexible enough to accommodate new information or variations in presentation of the same problem, without becoming a prolonged process.

When such a framework is not developed and utilized, ineffective problem-solving methods often evolve. Clinicians may be familiar with cases that have used the "long, drawn-out" approach (see figure 4-3, page 168) or the "shotgun" approach (see figure 4-4, page 169). Although the cause of the feeding problem may be determined, it may take a long time (and perhaps a lengthy hospitalization) or become costly in terms of the number of procedures and specialists.

Thus a system of problem-driven models has been developed to provide a framework for the comprehensive assessment of infant feeding problems. This system is flexible yet allows an organized and efficient evaluation process. Each model is based on a common presenting problem related to infant feeding.

1. Feeding-related apnea model

2. Feeding problem model

3. Respiratory compromise model

4. Poor weight gain model

In each model there is a set of primary evaluations that should be considered initially. The results of these evaluations may then suggest the need for second- or third-level evaluations. Using a hierarchical approach to evaluation maximizes the efficiency of the process. This approach also allows these models to be effective for simple feeding problems as well as those that are more complex.

Although not all infant feeding problems will fit neatly into one of these models, the problem-solving process that characterizes the models can be adapted to varying circumstances. These models do take into account the fact that many problems have varying presentations and that following different models may lead to the same diagnosis, though perhaps via different routes if the presenting problems differ. The CFEI plays a key role in the flexibility of this process, but only if the feeding specialist who does the evaluation is well trained in observation skills, has adequate background in understanding the nature of infant feeding and potential problems, synthesizes information sensitively, and works effectively within the larger medical team.

For each model, the key presenting problems will be described, the role of the CFEI will be discussed, and possible outcomes will be reviewed. Case examples will then be provided to illustrate the comprehensive assessment process utilizing these problem-driven models.

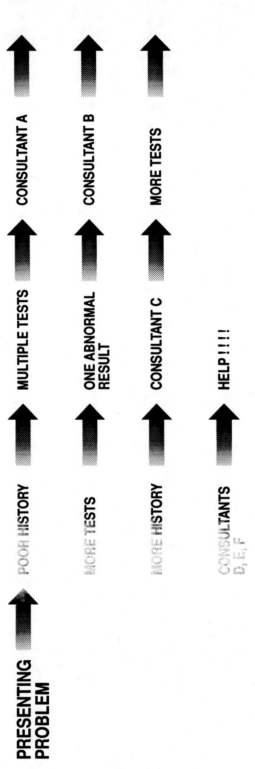

Figure 4-3 The "long, drawn-out" approach to assessment of infant feeding problems.

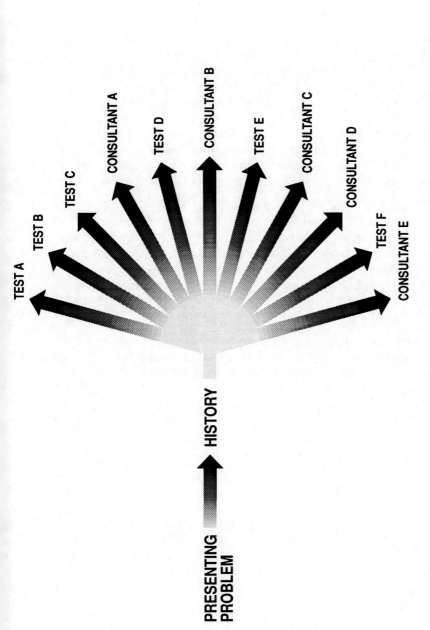

Figure 4-4 The "shotgun" approach to assessment of infant feeding problems.

Model 1: Feeding-Related Apnea Model

Key presenting problems: Apnea, cyanosis, oxygen desaturation, and/or bradycardia are seen at feeding time.

Role of clinical feeding evaluation: As there are *numerous* potential causes for the presenting problems seen in this model, and the presenting problems are potentially life threatening, it is crucial that the CFEI be carried out *early* in the assessment process. Only through this type of careful observation will it be clear whether the appropriate direction to follow is further evaluation of swallowing, evaluation of gastroesophageal reflux (GER), evaluating the presence of central apnea, or perhaps treating the problem immediately with techniques such as external pacing. If the presenting problem involves apnea, a multichannel pneumogram may be done simultaneously, looking for evidence of central or obstructive mechanisms. This can aid in interpretation of the CFEI.

During the CFEI, careful monitoring of the cardiorespiratory (CR) responses will be critical, and use of a CR monitor is recommended. Concurrent measurement of oxygen saturation is also highly recommended. When the presenting problems fall into this category, noting the timing of events as the baby becomes compromised is very important. This will be noted in some of the examples of this problem-solving model (cases 1, 3).

Possible outcomes: These might include but are not limited to central apnea; gastroesophageal reflux; tracheo-esophageal fistula; tracheal stenosis; poor coordination of sucking, swallowing, and breathing; or vascular ring around the trachea.

A variation of this model is the apnea model. The key presenting problems are apnea, cyanosis, and/or bradycardia that occur at non-feeding times. The underlying problem generally is either central apnea or obstructive apnea, the latter frequently related to gastroesophageal reflux. The diagnostic process typically does not include a CFEI, as the problems are not noted with feeding.

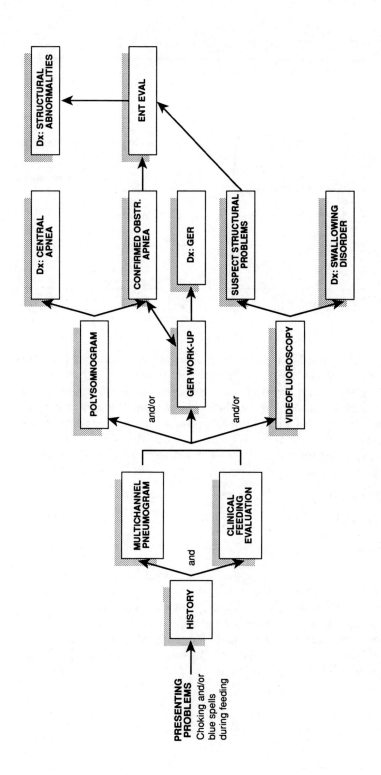

Figure 4-5 Feeding-related apnea model.

Case 1: Jason—Feeding-Related Apnea Model

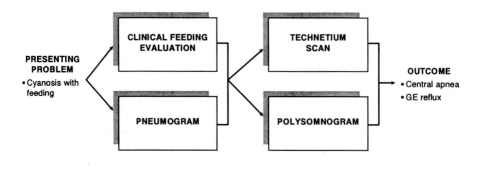

Figure 4-6 Case 1: Jason.

History: Jason (figure 4-6) was a 35-week premature infant. The pregnancy was uncomplicated until the spontaneous rupture of membranes at 35 weeks. Jason was then born in uncomplicated vaginal delivery. Apgar scores were 7 at one minute and 8 at five minutes. He required intubation for three days due to infant respiratory distress syndrome. Jason progressed to nipple feedings without difficulty. He was discharged home at 2 weeks of age. At 4 weeks of age (corrected age close to term) he became blue and limp during feeding on two occasions.

Presenting problem: Apnea and cyanosis during feeding.

Evaluations and findings:

Clinical feeding evaluation with oximetry: Jason demonstrated normal oral-motor skills, with good coordination between sucking, swallowing, and breathing. Some gulping swallows were noted during sucking pauses toward the end of feeding and were suggestive of GE reflux. He maintained adequate oxygen saturation throughout feeding, though as he fell asleep after the feeding, apnea and gradual oxygen desaturation were noted. A gradual oxygen desaturation in conjunction with the change to a sleep state is suggestive of central apnea disorder rather than GE reflux.

Two-channel pneumogram: Evidence of central and mixed apnea was present. Based on the clinical feeding evaluation and pneumogram results, a polysomnogram and technetium scan were planned.

Polysomnogram: Central apnea was diagnosed.

Technetium scan: Moderate GE reflux was diagnosed.

Treatment/management plan: The central apnea was treated with theophylline to stimulate respiratory drive. Home monitoring was provided. GE reflux was managed with upright positioning and thickened feedings (see page 340).

Summary: The clinical feeding evaluation was able to rule out problems such as poor coordination of sucking, swallowing, and breathing or inadequate oral-motor control. By observing the timing of the oxygen desaturation, and whether it was abrupt or gradual, potential causes could be inferred. Observations also suggested the presence of GE reflux. This information was then used by the physician to plan appropriate tests for further assessment.

Case 2: Alex—Feeding-Related Apnea Model

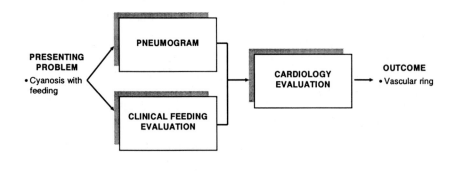

Figure 4-7 Case 2: Alex.

History: Alex (figure 4-7) as a full-term infant born after normal pregnancy, labor, and delivery. Apgar scores were 8 at one minute and 9 at five minutes. He was discharged home at 3 days of age. Feeding progressed slowly. Alex would begin a feeding with enthusiasm and interest but then fall asleep early in the feeding. On occasion he would finish the feeding without falling asleep. Weight gain was marginal. At 2 weeks of age, Alex was noted to become cyanotic regularly during feeding.

Presenting problem: Cyanosis during feeding.

Evaluations and findings:

Clinical feeding evaluation with oximetry: Alex had a strong suck with adequate oral-motor coordination. He showed good coordination between sucking, swallowing, and breathing early in the feeding. Respiratory rate increased dramatically during the first 5 minutes of feeding, from 50 to 80 BPM. Coordination between sucking, swallowing, and breathing became increasingly compromised, with coughing and choking noted. Intermittent oxygen desaturation to 70%, with cyanosis, was noted. It was apparent that some factor that was developing during feeding was compromising the respiratory patterns and coordination necessary for oral feeding.

Multichannel pneumogram: Periods of obstructive apnea were noted during feeding and effort, such as crying. No apnea was noted during sleep and there was no evidence of central apnea. These findings and the results of the clinical feeding evaluation suggested that a restriction to airflow was developing during periods of increased activity. Cardiology evaluation was planned to rule out the presence of a tracheal ring.

Cardiac evaluation: An aortic vascular ring was found circling the trachea. With increased activity and blood vascular flow, it constricted the trachea and restricted airflow. Since the infant's primary work is during feeding, the effects were first noted at feeding times.

Treatment/management plan: Cardiac surgery was performed to revise the aorta. Feeding resumed slowly, though by three weeks after surgery, Alex was nippling all feedings.

Summary: While the clinical feeding evaluation could identify aspects of the problem, it took a number of tests and specialists to determine the underlying cause of the feeding problem. The CFEI was valuable in determining the timing and relationship of events during feeding, to help support the concept that respiration was impaired during feeding. As Alex was a full-term infant, respiratory causes other than those associated with prematurity were suspected. In this case, after surgery therapeutic feeding activities were not needed to return to oral feeding. In other cases, feeding problems may persist, and further evaluation and intervention may be necessary.

Case 3: Allen—Feeding-Related Apnea Model

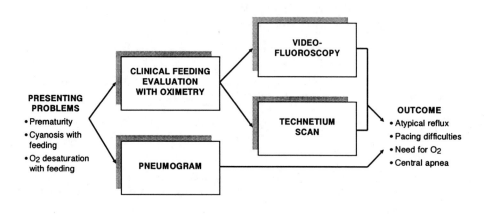

Figure 4-8 Case 3: Allen.

History: Allen (figure 4-8) was a 36-week premature infant born after a normal pregnancy, labor, and delivery. Apgar scores were 6 at one minute and 8 at five minutes. Dusky spells and oxygen desaturation were noted during early breast- and bottle-feedings. As these difficulties persisted, gavage feedings were begun. On day 6, feeding problems had not resolved and Allen was transferred to a tertiary-level pediatric hospital.

Presenting problem: Cyanosis and oxygen desaturation with feeding.

Evaluations and findings:

Clinical feeding evaluation with oximetry: Allen had a strong suck with adequate oral motor-control. Mild incoordination of sucking, swallowing, and breathing was noted with dysrhythmic respirations, gulping, and air swallowing. Mild oxygen desaturation was also noted during feeding. Strikingly, on two occasions as Allen's position was changed for burping, he became apneic, cyanotic, and bradycardic, requiring oxygen for recovery. As the most striking problems occurred with position change, GE reflux was suspected. The magnitude of the response, along with the difficulty coordinating sucking, swallowing, and breathing, also suggested the need for a VFSS.

Pneumogram: Though Allen was an "older" premature infant with less likelihood of ventilatory problems, his desaturations and feeding coordination problems led to a pneumogram. Central apnea and persistent oxygen desaturation were found.

VFSS: The oral phase was immature but adequate. The pharyngeal phase was normal. This VFSS was then modified to assess the esophageal phase. Poor esophageal motility was noted. Fluid pooled at the inlet of the stomach, and when Allen was repositioned to simulate the feeding experience, fluid quickly refluxed to the oropharynx. It appeared that poor esophageal motility was leading to an atypical type of reflux that occurred during feeding. With position changes, reflux triggered a vagally mediated response of apnea, bradycardia, and cyanosis.

Technetium scan: This was completed to assess the presence of more standard gastroesophageal (GE) reflux. It was negative for typical GE reflux and gastric emptying was normal.

Treatment/Management: Allen required theophylline for his central apnea, and supplemental oxygen was provided until it was clear that management of the central apnea would eliminate frequent oxygen desaturations. Since Allen's reflux was atypical and resulted in major compromise, special feeding and positioning techniques were developed. These are detailed in chapter 5, page 292.

Summary: In this case the timing of apnea and bradycardia during feeding was a key factor in expediently determining the cause of the feeding problems. This reinforces the importance of actually observing feeding and its problematic elements. Without such observation, Allen might have undergone many more tests and evaluations prior to determining the origin of the feeding problem. In addition, it points to the importance of trying to simulate actual feeding conditions, if possible, during evaluation procedures.

Case 4: Alyssa—Feeding-Related Apnea Model

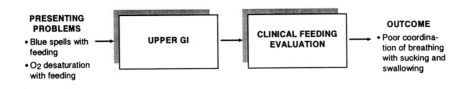

Figure 4-9 Case 4: Alyssa.

History: Alyssa (figure 4-9) was a term infant born after an uncomplicated pregnancy, labor, and delivery. She did well until 6 hours of life, when she was given a bottle of glucose water. She began coughing and sputtering and became cyanotic. Alyssa was fed again with oximetry at 12 hours of life. Coughing was again noted, with desaturation to 60% and a large emesis. A tracheal esophageal fistula was suspected.

Presenting problem: Coughing, cyanosis, and oxygen desaturation with feeding.

Evaluations and findings:

Barium swallow: A standard upper-GI study was performed. Anatomy of the pharynx and esophagus was found to be normal. Swallowing was also described as normal.

Clinical feeding evaluation with oximetry: As it was now unclear why this infant was experiencing feeding problems, a clinical feeding evaluation was requested to help assess the problem and determine the direction of further assessments. Sucking was strong and robust. Alyssa, however, demonstrated long periods of continuous sucking without evidence of respiration. The bottle was finally removed after she had completed 12 suck-swallow sequences without breathing. The same pattern was repeated several times. It was clear that Alyssa was having feeding-induced apnea due to her inability to coordinate breathing with sucking and swallowing. Although no desaturations were seen during this evaluation, allowing Alyssa to continue sucking and swallowing without breathing would have quickly led to desaturation.

Treatment/management plan: As determined during the clinical feeding evaluation, Alyssa responded well to the external pacing techniques described on page 253. Using these procedures, there was no further evidence of physiologic compromise during feeding.

Summary: This case illustrates that at times, even when the presenting feeding problem is significant physiologic compromise, the clinical feeding evaluation can determine the specific underlying problem and test the feasibility of treatment techniques.

Model 2: Feeding Problem Model

Key presenting problems: In this case the infant is unable to take food in the "normal" manner; either the baby cannot initiate feeding adequately early in life, or the baby feeds well for a time and then develops significant feeding problems or an inability to feed. In deciding to use this model, the problem is not only that the baby does not take an adequate quantity, but there will be something unusual about the way the baby feeds (for example, doesn't suck on the bottle, much loss of liquid, sucks on the bottle but gets no fluid, etc). This is not the baby who sucks well but only for a short time. If the feeding difficulties are not observed immediately in the newborn period, when the baby stops taking food there will be some sort of noticeable *change* in the way the baby feeds (for example, coughing, stridor, increased secretions, not sucking as well on the nipple).

Role of clinical feeding evaluation: The CFEI should again be carried out early in the problem-solving process, particularly if no medical diagnosis has been established, to allow careful observation of the feeding problems. Special attention should be paid to structural integrity, oral-motor control, and swallowing function. Respiratory control also should be monitored closely, because when there is no existing diagnosis with a component of respiratory compromise, this area may be overlooked when feeding problems arise.

Since many of the causes of this type of feeding problem have a neurologic basis, a careful neurologically based evaluation is appropriate. If the CFEI in any way suggests an unidentified neurologic basis for the feeding problems, the feeding specialist should not hesitate in making a referral for neurologic assessment. Failure to do this could lead to delays in making important medical diagnoses.

Often a medical diagnosis has been established prior to the CFEI (e.g., symptomatic Arnold-Chiari malformation in an infant with meningomyelocele, H-type tracheoesophageal fistula, cleft lip and palate, brainstem tumor, myopathy, etc). In this case the goal of the CFEI is primarily to help understand the specific nature of the feeding dysfunction and to assist with treatment planning.

Possible outcomes: Medical diagnoses that explain these feeding problems are often made. They may include myopathies, brain-stem tumors, unidentified clefts of the soft palate, cranial nerve damage, vocal-cord paralysis, or oral-motor control problems that turn out to be the first symptoms of cerebral palsy.

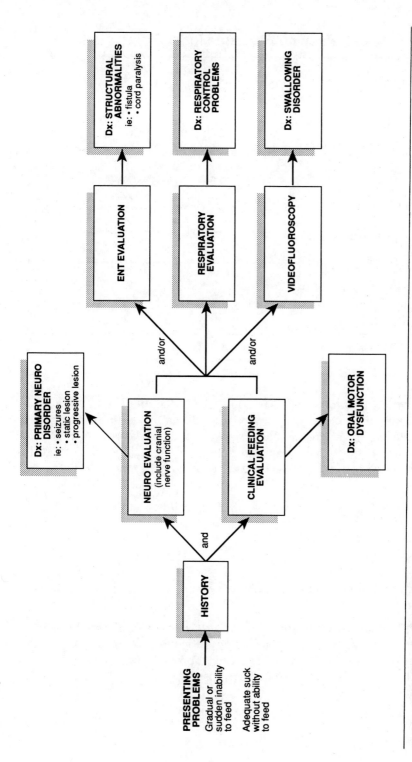

Figure 4-10 Feeding problem model.

Case 5: Mark—Feeding Problem Model

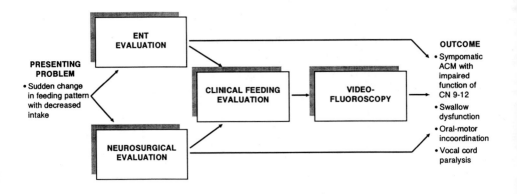

Figure 4-11 Case 5: Mark.

History: Mark (figure 4-11) was a full-term infant born with sacral-level meningomyelocele. This was repaired at 1 day of age. He then required shunting for hydrocephalus on day 6 of life. Mark was discharged home on day 11, feeding and gaining well. At 7 weeks of age he developed stridor and feeding difficulties, with markedly decreased intake.

Primary problem: This infant was feeding well but had a sudden change in feeding pattern and a reduction in intake.

Evaluations and findings:

Neurosurgical: An MRI was consistent with symptomatic Arnold-Chiari malformation and cervical compression. Surgical decompression was performed.

ENT: Bilateral vocal cord paralysis was noted prior to surgery and presumed to be a cause of feeding difficulties. Mark was kept NPO prior to surgery. While he showed improved vocal-cord movement after surgery, feeding problems persisted.

Clinical feeding evaluation: Poorly controlled tongue movements were observed, as well as minimal central grooving. Mark had difficulty initiating sucking, though facilitation techniques aided sucking. Intake was poor. Sucking and swallowing were poorly coordinated, with noisy breathing developing. This was suggestive of delayed or incomplete swallowing, so VFSS was recommended.

VFSS: Swallowing was markedly delayed and incomplete, with several small aspirations noted. This swallowing delay improved with chilled fluid but still placed Mark at high risk for aspiration.

Treatment/Management plan: Mark was made NPO to reduce the risk of aspiration. Nasogastric tube feed was instituted for primary nutrition. An oral-motor therapy program was begun to improve tongue movement and sucking. Small (5 to 10 cc) therapeutic oral feedings with chilled formula were allowed once per day to work on swallowing function and coordination of sucking, swallowing, and breathing.

Summary: Mark's feeding difficulties most likely reflect impairment of function in the lower cranial nerves, which can be produced by the Arnold-Chiari malformation. In this case the primary underlying cause was identified and managed by neurosurgeons. When feeding problems persisted, however, clinical feeding evaluation and subsequent VFSS could identify further impairments related to feeding and suggest therapeutic treatment techniques. It was hoped that with further recovery from the cervical decompression, with maturation, and with therapeutic activities these functions would improve. By 6 months of age, Mark had returned to full oral feedings.

Case 6: David—Feeding Problem Model

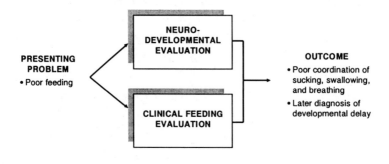

Figure 4-12 Case 6: David.

History: David (figure 4-12) was born at 37 weeks gestation after a normal pregnancy, labor, and delivery. Apgar scores were 8 at one and five minutes. He developed transient tachypnea of the newborn, requiring oxygen and observation. Oral feedings were delayed until 3 days of age and were slow to get started. David was discharged home on day 5. He was felt to be feeding adequately. At home, feeding was very frustrating for his mother. It appeared to her that David was often struggling to eat. Feedings took a long time and he fed frequently. Weight gain, however, was adequate. At 2 months of age, David was referred for a clinical feeding evaluation.

Presenting problem: By mother's report, David had never been able to feed in a normal manner.

Evaluations and findings:

Clinical feeding evaluation: Non-nutritive sucking was strong, and showed normal oral-motor control. David, however, demonstrated marked problems coordinating sucking, swallowing, and breathing. He had long sucking periods without adequate respiration (feeding-induced apnea). These were often terminated by coughing, choking, or gasping breaths. He became distressed with feeding, arching and pulling away. With persistence, he would finally take an appropriate volume of formula. External pacing techniques led to tremendous improvement in feeding.

Neurodevelopmental evaluation: David demonstrated emerging social responses, though with limited interest in his surroundings. He gave the impression of a cautious infant who was very slow to "warm up." The major motor concern was a strong extensor pattern of movement. The relationship of David's feeding problems to neurodevelopmental findings was unclear, though careful follow-up was planned.

Treatment/Management plan: External pacing techniques were used to improve the coordination of sucking, swallowing, and breathing. Proper positioning to minimize extensor movements was stressed. Feeding problems resolved. Neurodevelopmental follow-up was carried out.

Summary: The reason for David's feeding problems could be readily determined during the clinical feeding evaluation. Treatment techniques could be developed to minimize his problems in the coordination of sucking, swallowing, and breathing. Although two months of stress, arching, and irritability around feedings could certainly contribute to the findings of the neurodevelopmental evaluation, follow-up was warranted. At four months, feeding was progressing well, but there was increased evidence of neurodevelopmental dysfunction. David began regular outpatient developmental services and was later diagnosed with developmental delay. His feeding problems in the first months of life may have been an early reflection of these developmental problems.

Case 7: Lisa—Feeding Problem Model

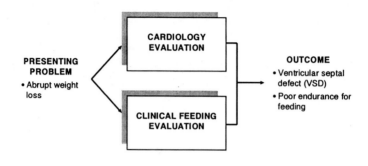

Figure 4-13 Case 7: Lisa.

History: Lisa (figure 4-13) was a full-term infant born following a normal pregnancy, labor, and delivery to a G_1 P_{1-2} healthy mother. She was discharged home at 2 days of age, breast-feeding and sleeping well. At 6 weeks she appeared to be feeding and gaining weight adequately. At 3 months, however, her weight gain had slowed dramatically and mother reported that she was now feeding poorly. Physical exam revealed mild respiratory distress and a slight heart murmur. Referrals were made for cardiology and feeding evaluation.

Evaluations and findings:

Clinical feeding evaluation: Lisa demonstrated normal oral-motor control and coordination of sucking, swallowing, and breathing. Sucking bursts, however, were punctuated by longer than average respiratory pauses. Sucking strength was average to weak, and Lisa stopped feeding after a short time, apparently due to fatigue. While interventions could have been developed to help increase intake, it was obvious that there was a specific problem compromising respiratory endurance and underlying the changes in Lisa's feeding performance. This needed to be identified before such interventions were attempted.

Cardiology evaluation: A ventricular septal defect (VSD) was identified, which was leading to congestive heart failure and inadequate energy for feeding.

Treatment/Management plan: The VSD was surgically repaired, and there was dramatic improvement in Lisa's feeding and weight gain. For some babies, however, feeding improvement might be more gradual following surgery. In these cases, the results of the clinical feeding evaluation would be important in maximizing oral feeding during this process.

Summary: Abrupt changes in feeding patterns often signify primary medical problems in a variety of systems. Clinical feeding evaluation should be well integrated with medical evaluations to insure proper medical attention to these problems.

Model 3:
Respiratory Compromise Model

Key presenting problems: Inadequate intake, coughing/choking with feeding, and color changes with feeding would be presenting problems in this model. Besides feeding difficulties, there is always a background of some sort of respiratory compromise, such as pneumonia, frequent upper-respiratory infections, bronchopulmonary dysplasia, infant respiratory distress syndrome, congenital heart disease, reactive airway disease, respiratory syncytial virus, or croup.

Role of clinical feeding evaluation: Because of the important interrelationship of respiration to infant feeding, when an infant with cardiorespiratory problems is not feeding well, evaluation often begins with the evaluation of respiratory function. If pneumonia or other acute respiratory illness is present, feeding will automatically be compromised and may explain the feeding problem. If oximetry or other pulmonary evaluation indicates the need for increased oxygen or adjustment of medication, the feeding problem may be easily resolved.

If the pulmonary evaluation does not point to a specific and treatable cause for the feeding problems, a CFEI is appropriate. The CFEI should focus in particular on the infant's respiratory support for feeding: RR, HR, O_2 saturation *with* feeding, and overall work of breathing. Indications of swallowing dysfunction or silent aspiration that could be causing or exacerbating respiratory problems should be noted. Babies with respiratory compromise may show poor coordination of sucking, swallowing, and breathing. Evaluation should focus on whether the suck/swallow/breathe incoordination results from increased respiratory rate, swallowing dysfunction, or poor central control of breathing/swallowing rhythms.

Evaluation of GE reflux may be indicated especially for babies with reactive airway disease, bronchopulmonary dysplasia, or swallowing dysfunction and aspiration. GE reflux is a potential cause or contributor to respiratory problems if aspiration of the ascending refluxed material occurs (see chapter 6).

Possible outcomes: The underlying cause of the problems in the respiratory compromise model may be silent aspiration, undetected or worsening heart disease, gastroesophageal reflux, or unrecognized swallowing dysfunction. Former premature babies with a history of lung disease may not be receiving adequate respiratory support (e.g., sufficient supplemental oxygen or medications) for the work of feeding.

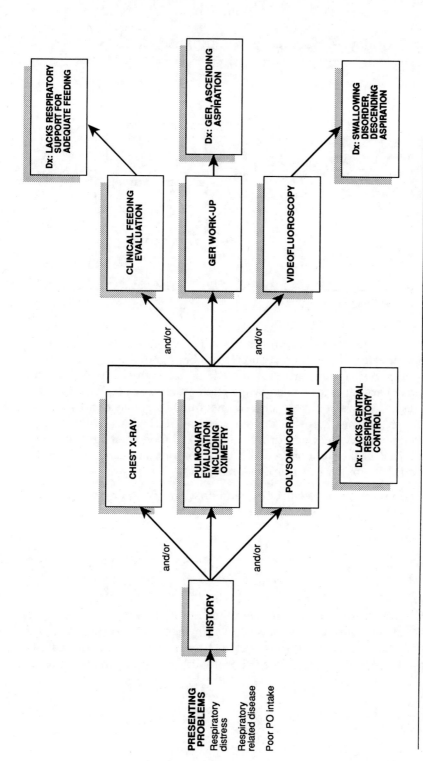

Figure 4-14 Respiratory compromise model.

Case 8: Jenny—Respiratory Compromise Model

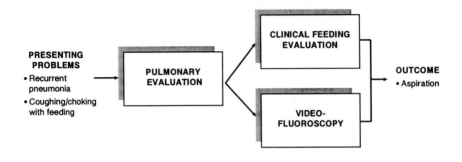

Figure 4-15 Case 8: Jenny.

History: Jenny (figure 4-15) was born in a small community hospital at 38 weeks gestation after an uncomplicated pregnancy, labor, and delivery. She developed pneumonia and respiratory complications in the newborn period, requiring antibiotics and supplemental oxygen. Feeding was marginal, with some gavage feedings required. Discharge home was at 11 days. Jenny developed pneumonia again at 2 and 4 months of age. Mother reported ongoing feeding difficulties, with frequent coughing and choking during feeding. At 5 months of age Jenny was referred to the pulmonary department of a tertiary-level hospital for evaluation of her recurrent pneumonia.

Presenting problem: Recurrent pneumonia and coughing and choking during feeding.

Evaluations and findings:

Pulmonary: Lung mechanics and pulmonary structures were adequate. Chest X-rays indicated chronic changes in the right upper lobe, consistent with aspiration. Jenny was referred for a CFEI and VFSS.

Clinical feeding evaluation: On the bottle, Jenny would suck vigorously for about a minute, pause to cough, then return to the bottle. This pattern was repeated throughout the feeding. She had already started receiving foods by spoon and showed little coughing on this texture.

VFSS: Jenny aspirated a small portion of every bolus during the swallow due to poor laryngeal elevation and closure. Coughing, in response to this aspiration, was inconsistent. During the study, several treatment techniques were tried to eliminate the aspiration. Strong forward neck flexion and thickened liquid seemed to be the most effective during the VFSS.

Treatment/Management plan: Jenny was fed using the techniques that appeared to eliminate aspiration during VFSS. Mother reported faster feeding times and minimal coughing, though some coughing persisted. Jenny once again developed pneumonia at $6\frac{1}{2}$ months of age, indicating that the feeding techniques were not adequately limiting aspiration. Tube feeding was then instituted, with very small therapeutic oral feedings allowed.

Summary: When an infant presents with recurrent pneumonia, with or without a history of coughing or choking during feeding, aspiration should be considered. Jenny coughed during feeding, but much of the aspiration was silent. In some cases, virtually all of the aspiration is silent. With a history of unexplained and recurrent pneumonia, a VFSS done in conjunction with a clinical feeding evaluation allows specific diagnosis of this problem. In this case, feeding modifications appeared to eliminate aspiration during the VFSS. This small sample, however, did not adequately reflect swallowing in all situations. Jenny's subsequent pneumonia indicated clinically significant aspiration was still present. Although it was not safe for her to continue as a fully oral feeder, in some cases feeding modifications are sufficient to control the problem.

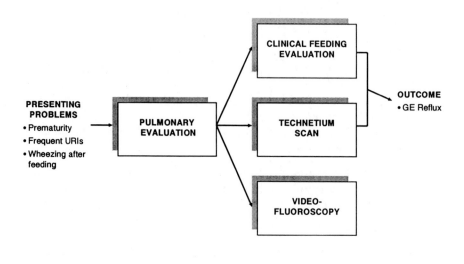

Figure 4-16 Case 9: Robert.

History: Robert (figure 4-16) was born prematurely, at 36 weeks gestation, following an otherwise uncomplicated pregnancy and delivery. The neonatal course was uneventful, though he required supplemental oxygen for three days. Bottle-feeding was introduced slowly and was well established prior to discharge at 3 weeks of age. Over the next three months, no specific feeding problems were noted, though Robert had frequent upper respiratory infections and sounded wheezy between feedings. He was admitted to the hospital for evaluation of his respiratory symptoms and suspected swallowing dysfunction.

Presenting problem: Recurrent respiratory illness and suspected swallowing dysfunction.

Evaluations and findings:

Pulmonary evaluation: This evaluation revealed normal oxygen saturations at rest and with feeding, though breath sounds were coarse. Chest X-ray findings showed changes in the right upper lobe that were suggestive of aspiration.

Clinical feeding evaluation: Oral-motor control and coordination of sucking, swallowing, and breathing were normal. Mother described behaviors at home that were indicative of GE reflux. Although these behaviors were not seen during the feeding evaluation, they were also reported by hospital nurses. No observations were made that suggested swallowing dysfunction. The history of recurrent respiratory infections and pulmonary changes, however, indicated the need for a complete swallowing evaluation.

VFSS: All phases of swallowing were normal. Reevaluation at the end of feeding did not reveal changes in performance with fatigue.

Technetium scan: Marked GE reflux was found, leading to the hypothesis that Robert was aspirating only in conjunction with episodes of GE reflux.

Treatment/Management plan: Strict treatment for GE reflux was instituted, including upright positioning, thickened feedings, and medication to reduce the stomach acidity (see page 340). Pulmonary status improved and recurrent respiratory illnesses ceased.

Summary: When aspiration is suspected based on compromised respiratory status, ascending as well as descending aspiration must be considered.

Case 10: Mary—Respiratory Compromise Model

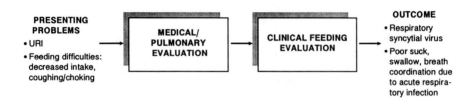

PRESENTING PROBLEMS	MEDICAL/ PULMONARY EVALUATION	CLINICAL FEEDING EVALUATION	OUTCOME
• URI • Feeding difficulties: decreased intake, coughing/choking			• Respiratory syncytial virus • Poor suck, swallow, breath coordination due to acute respiratory infection

Figure 4-17 Case 10: Mary.

History: Mary (figure 4-17) was a term infant, born without complications. At 6 weeks of age she was feeding and gaining well, without evidence of medical problems. She developed a runny nose at 2 months of age, which was felt to be a cold, since her older brother also had a cold. The runny nose persisted and Mary began coughing, sputtering, holding her breath, and gasping for air with feedings. This alarmed the parents, who brought her to the emergency room of a pediatric hospital.

Presenting problem: Coughing and choking during feeding, in association with symptoms of mild upper respiratory infection.

Evaluations and findings:

Medical/pulmonary evaluation: Physical examination revealed more significant respiratory distress, so oximetry, cultures of nasal secretions, and chest X-rays were ordered. Respiratory syncytial virus was diagnosed and appropriate medical treatment provided. Oral feeding was not allowed during the acute phase of the recovery process. As respiratory status improved, oral feeding was begun, and coughing, choking, and breathing difficulties were again noted. Clinical feeding evaluation was requested to evaluate for further feeding-related problems.

Clinical feeding evaluation: Mary had adequate oral-motor control and produced a strong suck. Respiratory rate was 65 to 70 BPM at rest, with some increased work of breathing indicated by intercostal retractions. Rhythm of sucking, swallowing, and breathing was erratic. There were some very short sucking bursts and some longer sucking bursts punctuated by individual breaths but ending with small gasps for air. Coughing was intermittent, generally occurred during sucking pauses, and was felt to be related to the presence of pulmonary secretions. It appeared that while Mary's pulmonary status had improved on X-ray and clinically, it had still not returned to baseline function and was therefore interfering with oral feeding.

Treatment/Management plan: The expectations for oral feeding were reduced, and Mary was offered small amounts of formula orally throughout the day. Feeding was terminated if increased work of breathing was noted, or if gasping for air was frequent. The balance was given by gavage tube, primarily at night. Within a week, as pulmonary recovery was more complete, Mary was fully nipple feeding with only occasional difficulty.

Summary: Despite clinical improvement after a major respiratory illness, recovery of feeding performances may proceed slowly. Even small residual pulmonary changes can compromise feeding in the infant.

Case 11: Emily—Respiratory Compromise Model

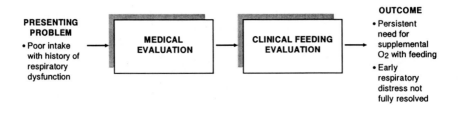

Figure 4-18 Case 11: Emily.

History: Emily (figure 4-18) was born at 34 weeks gestation to a mother who had been hospitalized for premature labor since 32 weeks gestation. Emily developed respiratory distress syndrome at birth and required intubation for 11 days and supplemental oxygen for three additional weeks. Nipple-feeding was introduced at 36 weeks gestation, with slow, steady increases in intake. By 38 weeks gestation, Emily had been weaned from her oxygen and had just begun to take all of her feedings orally when she was discharged home. She saw her pediatrician two weeks after discharge and had not gained weight since leaving the hospital. Mother reported that she often fell asleep before finishing her feeding and was often difficult to arouse for feeding.

Presenting problem: Poor intake in an infant with a history of respiratory dysfunction.

Evaluations and findings:

Medical evaluation: No concerning findings were noted on basic physical examination. Oximetry was within normal limits when briefly tested with the infant at rest.

Clinical feeding evaluation with oximetry: Despite normal readings at rest, the history suggested that oxygen saturations with work should also be assessed. Emily needed to be aroused prior to feeding, though sucking was strong and well coordinated with swallowing and breathing. Again, oximetry was normal prior to feeding. As the feeding progressed, however, Emily slowly became desaturated to the low 80s, and remained at that level until ceasing to suck.

Treatment/Management plan: Emily was given supplemental oxygen only during feedings. Intake and weight gain improved. Equipment was supplied so that Emily could receive oxygen at home. She was then slowly weaned over the next three weeks and showed no further feeding problems.

Summary: Even though the presenting problem might appear to be poor weight gain, if the infant has any history of respiratory problems, the respiratory compromise model should be used to evaluate feeding dysfunction. This case is an example of the differences in demand on the respiratory system and differences in oxygen saturation that may be observed between periods of relative inactivity and the work of feeding. When weaning from supplemental oxygen, some infants may be able to maintain oxygen saturations at rest but may have insufficient respiratory reserve for feeding. Evaluation of respiratory support needs to occur in both conditions.

Model 4: Poor Weight Gain Model

Key presenting problems: Poor weight gain for unknown reasons is the primary problem. Generally there is not an associated diagnosis. This infant may be labeled as failure to thrive (FTT), or may not completely fit the criteria and so would be considered "pre-FTT."

Role of clinical feeding evaluation: A nutritional assessment is key at the start of this model. It includes a food record, careful evaluation of growth parameters on an appropriate growth grid, and anthropometric measurements if possible. The nutritional assessment should determine if the child is (1) truly not gaining weight appropriately or (2) not getting adequate calories. If the child is getting adequate calories and not gaining weight, further medical workup for metabolic problems should be considered. If the child is not getting adequate calories, a CFEI can provide a basis for either problem identification or suggestions for further evaluation. The CFEI on this infant should focus on the psychosocial dynamics of the feeding situation while looking for evidence of oral-motor, neurologic, respiratory, and/or structural problems. In this model the CFEI plays a role similar to that in the feeding problem model. The CFEI will reveal oral-motor, swallowing, or coordination difficulties that may be at the root of the growth failure. In close conjunction with the CFEI, a full psychosocial evaluation by a social worker or psychologist is frequently warranted.

Possible outcomes: Metabolic problems, lack of parental knowledge or skill in infant feeding, oral-motor dysfunction, previously unrecognized developmental delay, swallowing dysfunction.

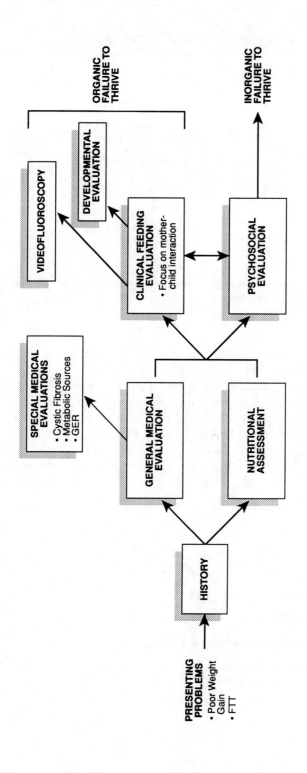

Figure 4-19 Poor weight gain model.

Case 12: Jonathan—Poor Weight Gain Model

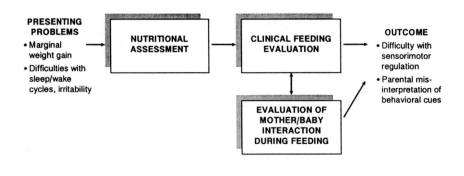

Figure 4-20 Case 12: Jonathan.

History: Jonathan (figure 4-20) was the first-born child of a professional couple who had tried for several years to conceive. He was born at 38 weeks gestation with birth weight at the 25th percentile. Jonathan was breast-fed, though latch-on was often difficult. Although he appeared eager to feed, unsuccessful attempts to latch-on led to frenzy and irritability. Mother would then give him a pacifier, and Jonathan would suck strongly and fall asleep. Weight gain was poor. Jonathan also startled easily, cried frequently, and was difficult to burp. Sleeping patterns were irregular, with Jonathan awake frequently at night.

Mother became increasingly frustrated with Jonathan's behavior and with her own inability to meet his needs. After daily contact with the family pediatrician and continued poor weight gain, at 4 months of age Jonathan was referred to the Growth and Development Clinic at a pediatric hospital.

Presenting problem: Poor weight gain

Evaluations and findings:

Medical evaluation: All tests were negative.

Nutritional assessment: Growth was at the 10th percentile, and intake was not adequate for growth.

Clinical feeding evaluation: Breast-feeding was characterized by frenzy on the part of the mother and infant. Jonathan arched, rooted excessively, and thrashed his arms about as he attempted to latch-on to the breast. Mother responded by walking and jiggling him until he latched-on. Walking and bouncing was continued throughout nursing, sometimes leading to Jonathan losing the nipple. The process would then begin again. When on the breast, Jonathan demonstrated normal sucking, with good coordination of swallowing and breathing.

Mother-baby interaction: Jonathan was a hyperalert infant who appeared to be easily disorganized by internal and external stimuli. Mother was particularly anxious and responded with a flurry of activity when Jonathan began to fuss. Although she would use appropriate calming strategies, they were used rapidly, without waiting long enough for the baby's response.

Treatment/Management plan: The basis of the feeding problem appeared to be in the interaction between an infant with difficulty in sensorimotor responsivity and regulation, and an anxious mother not able to read and respond appropriately to her infant's cues. A treatment plan was developed to delineate the most effective calming strategies for this baby during feeding and other times throughout the day. Mother was trained to read the baby's behavioral cues so she could assess his state and the effect of her actions on his ability to self-regulate. Support was also provided so that she had the stamina to deal with this difficult baby. The interaction improved, feeding became a more pleasurable experience for mother and infant, and Jonathan's weight slowly improved.

Summary: The impact of the mother-infant relationship on the feeding process should never be underestimated. While it appears dramatic in this case, at other times the effect can be more subtle, though equally important.

Case 13: Cassandra—Poor Weight Gain Model

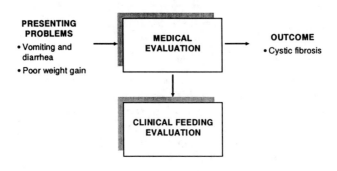

Figure 4-21 Case 13: Cassandra.

History: Cassandra (figure 4-21) was born at term without complications. Weight gain had been marginal despite mother's report of adequate breast-feeding. At 4 months of age she developed diarrhea, then vomiting and a dry cough. These symptoms resolved slowly over four weeks, though Cassandra showed no weight gain during this time. Her weight was now below the 5th percentile, and she was admitted to the hospital for evaluation of failure to thrive.

Presenting problem: Poor weight gain, though with associated medical complications of prolonged diarrhea and vomiting.

Evaluations and findings:

Nutritional assessment: Daily weights and pre- and post-breast-feeding weights revealed very inadequate intake.

Medical evaluation: A number of tests were ordered, including a sweat chloride test. This was positive, leading to a diagnosis of cystic fibrosis. Further tests found gastrointestinal malabsorption, a problem common in cystic fibrosis and a contributor to poor weight gain.

Clinical feeding evaluation: While the primary reasons for this infant's poor weight gain had been determined, clinical feeding evaluation was completed to help determine strategies to maximize oral intake. During breast-feeding, Cassandra latched-on well, demonstrated normal oral-motor control, and showed coordination of sucking, swallowing, and breathing. However, she did fatigue quickly.

Treatment/Management plan: Management included medication for a lung infection, enzymes to improve absorption, and methods to supplement nutritional intake. Supplemental bottles were attempted but refused. A feeding tube device to supplement breast-feeding (see chapter 8) was then utilized, with only a small improvement in oral intake. Nighttime continuous drip gavage feedings were necessary for adequate nutrition.

Summary: In this case, poor weight gain was secondary to a medical condition. The feeding specialist was able to develop strategies for supplementing nutrition while maintaining some level of oral feeding.

Case 14: Roger—Poor Weight Gain Model

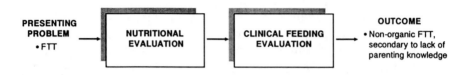

Figure 4-22 Case 14: Roger.

History: Roger (figure 4-22) was an otherwise healthy 3-month-old infant admitted to the hospital because of failure to thrive. Since birth his weight had steadily declined from the 50th percentile to the 5th percentile. He was the first child born to a 17-year-old mother with limited resources.

Presenting problem: Failure to thrive

Evaluations and findings:

Nutritional evaluation: Mother reported feeding Roger often, yet would not keep regular feeding records at home. It was hoped that in the hospital, intake could more accurately be assessed. During the first 24 hours in hospital, Roger took normal volumes, with a small weight gain noted the next day. He continued to feed well and showed nice weight gain over the next two days. It was clear that Robert could gain weight in the hospital. The reasons for poor weight gain at home were still not clear but pointed to some aspect of the home environment.

Clinical feeding evaluation: Robert had a strong, well-coordinated suck, and showed normal feeding for the nurses and feeding specialist. The nurses reported that he also took the bottle well for mother when she was present. During a feeding session with mother, Roger fed well and took an adequate amount. In discussing factors surrounding the feeding situation at home, however, it became clear that mother was often too "busy" with other things to hold Roger during feeding. She frequently propped his bottle. When asked how she knew he had enough, she reported that when he "pushed" the bottle over she was sure he was telling her that he was finished, though this usually happened two to three minutes into the feeding.

Treatment/Management plan: This infant clearly did not have a problem feeding. However, the mother had very inappropriate expectations about feeding and about her son's ability to communicate to her. Basic feeding techniques were carefully reviewed and social workers became actively involved in helping locate services for the mother to aid her in developing parenting skills. In-home follow-up by a public health nurse was provided.

Summary: In this case, the reason for the infant's failure to thrive seems painfully simple. To fully evaluate this problem it was first necessary to determine if the baby could gain weight. Hospitalization was required, since the mother was not able to keep accurate diet records at home. In addition, his feeding skills with health-care providers, in contrast to his skills with his mother, needed to be observed on a regular basis. As the mother felt more comfortable with and trusting of the medical staff, the true nature of the feeding problem was revealed and appropriate intervention begun.

Developing a Treatment/Management Plan

Without going through the process of determining the specific cause, or causes, for the feeding problem, any treatment or management program is likely to be ineffective. In some cases it may even be dangerous when it wastes time in identifying the actual problem and the baby has suffered a lack of nutrition, or when aspiration is present. Once the underlying cause for the feeding problem has been determined, and its interaction in the feeding process is understood, however, developing an effective treatment or management plan becomes a relatively straightforward process. This will be discussed in chapter 5.

5 Therapeutic Treatment Strategies for Infant Feeding Dysfunction

General Treatment Considerations

Developing and implementing a treatment or management plan for an infant's feeding dysfunction is the final step in the problem-solving process described in chapter 4. First the feeding problem is identified. Then the underlying reason for the feeding difficulty is determined based on the observations and interpretation of the CFEI (see chapter 3), as well as the results of related tests and procedures (see chapter 2), and/or other medical consultations. A **clear understanding** of the underlying cause or causes for the feeding problem should lead directly to selection of the most appropriate, and likely most effective, feeding plan. While at times a simple modification may solve the feeding problem, at other times a number of modifications or changes may be necessary to deal effectively with more complex feeding difficulties.

Any feeding plan developed for an infant must meet three criteria:

1. It must be safe. It should support and maintain the baby's health.

2. It should strive to maintain optimal nutrition.

3. It should be farsighted. The implications of the current treatment on future feeding and oral functions (such as speech) must be considered.

Although the infants discussed in this text have "feeding" problems, the clinician must not see the sole goal and benchmark of success as achieving full oral feeding. The feeding specialist and infant are successful if a plan is developed that meets the three criteria described above. Often this involves making decisions whereby all (or part of) the infant's nutrition is by non-oral means. For example, if an infant with chronic aspiration has not responded to conservative treatment, a feeding plan that provides nutrition by gastrostomy, along with non-nutritive oral-motor and oral-tactile stimulation, is far more successful than maintaining oral feedings that lead to chronic pneumonia and poor weight gain.

Treatment versus Management

A feeding plan may be composed of treatment strategies and/or management strategies. Utilizing treatment strategies suggests that the goal of the intervention is to improve a problem or condition underlying the feeding dysfunction. For example:

- A baby who is having apnea and bradycardia during feeding as a result of oxygen desaturation is treated with supplemental oxygen during feeding. This improves the underlying problem of oxygen desaturation.

- A baby who has an inefficient suck due to excessive jaw movement is treated with selected oral-motor techniques that provide external stabilization to the jaw. This reduces the amount of jaw movement and produces a more efficient suck.

Selecting a management strategy suggests that the underlying cause of the feeding problem cannot be modified by treatment techniques at this time. The symptomatology, however, must be addressed in order to maintain the infant's health and nutrition. In some cases this is a strategy used to "buy time" until the underlying problem changes through maturation or medical improvement. For example:

- An infant with aspiration during the swallow does not show improvement in respiratory symptoms despite strict use of techniques to improve the swallow. Therefore a gastrostomy is placed. The swallowing dysfunction was not improved satisfactorily to make the feeding safe, so the gastrostomy is used to manage the baby's nutrition and respiratory health.

- A baby with BPD, on oxygen by nasal canula, with good oral-motor skills, fatigues prior to taking the required feeding amount by nipple. Additional oxygen at feedings does not improve performance, so nasogastric feedings are used to provide the balance of the calories. As the factors underlying the fatigue could not be modified, supplemental nasogastric feedings are used to maintain adequate nutrition until the respiratory status improves and allows full oral feeding.

The use of management techniques does not preclude the use of treatment techniques. Often the overall feeding plan *must* include both management and treatment techniques to meet the third criterion listed above—planning for feeding and oral functions in the future. Particularly when non-oral feedings are needed, the feeding plan may include treatment techniques to maintain and improve oral-motor skill and/or tactile responses.

The options for treatment and management of infants with feeding problems fall into several categories. These include medical techniques (medications, changes in amount of supplemental oxygen, use of nasogastric tubes, etc.), surgical techniques (including repair of anatomical anomalies, placement of gastrostomies, etc.), and therapeutic techniques to modify the feeding situation. This chapter will focus on the latter category, discussing techniques that could modify state; posture and position; swallowing; oral-motor control; coordination of sucking, swallowing, and breathing; and tactile responses. The relationship of these therapeutic treatment techniques to other methods of treating and managing feeding will also be addressed.

It is anticipated that the techniques presented here would be used by occupational therapists, speech therapists, physical therapists, and/or nurse specialists, all of whom should have training and experience with infant feeding problems. While these care providers would be responsible for determining appropriate techniques, then initiating and monitoring their use, often the therapeutic treatment techniques will be carried out by other caregivers, particularly parents. Information on maximizing the effectiveness of transferring these techniques to a variety of caregivers is included.

Preparation for Treatment

Many of the techniques discussed in this chapter will be used as specific treatments at the time of an infant's feeding. These techniques often target components of the suck/swallow/breathe triad. Limiting treatment considerations to these techniques, however, is to limit the potential effectiveness of the treatment. In infant feeding there is an interplay among physical, psychosocial, behavioral, and physiologic factors. For successful feeding the "whole baby" must be considered within the context of the feeding milieu, which encompasses the feeder and the feeding environment.

Although these multiple factors must be considered during the actual feeding session, for maximal effectiveness a therapeutic feeding program will also address aspects of the baby, or elements of the feeding milieu, which need modification to support the ultimate feeding goals but require preparation prior to initiating feeding.

Preparing the Infant
Activities to "prepare" an infant for feeding may occur in a number of areas including state, overall tone and movement, and tactile responses. Specific treatment strategies addressing each of these areas are included in this

---

chapter. While a small number of researchers have addressed the effect of such preparations on feeding in premature infants,[1,2] the results are not definitive and do not indicate how an individual infant will respond to this component of the treatment plan. Therefore, the feeding specialist must carefully consider each infant's particular need for such preparations and make a conscious decision to include or exclude them when developing a feeding plan.

If it is determined that an infant will benefit from preparation in any of the areas listed above, the complexity of the activities and the amount of time spent should be matched to the ability and time constraints of the feeder. The feeding specialist might provide a fairly complex preparation but suggest a less complex procedure for a busy nurse. At the same time the therapist might teach a very invested mother a number of preparation techniques, particularly if they make a significant change in the quality or quantity of feeding. A mismatch between treatment activities and the feeder's skills or needs will result in the program being carried out incorrectly or not at all.

Preparing the Environment

The characteristics of the environment should support the optimal feeding state, take into account the infant's ability to cope with stimuli in the environment, and allow the therapist to make necessary observations during feeding. Factors to consider include visual stimuli and light, noise, and temperature.

Visual stimuli: The amount and type of visual stimuli can affect a baby's state and feeding. A well-lit room may assist in arousal of a sleepy baby by increasing the visual stimuli. A dimly lit or darkened room may be needed to maintain a calm state in a hypersensitive baby. As babies mature and their visual field expands, some babies may have a harder time remaining focused on feeding should the environment be visually stimulating. On the other hand, visual stimuli that focus a baby's attention away from the feeding process may decrease oral hypersensitive responses. Some babies may be more willing to feed when provided with visual entertainment or distraction.

Noise: The amount and level of noise in the room can influence a baby's state control and thus feeding behavior. In an effort to deal with constant noise a baby may tune out stimuli and therefore be unavailable for feeding or interaction. Frequent startling to loud noises is very disruptive to smooth feeding. Once the baby is home from the hospital, the loud and often unpredictable noises of siblings can be a disorganizing factor.

When treating babies with disorders in the suck/swallow/breathe triad it is essential to be able to hear the baby's swallows and breaths in order to monitor the effectiveness of treatment or make changes as needed. Thus, an environment with minimal ambient noise should be selected.

Temperature: In general, warm temperatures are more relaxing and induce calmness or sleep, while cooler temperatures are more alerting. Any temperature, however, that is outside of the infant's comfort zone in either direction may distract from the feeding. Temperature can be manipulated by changing the air temperature or adjusting the amount of clothing or blankets. Caution is indicated in manipulating the temperature for very small babies, as discussed on page 213.

Preparing the Feeder

The person feeding an infant communicates to that infant throughout the feeding session by the way he or she handles and moves the baby, looks at the baby, talks to the baby, and responds to the baby's behaviors. If a clinician is rushed and frazzled, this is communicated to the infant and may add to the infant's disorganization. If a parent lacks confidence in his or her ability to feed successfully, the baby may not be given clear handling to guide the feeding.

Often treatment can be improved by first preparing oneself for feeding an infant. This might include taking a minute prior to approaching the baby to clear away distracting thoughts, use simple relaxation techniques to reduce stress, and prepare to focus entirely on the baby. It may be helpful to develop a mind-set for treatment, reviewing the goals for the feeding and the techniques that will be used. Visualizing the baby as being successful in the feeding may also be helpful. This preparation helps the feeder to lead the infant through the feeding—not in a rigid way, but flexibly responding to communication from the infant to take it in the direction established as the goal for that feeding.

State

For successful feeding, the infant must be in an optimal state of alertness or receptivity. Of the six levels of state proposed by Brazelton (see page 94),[3] feeding is possible in the drowsy/semi-dozing, quiet alert, and active alert states. For a particular baby, however, there may be one state that is best for feeding. The feeding specialist must determine whether state is a critical factor in successful feeding for an infant, and which state provides optimal results. For example, a hypersensitive, easily disorganized baby may show better feeding behaviors in a drowsy state than when active and alert. A very sleepy baby may show adequate intake only when a very alert state is maintained throughout most of the feeding.

During a feeding session, the baby must first be brought to the optimal state; then that state must be maintained throughout the feeding. To bring the baby into the desired state, it may be necessary to use a wide variety of techniques and to use them frequently. Using fewer and lower-amplitude techniques generally will maintain the state the therapist has chosen.

When selecting techniques, keep in mind that each infant will respond differently to a particular technique. The feeding specialist must match the methods that are chosen for modifying state to the individual infant. In addition, each caregiver will implement the same technique slightly differently, potentially eliciting a different response from the baby. Therefore it is often necessary for different caregivers to try a number of techniques to determine which will achieve the desired result.

The baby's pattern of states, transition between states, and stability of state may also be an indication that something in the environment is stressful. Before working to modify the infant's state the feeding specialist must determine whether any such stressors are present and, if so, attempt to eliminate or modify them. For example, an infant may be difficult to arouse. This infant may appear to be sleeping but is actually using sleep to "tune out" the stressors of excessive light and noise. Reducing the light and noise may produce a more optimal state for feeding.

State is also related to the infant's neurologic and medical status. Infants with neurologic damage or pain from medical conditions may show patterns of state that are not compatible with feeding but are beyond the realm of the clinician to modify successfully with the techniques covered below.

Arousal

These techniques are designed to bring the infant from a sleepy or semi-drowsy state to a calm, alert state. In this state, the baby's eyes are open and attentive; the face is calm and the movement is smooth and well modulated. Most arousal techniques are applied with variability, are not predictable, and may not be rhythmic.

Treatment Techniques
Movement: Vestibular or movement stimulation can have a strong alerting effect. Just picking up a baby can sometimes cause the baby to open the eyes and begin to awaken. Being in an upright position may increase alertness in neonates.

- Movement stimulation can occur in any direction: sideways, up/down, or in an anterior/posterior direction.

- Movement should be unpredictable or with uneven rhythms to encourage alerting.

- Gentle, firm bouncing in an up-and-down direction while firmly supporting the head can cause arousal, as well as have an organizing effect.
- Rocking the baby from side to side or in a rotary direction while supporting the head may help arouse the baby.

Auditory: The pitch and animation of the voice may be useful in encouraging alerting.

- Vary the pitch, tone, and rhythm when talking to the baby.
- Progressing from a quiet, monotone voice to a louder, enthusiastic voice can stimulate alerting.
- Lively music may improve arousal.

Tactile: Touch, particularly light touch, can have an alerting effect on a baby. When tactile stimulation is combined with movement stimulation the effects of both modalities may be enhanced.

- Tickling or stroking the palms or soles of the feet can bring a baby to, or maintain, an alert state.
- Stroking the baby's head or putting a cool washcloth on the face can wake a sleepy baby.
- Cooler temperatures can help alert a baby. A baby who is too warm and snug may want to stay asleep rather than wake up to eat. Changing the baby's clothes or diaper, or unbundling the baby, can be helpful.

  Care must be taken, however, not to expose small, sick babies to hypothermia. Many babies receiving intervention for feeding disorders are still in isolettes and therefore have difficulty maintaining their own body temperature. While some change in temperature may assist the eating process, making the baby cold can result in using more energy keeping warm than is gained during eating or can lead to other physiologic changes such as bradycardia. Caution, therefore, must be exercised when using temperature change as an arousal technique.

Calming

Calming techniques are used to bring an irritable, crying, hyperstimulated, disorganized, or easily startled baby to a well-modulated, calm alert state. Usually these techniques involve limiting or toning down the amount of stimuli impinging on the baby. Containment and rhythmicity are key components of calming techniques. It is important to begin by applying only one stimulus at a time. Combining stimuli may result in overstimulation and/or tuning out.

Treatment Techniques

Tactile: Firm, deep pressure and containment are the elements of tactile input that produce calming effects.

- Swaddling (figure 5-1) is an extremely useful calming technique. Not only does swaddling provide physical containment to a baby whose movement may be tonic, disorganized, or frequent, but the firm proprioceptive and deep pressure contact provided by the blankets may provide a calming, integrating force. A baby who responds to environmental sounds through frequent Moro reflexes or who has intermittent flailing extensor thrusts will benefit from swaddling. When swaddled, the arms should be together in the midline and the hips flexed. The head can be covered by the blankets for additional containment if needed.

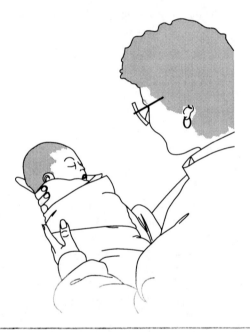

Figure 5-1 Swaddling provides proprioceptive and deep pressure contact, in addition to physical containment, to promote calming.

- Swaddling the baby with a small roll beneath the feet for the baby to grab with the toes may provide an additional point of centering and calming.

- Holding the baby in a well-flexed, somewhat vertical position can decrease a tendency toward excessive extension that may be present in a disorganized baby.

- Therapists need to use their own body language to convey a sense of stability and calmness. By posture and firmness of holding, the therapist should tell the baby, "It is all right, you can calm yourself down, I will help you do it."

- Infant massage prior to a feeding session may also be a useful tool to calm the disorganized baby.[5,45]

Movement: When provided in a rhythmic manner, vestibular stimulation has been shown to have a calming effect. The movement stimulation should be constant and predictable. Some babies will calm to fast, rhythmic movement, whereas others calm better to slow, rhythmic movement.

- In a swaddled position, strong, rhythmic vertical bouncing or rocking can be used to calm a baby.

- The therapist often needs to be standing to provide the most effective movement stimulation for calming. Rocking, bouncing, or jiggling are perceived by the baby differently when the caregiver is sitting as compared to the same stimuli being applied when standing.

Auditory: Decreasing the auditory input to a baby while feeding can assist in calming. Auditory input can be distracting and thereby disorienting to some infants.

- Some babies will feed better if they are not spoken to while feeding.

- Using "white noise" may block out extraneous, unpredictable noises and allow the baby to maintain an even state.

- Rhythmic, repetitive music may also provide a calming influence.[4]

Tone, Posture, and Position

The quality of muscle tone throughout the body and the resulting posture of the infant are interrelated with the baby's state, physiologic control, and oral-motor control during feeding. Optimally, each of these parameters supports the others in the feeding process. Conversely, deviations in any one of these areas can negatively impact the other parameters, further compromising the feeding. For example, a hypertonic baby may have rigid posture and poorly graded movement, which make relaxation and maintenance of quiet states difficult. The infant, therefore, is unable to maintain an appropriate state for feeding. Or an infant with bronchopulmonary dysplasia may show resting and active postures with excessive neck extension as a result of prolonged intubation for ventilation. When this baby is finally able to feed orally, neck hyperextension contributes to inefficient tongue movement and excessive jaw movement, limiting oral intake.

Although there is wide variation in "normal" postural muscle tone that will support feeding, there should be a balance of function between flexor and extensor muscle groups, movements should be smooth and well modulated, and there should be an appropriate amount of movement. An infant's muscle tone can also influence the feeding position, where alignment of the head, neck, and trunk are crucial components. Characteristics of the optimal feeding position (see figure 5-2a) include:

- An overall feeling of flexion
- Orientation of the head and extremities about the body midline
- Shoulders symmetric and forward with the arms flexed and toward the body midline. (Infants below two months of age may normally demonstrate some shoulder elevation, though older infants should maintain a neutral shoulder position with an elongated neck.)
- Hips flexed from 45° to 90°
- Neutral anterior-posterior alignment of the head and neck, though slight flexion or extension may have therapeutic benefit in some cases

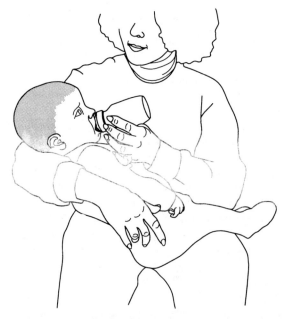

Figure 5-2a The optimal feeding position emphasizes flexion, midline orientation, and neutral alignment of head and neck.

The alignment of the head and neck to the trunk is a key component of the feeding position. While slight modifications may prove therapeutic for an infant, improper alignment may be a major contributor to feeding dysfunction (see figure 5-2b, c).

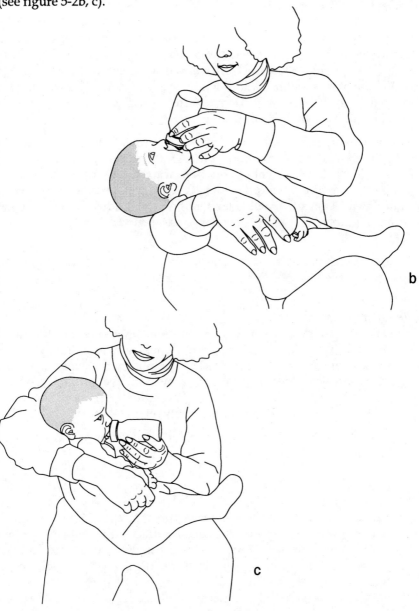

Figure 5-2b, 5-2c Without attention to the head and neck alignment, excessive extension (b) or flexion (c) can result.

Excessive head and neck extension is generally counterproductive to efficient feeding. When the head is in a hyperextended position, the ability of the larynx to elevate and seal off the airway is impaired. Not only is movement of the larynx difficult in this position, but the larynx must travel further to close off the airway during a swallow. If laryngeal closure is then insufficient, penetration or aspiration may result. Excessive neck extension during feeding may also cause the bolus of liquid to move back in the mouth too quickly, before the baby has had sufficient time to organize the oral phase of swallowing. Additionally, marked neck extension may lead to tongue protrusion or retraction patterns, as well as excessive jaw movement, resulting in inefficient sucking.

Similarly, excessive neck flexion may be dangerous during feeding. Bosma suggests that stable maintenance of the pharyngeal airway in infants is related to the development of craniocervical postural control.[6] The very small or premature infant may not yet have developed the craniocervical control to assist in adequately maintaining a stable airway. The infant then becomes vulnerable to airway collapse and apnea due to excessive neck flexion.[7]

Treatment techniques are available to the clinician to modify tone and posture, as well as position, to help increase the effectiveness of oral feeding.

Treatment Techniques

Movement activities: When abnormal muscle tone is present throughout the body, providing handling or movement activities that modify the muscle tone prior to feeding is a key component of the neurodevelopmental treatment techniques utilized by many therapists. It is beyond the scope of this text to describe the multiple strategies that have been proposed to achieve this goal, but many references are available.[1,4,8-12]

In selecting this approach as a treatment component for infant feeding dysfunction, several factors must be considered. Although these techniques were developed to manage tonal problems related to central nervous system disturbances, in infants with feeding problems, tonal variations may stem from other sources. In particular, stress from medical conditions and/or environmental stimuli impinging on the immature nervous system may be communicated as abnormal patterns of tone and movement. As long as the underlying stressor remains present, handling techniques may have little impact on modifying the tone or posture. On the other hand, if the deviant motor patterns developed originally in response to stress have become "habits of movement" for the infant, and the stressors are no longer present, handling techniques to modify the tone and movement patterns may be useful.

The decision to include handling activities in preparation for feeding must be a carefully considered treatment decision. It will depend on the degree of muscle tone abnormality, as well as its hypothesized source. Most importantly, however, it will depend on its contribution to the infant's feeding problems. If preparatory handling activities are not considered because they are not a treatment to the mouth and thus not felt to be "feeding related," or because of time limitations, achievement of maximal change in feeding function may be sacrificed. On the other hand, our experience suggests that in practice only a small percentage of very young infants with feeding dysfunction have the type of tonal problems that require preparatory handling. For the majority of babies, appropriate motoric support through correct positioning during feeding is adequate.

Feeding positions: A wide variety of positions may be used in feeding the infant. The positions described below are a representative sample, though not inclusive. The positive and negative characteristics of the positions are described to aid in selecting an appropriate position, not just a convenient position. It is hoped that when any position is selected, careful consideration is given to the particular characteristics that position brings to the feeding session.

- **Standard** (figure 5-3): This position is comfortable for most feeders. It can allow a very upright position. The degree of trunk flexion can vary, though it is easy to allow excessive trunk and neck flexion. Some feeders may find it difficult to control neck extension adequately.

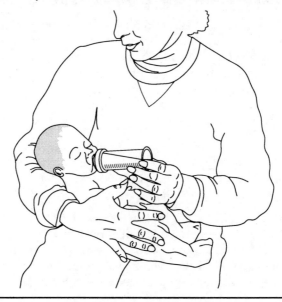

Figure 5-3 The standard cradled position for feeding an infant.

- **En face** (figure 5-4): In this position, maximal control of the head is possible. It is difficult, however, to provide adequate trunk support for a more upright position, unless the baby is quite small.

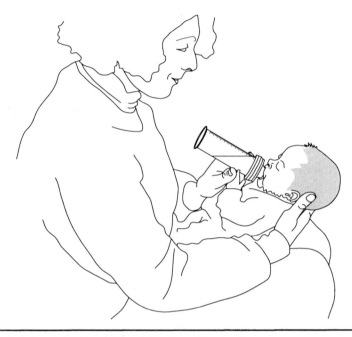

Figure 5-4 The infant is positioned "en face" for feeding.

- **Supine in lap** (figure 5-5): When the baby is in this position, the feeder has both hands free, but it may be difficult to control side-to-side head movement. The trunk is straight and well supported, and the head is in a neutral anterior-posterior position. The feeder must be careful to keep the head from extending over the knees. It is a good position for tube feeding as the feeder's hands are free to hold a pacifier for non-nutritive sucking while giving the tube feeding.

- Sidelying on lap (figure 5-6): In this position, the trunk is straight and well supported. This may help a retracted tongue come forward. The feeder must be observant so that the head does not move into excess extension.

- **Bringing head into greater flexion:** This positional adjustment may be used in conjunction with most of the basic positions. It may facilitate sucking and lip seal. Swallowing dysfunction secondary to poor laryngeal elevation may be improved as laryngeal movement, closure, and airway protection are enhanced.

- **Bringing head into slight extension:** This positional adjustment may also be used in conjunction with most of the basic positions. It may assist breathing for babies with respiratory problems by increasing the diameter of the pharyngeal airway (see chapter 1).

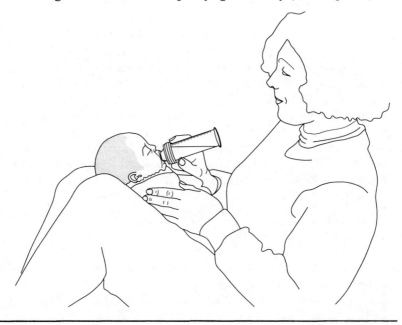

Figure 5-5 The baby is fed while inclined on the lap.

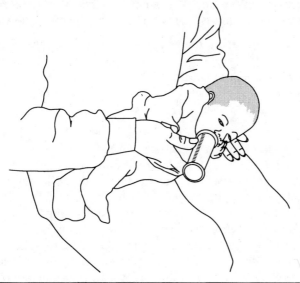

Figure 5-6 An infant is fed in sidelying.

Swallowing

Disorders in swallowing function are being diagnosed more frequently in infants. Swallowing disorders can result from poor organization of the bolus in the oral phase, delay in initiation of the swallow reflex, abnormalities in pharyngeal protective mechanisms, or incoordination of pharyngeal or esophageal peristalsis. While clinical evaluation may suggest swallowing dysfunction, the most accurate method of diagnosing a swallowing disorder is the videofluoroscopic swallowing study (VFSS) (see chapter 2). Only with a VFSS can the specific type of swallowing disorder (or combination of disorders) be clearly identified. As treatment varies for each swallowing disorder described below, accurate diagnosis of the mechanism of swallowing dysfunction is crucial to successful treatment. Caution and close medical supervision are also advised when treating swallowing dysfunction, since aspiration (possibly leading to respiratory compromise) is a frequent consequence of swallowing disorders.

Delayed Swallow Reflex

The swallowing reflex is generally initiated when the bolus reaches the area of the faucial arches. In infants, there may be some very brief pooling in the vallecular space, but generally the swallow is triggered before significant pooling occurs. When swallowing is dysfunctional, the amount of delay in initiating the swallowing reflex can vary from a fraction of a second to greater than 10 seconds.[13] When marked delay is present, material may reach and pool in the pyriform sinuses prior to the initiation of swallowing.

The longer the delay in triggering the swallowing reflex, and the farther the bolus travels down into the pharynx, the greater the risk of aspirating all or part of the bolus before the swallow. When a swallow has not been triggered, the airway remains open, increasing the risk that material in the vallecular or pyriform sinus may spill over into the open airway.

Treatment Techniques

Thermal stimulation with oral feeding: One method to decrease the delay in swallowing reflex is through thermal stimulation. Logemann has described a procedure of thermal sensitization with adults whereby ice-cold stimulation is applied to the faucial arches by rubbing them with a chilled 00 laryngeal mirror.[14] Immediately following this stimulation, the swallowing reflex was triggered more quickly. As this method of stimulating the faucial arches would be impossible with infants or young children, an alternative method is to provide cold stimulation by feeding refrigerator-chilled formula or semisolids.

The use of refrigerator-chilled liquids and foods advances the procedure of Logemann one step further. The effectiveness of the thermal sensitization seemed to diminish over subsequent swallows and was most effective in swallows just after the thermal stimulation.[15] By using chilled foods, the thermal sensitization is ongoing and therefore can more effectively improve the speed of the swallowing reflex.

In our experience, dramatic improvement has been noted using this technique. A number of infants with aspiration resulting from marked delays in the pharyngeal swallow have been fed chilled formula without further evidence of aspiration, clinically or radiographically. Most young babies will take chilled formula without complaint, though older babies (6 months or older) may refuse bottles at temperatures that they are not accustomed to. Gradually introducing chilled formula may be useful, if it is safe for the infant to make a slow transition. Chilled semisolids are generally introduced without difficulty.

Case example:
Cassie was a full-term infant born with meningomyelocele, which was repaired immediately. She required shunting for hydrocephalus at 6 days of age. She recovered without problem and was discharged to her home.

At 7 weeks of age, breathing became stridorous and feeding difficulties arose. Evaluation revealed a functional shunt, but slight vocal-cord paralysis associated with symptomatic Arnold-Chiari malformation was observed. Neurosurgery elected to observe her course and did not pursue surgical management.

While her stridor resolved, feeding problems persisted, with inadequate intake. Evaluation suggested the presence of swallowing dysfunction, as her breathing became noisy and wet-sounding during feeding. VFSS revealed delay in swallowing of up to 30 seconds. Formula pooled throughout the pharynx during this time, leading to the risk of aspiration. Under the fluoroscope, she was given ice-cold barium. Swallowing was markedly improved with only slight hesitation noted in the triggering of her swallow. Cassie was then fed refrigerator-chilled formula. Intake improved; there was no longer clinical evidence of a delay in swallowing and no evidence of aspiration.

Thermal stimulation during non-nutritive sucking: In a baby who is non-orally fed, the speed of the swallowing reflex may be improved by having the baby suck on a frozen pacifier. Many pacifiers are hollow. This space can be filled with water, frozen, then given to the baby to suck on. Hypothetically, the frozen pacifier will chill the baby's secretions, providing thermal sensitization to the swallow. Since the ice within the pacifier tends to melt quickly from the warmth of the baby's mouth, several frozen pacifiers may be needed for a treatment session.

Improve bolus formation in the oral phase: In the oral preparatory phase of swallowing, the role of the tongue is to form the bolus and hold it in the mouth prior to the initiation of the swallow. If there are problems with tongue control, the bolus may spill over the posterior portion of the tongue in a piecemeal fashion that does not trigger the swallow in a timely manner. If swallowing delay is caused by this mechanism, treatment must focus on improving oral preparation of the bolus. Three methods might be considered.

- **Provide single boluses:** This can be accomplished by giving a single suck from a bottle then pausing to allow organization of the swallow. Having the baby suck on an open nipple and dripping small amounts of fluid slowly into the nipple is one way to provide single boluses. Another option is to have the baby suck on a pacifier, then place a single bolus in the corner of the mouth with a soft eyedropper. In each case it is necessary to establish sucking to assist in producing the tongue movements needed to move the bolus to the back of the mouth in a cohesive manner. Single boluses should be 0.1 to 0.5 cc in size.

- **Provide small boluses:** Reducing the bolus size when giving single or multiple nutritive sucks will facilitate organization of the bolus prior to the swallow. To control the bolus size, a soft dropper may be used for single nutritive sucks, as described above, or a "pacifier trainer" may be used (figure 5-7). In this method a 5 fr. gavage feeding tube is attached to a 20 cc feeding syringe. The liquid is drawn up through the tube into the syringe to create a closed system. The feeding tube is then taped to the baby's pacifier of choice. Alternately, the tube can be inserted into the corner of the baby's mouth while the pacifier is in the mouth. Due to the small size of the feeding tube, babies generally do not notice the tube and will continue sucking. As the baby sucks, very small boluses of liquid are squeezed through the syringe into the baby's mouth at a rate appropriate for the infant. Pacifiers should not be modified so that liquid fills the bulb portion and is then sucked out. The feeding specialist is not able to adequately control the flow of liquid out of the pacifier, and in this configuration the bulb of the pacifier cannot be thoroughly cleaned and dried, potentially allowing bacterial growth.

- **Thicken the liquid:** Thickening the baby's milk slightly with dry baby cereal or commercial thickeners allows the liquid to form a more cohesive mass. It may move more slowly during the oral preparation phase and is easier for the tongue to maintain as a single bolus prior to triggering the swallow. Using one tablespoon of baby rice cereal to two ounces of liquid often provides adequate thickening.

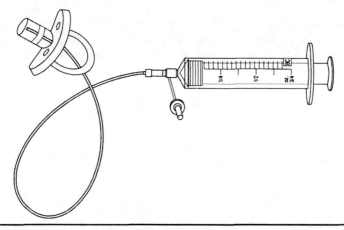

Figure 5-7 The "pacifier trainer," fabricated from a pacifier and small feeding tube allows the infant to receive very small, controlled boluses of fluid during sucking.

Aspiration during the Swallow

Aspiration during the swallow is usually caused by reduced or insufficient laryngeal elevation and closure; part of the bolus seeps under the epiglottis and into the airway prior to sufficient closure of the larynx.

Treatment Techniques
Treatments for aspiration during the swallow are aimed at improving laryngeal elevation and changing the viscosity of the bolus so that it is less likely to seep into the supraglottic space.

Improving laryngeal closure: Strong forward head flexion or chin tucking changes the relative position of the larynx so that less elevation is needed for complete closure. Flexing the head forward, the hyoid and larynx move slightly upward. From this "pre-elevated" position, the distance the larynx needs to travel may be shortened. The larynx may then be better able to move fast enough to close the airway.[14] Forward head flexion can be accomplished by using the feeder's arm or chest to support the infant's head in the appropriate position. Using an angled-neck bottle such as the Corecto® (Corecto Products Company, P.O. Box 1014, Atlanta, GA 30301) or Degree® bottle (Degree Baby Products, 20426 Corisco Street, Chatsworth, CA 91311-6121) can assist in maintaining adequate neck flexion (see figure 5-8, page 226).

Normally the position of the larynx changes, becoming lower, at 5 to 6 months of age. Infants who demonstrate problems with laryngeal elevation should be reassessed carefully at this time. They may have more difficulty with laryngeal elevation due to the increased distance the larynx needs to travel, and previously effective treatment techniques may no longer be effective. Since maintaining forward head flexion is difficult during cup drinking, careful reassessment of this type of swallowing dysfunction is indicated prior to initiating cup drinking. A cut-out cup or straw can assist in maintaining neck flexion when transitioning away from the bottle.

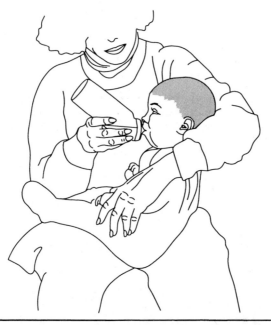

Figure 5-8 Using an angled-neck bottle allows the infant's neck to be strongly flexed during feeding.

Thickening feedings: Thickening the baby's food may create a more cohesive bolus that does not seep under the epiglottis and enter the larynx during the swallow. In addition, a thickened bolus may move through the pharynx more slowly, so there is more time for adequate laryngeal elevation to occur. While minimal thickening may help (one tablespoon rice cereal to two ounces formula), more marked thickening may be necessary. When any additives are suggested for a young baby's formula, medical and nutritional consultation is imperative so that caloric needs, fluid needs, and nutritional needs are met.

Strained baby food may also be an appropriate consistency. Even if changes in head position or viscosity of the fluid do not make it safe to swallow liquids, a baby may be able to safely swallow pureed foods. If developmentally appropriate, allow the infant to take semisolids by spoon, but utilize non-oral feeding methods for liquids (see page 266).

Aspiration after the Swallow

Aspiration after the swallow is usually secondary to residual liquids or solids remaining in the pharynx following the completion of the swallow. This material is then inhaled or aspirated into the airway. The residue may result from decreased pharyngeal peristalsis, dysfunction of the cricopharyngeas muscle, or inadequate generation and maintenance of pressure gradients to propel the bolus through the pharynx.[14] Infants with residue following the swallow often present with extremely noisy, wet-sounding breathing that is worse following feeding. They are literally breathing through the material in their hypopharynx, whether this be formula or their own secretions.

Treatment Techniques

Modify food consistency. Treatment of aspiration after the swallow is extremely difficult. For some babies, pharyngeal peristalsis may be better on one texture than another, so the residue left after the swallow may be less. For example, an infant may have less residue with thin liquids than with thickened liquids or foods, as it may be easier for the pharyngeal muscles to propel the thin liquids through the pharynx. On the other hand, for some infants thicker foods may form a more cohesive bolus and therefore move more effectively through the pharynx.

Encouraging "dry" swallows. Sometimes, giving one or two boluses of thicker substances, followed by several boluses of thinner liquids, helps to clear the pharynx. Another technique is to allow the baby to suck on a pacifier following oral feeding or after single boluses. This may provide additional "dry swallows," which may improve pharyngeal clearance. Maintaining the head in a flexed position (chin tucked, neck elongated) will maximize the effects of the "dry swallows."

Improve pharyngeal pressure. In some cases, residue and aspiration after the swallow is secondary to inadequate generation and maintenance of pressure gradients that help propel the bolus through the pharynx into the esophagus. Pressure can be inadequate when the valves that assist in sealing the oral and pharyngeal cavities do not function adequately. In particular, if the soft palate does not elevate and seal sufficiently, pharyngeal pressure may be inadequate. This can lead to poor clearance of the bolus during the pharyngeal swallow. When the soft palate is not fully elevated, food can also escape into the nasopharynx.

Shelly and Boxall have described the use of a palatal training appliance (PTA) to assist with velar function.[21] The PTA is similar to a palatal obturator, with the addition of a U-shaped wire on the distal aspect that extends to the base of the uvula (see figure 5-9, page 228). Through pressure and tactile input, the device is felt to facilitate palatal elevation. Experimenting clinically with this device on a small number of babies with poor

---

velar elevation, incomplete pharyngeal swallow, and subsequent aspiration, we have seen improved elevation of the soft palate, improved pharyngeal clearance, and decreased aspiration after the swallow. With this device these infants have continued to be fed orally.

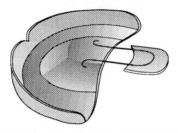

Figure 5-9 A palatal training appliance can assist with velar function.

Decision Making regarding Oral Intake When Aspiration Is Observed

As imaging techniques improve, increasing our ability to clearly identify infants who aspirate or are at high risk for aspiration, making decisions on feeding management in these babies becomes more complex. While it appears that it may be normal to aspirate a certain unquantified amount of secretions, it is also clear that chronic aspiration (or even single episodes) of other substances can lead to respiratory infection and possibly chronic pulmonary changes.[16]

In making feeding decisions when aspiration is present, several factors must be considered. First is the degree of swallowing dysfunction and/or the amount of aspiration, along with its response to treatment. This is best determined by VFSS. The infant with delayed or incomplete swallowing may not demonstrate frank aspiration during VFSS; nevertheless, that infant is at increased risk due to liquid pooling in the laryngeal vestibule during breathing. The infant with supraglottic penetration but no true aspiration is also at high risk for actual aspiration, as liquid is regularly entering the larynx. Changes in head position or timing of respirations may cause an episode of penetration to become true aspiration. In each of these cases, however, the amount of material that is actually aspirated may be less than the amount that occurs with chronic microaspiration or intermittent frank aspiration. Theoretically, the smaller the total amount of foreign material entering the lungs, the more likely that it will be handled by "pulmonary toileting" mechanisms and the less likely that it will cause respiratory disease. For this reason it is important to use VFSS to gain a clear picture of the amount of actual or potential aspiration *and* to determine if there are feeding modifications that appear to improve swallowing and reduce aspiration.

THERAPEUTIC TREATMENT STRATEGIES

The second consideration is the baseline pulmonary or respiratory status of the infant. While aspiration may compromise healthy respiratory function, lungs that are already damaged by BPD or some other primary pulmonary problem are even more susceptible to deterioration from small amounts of aspirated foreign material. In these cases even a single episode of aspiration can quickly lead to respiratory infection, and chronic microaspirations can make improvement in pulmonary status difficult to achieve. For infants with pulmonary dysfunction, even minimal aspiration cannot be tolerated without risk of major medical compromise. On the other hand, the infant with healthy lungs and low-level aspiration may be able to continue a certain amount of oral feeding without respiratory problems. Even without VFSS evidence confirming aspiration, when an otherwise healthy infant has a history of frequent pneumonia or respiratory illness, aspiration must be considered as a possible cause. In this case, management for aspiration may be indicated to look for clinical change that could help in differential diagnosis of the underlying problem.

When an infant aspirates or is at risk for aspiration, eliminating all oral feedings is often the initial response, for fear of pulmonary damage. Other options that may be considered are described below. The amount of aspiration and the baby's pulmonary status will be the key factors in determining the appropriate strategy. Regardless of the management plan that is selected, two confounding factors must be considered. These are the infant's own secretions and the presence of gastroesophageal reflux.

Despite eliminating all oral feeding, infants must still manage their own secretions. In the face of severe swallowing dysfunction and aspiration, the infant may aspirate enough of its own secretions to cause respiratory infection and pulmonary compromise as described above. If the degree of medical compromise is significant and the swallowing dysfunction is felt to be long term, options to manage the secretions may be considered. These include use of pharmacologic agents that reduce the amount of secretions and thus the amount of secretions that are aspirated. In more significant cases surgical procedures may be used to close off the airway and allow secretions to travel through the pharynx and esophagus without the possibility of aspiration.[38] A tracheostomy must then be placed to create an open airway.

When gastroesophageal reflux (GER) is present in a baby who aspirates, even when descending aspiration of swallowed food is eliminated by terminating feeding, ascending aspiration of refluxed material may still be present. Again, aspiration from this mechanism can cause ongoing respiratory compromise despite elimination of oral feeding. Chapter 6 provides a complete discussion of this interaction and possible management strategies for GER.

Eliminate oral feeding: In infants with significant aspiration or severe lung disease, eliminating oral feeding may be the only option that allows adequate nutrition and maintenance of healthy pulmonary status. In the infant who is fully nourished by non-oral means, it is imperative to establish an ongoing oral therapy program. The goals of the program would include maintaining oral-motor skills for possible return to oral feeding and for later speech, as well as minimizing development of oral-tactile aversions that could interfere with oral hygiene and return to oral feeding. Encouraging non-nutritive sucking on pacifiers, mouthing of fingers and toys, and direct tactile stimulation with touch/pressure and vibration are useful. Further suggestions are provided on page 247.

Case example:

Trevor was an infant who developed apnea associated with feeding and at nonfeeding times early in infancy. Marked central apnea and gastroesophageal reflux (GER) were diagnosed and appropriate treatment instituted. As he became older, significant delays in development were noted and a rare syndrome was diagnosed. With oral feeding by bottle and spoon he was marginally able to meet nutritional needs. Respiratory illness and pneumonia were common.

At 1 year of age, he was admitted to a pediatric hospital for treatment of a major respiratory illness. He continued to have marked GER, and VFSS revealed significant swallowing dysfunction, with consistent aspiration. Oral feeding was discontinued and a gastrostomy was placed. Surgical management of GER was considered due to the high risk of aspiration of refluxed material but was rejected. Strict upright positioning was instituted, along with continuous drip feedings to minimize the amount of gastric contents.

Respiratory status improved, and these improvements were maintained. Despite the mother's enjoyment of oral feeding and reluctance to give up this interaction, she was pleased with Trevor's improved medical status. Activities were identified to replace the interactions that were lost when oral feeding was terminated.

An oral therapy program, focusing on non-nutritive activities, was developed. These included maintaining tactile awareness and acceptance of pressure, texture, and taste. As Trevor remained stable, swallowing activities using small amounts of chilled, thickened liquid (determined by VFSS results) were instituted.

Therapeutic swallowing trials. For some infants who are managed in this manner, it may be desirable to continue to work on facilitation of swallowingwhileawaiting improvement. Typically a larger amount of material than can be obtained through saliva alone is needed. Substances containing proteins and sugars (e.g., formula, fruit juices, glycerine swabs) act as a growth medium for bacteria in the lungs, should they be aspirated. Therefore, they are generally not appropriate for therapeutic swallowing trials in this group of children. Sterile water and saline have been suggested as alternatives. These two substances react differently in the lungs than do proteins or sugars and trigger different pulmonary defense responses. Although normal saline is the least irritating substance to the lungs if aspirated, protective laryngeal reflex responses (i.e., cough, swallow) are less dramatic than with water.[17-20] Sterile water, if aspirated in small amounts, may be no more irritating to the lungs than the infant's own secretions; yet it is more likely to trigger a cough and provide feedback about the functioning of the swallowing mechanism.

Weighing all options, it appears that the safest choice for therapeutically facilitating swallowing in infants who may aspirate some material is to use small amounts of sterile water. Sterile water has a good chance of eliciting protective mechanisms like the cough and functional skills like the swallow; yet it does not appear to expose the infant's lungs to excessive trauma. Use of any substance to maintain or improve swallowing abilities in the infant who aspirates needs to be undertaken with careful medical supervision before the initiation of the procedure and throughout the course of treatment. If at any point a deterioration in respiratory status is observed and could potentially be linked to aspiration, this intervention should be curtailed.

Small therapeutic feedings: Infants with less severe aspiration and reasonable pulmonary status may receive primary nutrition by non-oral means but may be able to take controlled amounts of food orally without compromising their health. The focus of these feedings is therapeutic; to maintain or improve oral and swallowing control so that in the future the baby may be more fully orally fed. A therapeutic oral feeding program would use food types/textures and treatment techniques that reduce aspiration as confirmed by VFSS. Initially, a very conservative, small amount of food is given orally. As the infant is medically stable at one level of oral feeding it can be increased gradually, always maintaining a stable medical status before advancing the program. Close medical supervision is essential.

Case example:
Ashley, who was a former 32-week SGA premature infant, was referred at 5 months of age for a feeding and swallowing evaluation secondary to recurrent respiratory infections. Her clinical feeding evaluation showed weak sucking due to excessive jaw excursion and mild tongue

thrust. These problems responded well to the oral facilitation techniques of jaw control and downward pressure on the tongue.

The VFSS showed a normal swallow at the start of the feeding. As the feeding progressed, however, Ashley had increasing delay in triggering her swallow and aspiration during the swallow was noted. This clinical picture of aspiration toward the middle or end of feeding is referred to as fatigue aspiration.[39] Therapeutic modifications to the feeding were not successful in eliminating the aspiration. As no aspiration was seen during the first two ounces of feeding, Ashley was allowed to nipple feed the first two ounces of each feeding. The remainder of her feeding was supplemented by gastrostomy feedings until she had sufficient maturation so that she no longer exhibited delayed swallowing and aspiration.

Full oral feedings using therapeutic techniques: In some cases the VFSS demonstrates aspiration or high risk for aspiration; however, modifications to the characteristics of the food or the baby's position appear to eliminate aspiration. For these infants, if they are medically stable enough to be exposed to the risks of failure, full oral feeding may be attempted, with careful attention to using the appropriate therapeutic modifications. Close medical supervision is important. Any deterioration in health status felt to be related to aspiration would indicate the need for reevaluation. In this case it is likely that full oral feeding would be discontinued and some form of non-oral feeding (as discussed in strategies one and two above) would be initiated.

Case example:
Kristie was a 7-month-old girl admitted to the hospital with a respiratory infection. Earlier medical care had been scarce, but her history suggested recurrent respiratory infections. While hospitalized it was noted that she frequently coughed with feeding. Evaluation revealed good oral feeding skills for the bottle and spoon but coughing episodes toward the end of some feedings. While the coughing was not consistent, in conjunction with the history of respiratory illness, a VFSS was undertaken.

VFSS initially demonstrated normal swallowing skills. Because of the timing of the coughing in the feeding, however, Kristie completed a bottle of formula and was then reevaluated. At this time, numerous episodes of silent aspiration were seen during the swallow. Marked neck flexion and thickened fluid appeared to eliminate the aspiration. Kristie was then routinely fed in this manner. She demonstrated no problems during her hospital stay and had no recurrence of respiratory illness up to six months later.

Oral-Motor Control

Difficulties in basic motoric control of the tongue, lips, cheeks, and jaw can significantly affect feeding and swallowing abilities. In this text, the treatment techniques presented will relate primarily to the movements of these structures during sucking. Treatment techniques related to the acquisition of mature spoon skills, cup drinking, chewing, and self-feeding skills will not be discussed. Information regarding treatment techniques for those skills is available in other references.[4,8-10]

Problem: Oral-Facial Hypotonia

Oral-facial hypotonia leads to poor stability in the oral-facial area, contributing to abnormal control of the tongue, jaw, lips, and cheeks.

Causes and Contributing Factors

- Premature infants are known to have hypotonic oral-facial tone.

- Oral-facial hypotonia may be part of an overall picture of hypotonia seen in association with some medical conditions (e.g., Down syndrome) or other neurologic abnormality.

- Weakness may be associated with hypotonia and/or look like hypotonia in the young infant. Weakness may be secondary to compromised medical status or poor nutrition, or may be neurologically based, as in myopathies.

Treatment Techniques

Infants may or may not respond to treatment aimed at modifying decreased oral-facial tone, depending on the degree of tonal dysfunction and the source of abnormality. While these techniques may be helpful for some infants, modifying positioning and using techniques to compensate for low oral-facial tone may show greater results. The area of the face/mouth where these techniques are used will be based on the infant's specific motor and feeding problems.

Tapping: Firm tapping directly to the lips, cheeks, and tongue may increase postural tone in these areas.

Vibration: The clinician holds a commercial vibrator, then places a vibrating finger on the lips, cheeks, or tongue to build tone (see figure 5-10, page 234).

Quick stretch: Leonard et al. found that providing quick stretch over the area of the masseter and buccinator muscles during a sucking pause of greater than two seconds resulted in faster and greater intake.[22] Similar procedures may also be useful on the lips or tongue.

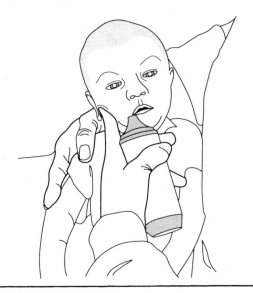

Figure 5-10 A small vibrator may be used to build lip and cheek tone.

Problem: Oral-Facial Hypertonia

Increased oral-facial tone may result in abnormal movement patterns of the tongue, jaw, and/or lips. Hypertonia may eventually lead to abnormal alignment of the oral-facial structures.

Causes and Contributing Factors
- Neurologic insult or abnormality can lead to increased oral-facial tone as part of an overall pattern of increased tone. A baby stressed by the environment or by medical problems may respond with hypertonic postural patterns, including elements of oral-facial hypertonia.

Treatment Techniques
Preparatory movement: The infant with marked hypertonicity, particularly originating from neurologic abnormality, will probably benefit from some preparatory neurodevelopmental handling to reduce overall tone and improve body alignment. There should be a strong emphasis on the head, neck, and shoulders. Positioning will then be crucial to maintain the effects of this handling.

Firm pressure: Using the fingers, the therapist may apply firm pressure along the sides of the nose and mouth or above and below the lips. This may help reduce tone in these structures.

Shaking/Vibration: Tone may be reduced by sandwiching the cheeks or lips between two extended fingers. Rapid shaking or vibration with slight traction is then provided (figure 5-11).

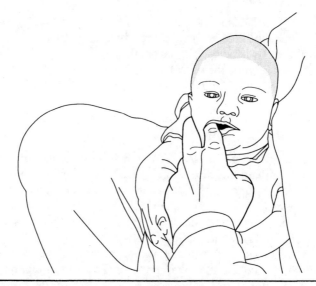

Figure 5-11 Extended fingers sandwich the cheeks when shaking or vibrating to reduce tone.

Problem: Tongue Retraction

The retracted tongue is pulled into or falls into the posterior portion of the oral cavity. In this position there is less contact between the tongue and the nipple, leading to ineffective use of the tongue during sucking. The tongue may not be able to produce an adequate central groove; thus, preparation of the bolus for swallowing may be difficult. If the tongue is sufficiently retracted, it may impinge on the pharyngeal airway and can become a consistent or intermittent obstruction to breathing.

Causes and Contributing Factors
- Hypertonicity may contribute to an active type of tongue retraction.

- Neck hyperextension can functionally pull the tongue into a retracted position.

- In the hypotonic infant, the tongue may be passively retracted. It can also be actively retracted as the infant seeks a point of tongue stability.

- A retracted tongue is typically seen in association with micrognathia and in the Pierre-Robin malformation sequence. In these cases, the infant is at particular risk for obstruction (see chapter 6).

Treatment Techniques
Postural support: When neck hyperextension is present, positioning to improve head and neck alignment is an important starting point. If neck hyperextension is part of an overall pattern of hypertonicity,

---

handling activities to normalize body tone, particularly in the neck and shoulders, may be useful. If a small, weak, hypotonic infant is seeking postural stability through tongue retraction, better postural support through positioning is needed. A well-supported, semi-upright position with neck elongated, chin slightly tucked, and shoulders symmetric and toward the body midline will assist in bringing the tongue toward the front of the mouth.

Modifying tone of the tongue: When the tongue is actively retracted, tone can be reduced and the tongue relaxed by various movements to the tongue. Movements should begin with the therapist's finger in a midline position on the tongue, and movement should always be proximal to distal. It may be difficult to position the finger on a very retracted tongue. Gently work the finger between the lateral gum ridge and then onto the top of the tongue. Shaking, jiggling, tapping, and stroking the tongue may be useful movements. Care should be taken to monitor the baby's response to this procedure so that the intensity of the stimuli can be graded to the baby's level of tolerance. In addition, vibration of the finger, or through the finger with a commercial vibrator, may be useful (see figure 5-10, page 234).

Longer nipple: When the tongue is not brought forward adequately by the above techniques, choosing a nipple with a slightly longer profile may provide greater contact on the tongue and promote more effective tongue movements during sucking.

Problem: Lack of Central Grooving of the Tongue

The central groove, formed along the median raphe of the tongue, creates a channel for liquid to travel from the anterior to the posterior portion of the mouth. When this is not well formed, food and liquid can spill over the sides of the tongue and move in a poorly coordinated manner to the oropharynx. In the posterior portion of the central groove the tongue organizes the bolus and holds it until swallowing is initiated. When the central groove is poorly formed, the tongue cannot adequately assist with the oral preparatory phase of swallowing, perhaps leading to delays in initiating swallowing and increasing the risk of aspiration. In addition, inability to form a central groove is associated with ineffectively coordinated tongue movement and difficulty producing negative pressure suction.

Causes and Contributing Factors
- Lack of central grooving is often seen in a tongue that is tight, bunched, humped, and/or retracted.

- A tongue that is hypotonic may lack sufficient internal stability to curve and form a central groove.

Treatment Techniques

The primary method of facilitating formation of a central groove in the tongue is through proprioceptive input. If the tongue is also retracted, however, treatment must first address this problem using the techniques described above for tongue retraction.

Proprioceptive input: Downward pressure to the midline of the tongue provides proprioceptive input regarding proper position in the mouth and encourages central grooving. Slight stroking forward combined with downward pressure may help initiate appropriate sucking patterns. This technique can also be used to build tone in the tongue that shows poor central grooving due to hypotonia or flaccidity. Downward pressure can be applied with a finger prior to feeding or with the nipple during feeding. A firm, straight nipple with a round cross section will provide more appropriate proprioceptive input and tongue shaping than a broad, flat nipple (see chapter 7).

Problem: Excessive Tongue-Tip Elevation

The tip of the tongue is elevated against the hard palate, just distal to the alveolar ridge. Insertion of the bottle nipple or breast is difficult. At times the baby may appear to be sucking, but no liquid flows, since the nipple is actually underneath the tongue.

Causes and Contributing Factors

- This pattern is common in premature babies, particularly around the time they are beginning to nipple feed.

- Tongue-tip elevation may be used as a means of stabilization when there is decreased tone and stability in the head, neck, and trunk— such as when hypotonia, neck hyperextension, or hypertonia is present.

Treatment Techniques

Postural support: Providing a stable feeding position that decreases head/ neck extension and encourages neck elongation and forward head flexion may be useful. If hypertonicity is contributing to tongue-tip elevation, preparatory handling activities should be considered to normalize the overall tone.

Facilitation of tongue movements: Quick swiping or vibration to the tip of the tongue followed by downward pressure into the tongue will help bring the tongue down in the mouth.

Assist with mouth opening: Stimulation to the lips and slight downward pressure on the jaw encourage greater jaw opening, bringing the tongue tip down for easier nipple placement.

Problem: Tongue Protrusion

The front edge of the protruded tongue often sits on the lower lip, below the nipple, during sucking. In this position it interferes with lip activity and adequate seal around the nipple. The protruded tongue may not be able to move well, and a "lick-suck" pattern will be seen as the infant generates greater compression than suction.

Causes and Contributing Factors
- Hypotonia and/or weakness often result in a "passive" protrusion; the tongue simply hangs out of the mouth.

- Problems with organizing appropriate tongue movements may result in "active" protrusion, as the infant searches for a method of expressing liquid from the nipple.

- Increased neck extension can lead to the development of active tongue protrusion as the infant thrusts the tongue forward, attempting to latch-on to the nipple.

- Increased tone may contribute to the development of tongue protrusion as it is manifested in increased neck extension and/or difficulty organizing tongue movement.

Treatment Techniques
Postural support: If active or passive neck hyperextension is present, the feeding position will need to be modified to bring the head into a neutral or slightly flexed position and provide stable support to the head. If strong extensor tone contributes to this pattern, neurodevelopmental handling to reduce the extensor tone may be useful.

Building tone in the tongue: The hypotonic, protruding tongue requires increased sensory input to increase its tone. Firm tapping to the midline of the tongue moving from the tip toward the base may help bring the tongue further into the mouth. Stimulation should not be provided from the base to the tip, as this may encourage more protrusion.

Facilitating appropriate tongue movements: When tongue protrusion results in a compression pattern dominating sucking, techniques to facilitate normal tongue movement may be necessary. Firm, downward pressure to the tongue midline (possibly including forward stroking) will improve central grooving and increase negative pressure suction, leading to a more efficient suck. A firm, straight nipple with a round cross section can also put strong pressure on the tongue in midline, facilitating better sucking patterns. A broad, flat nipple, however, may encourage thrusting or compression and is not recommended for an infant with this problem. As the clinician's finger can provide stronger input than a bottle nipple, it may be necessary to use techniques to facilitate an appropriate sucking pattern on the finger before moving to the nipple.

Facilitating lip activity: If the lips have not been actively involved in producing a seal around the nipple, using the thumb and index finger to provide pressure over the fat pads during sucking may facilitate better lip seal (see page 244).

Problem: Lack of Spontaneous Mouth Opening

When an infant does not spontaneously open the mouth, the feeder is unable to place the nipple easily and initiate feeding.

Causes and Contributing Factors
- State of alertness may affect how readily a baby will open its mouth for feeding.

- Neurologic insult resulting in marked hypertonia may lead to a clenching pattern in the jaw, which inhibits spontaneous mouth opening.

Treatment Techniques

Prepare the baby's state: Arousal techniques (described on page 212) may be needed to alert the baby and elicit more spontaneous mouth opening.

Elicit the rooting reflex: Mouth opening is a crucial component of the rooting reflex; therefore, stimulating this reflex may facilitate a mouth opening response.

Assist mouth opening: For some infants, gentle downward pressure and traction to the jaw may help open the mouth. This technique is particularly useful in eliciting the wide mouth opening necessary for breast-feeding.

Inhibit jaw clenching: Overall preparation and reduction of postural tone may be necessary prior to direct treatment to the mouth. Jaw clenching may be reduced by vibration to the mouth. Hold the mandible between the thumb and index finger and provide extremely small-range, low-amplitude, side-to-side movement of the jaw.

Touch/pressure to the gums is another useful technique. It can be applied by firmly stroking the outer portion of the gum ridges. Start at the middle of the mouth and firmly stroke toward the back of the gums on one side. Return to the midline and repeat two or three times. Apply stimulation to all four quadrants of the mouth. Pause between quadrants, allowing the baby to swallow.[4,8,32] In cases of severe neurologic involvement, jaw opening may need to be included in an overall passive range-of-motion program.

Problem: Weak Suck

A weak suck often results in inefficient feeding. While the motoric components of sucking may be well organized, a weak suck generates inadequate pressure and liquid flow.

Causes and Contributing Factors

- Overall weakness from medical or nutritional compromise, immature muscular development (as in the premature infant), or conditions that result in muscular weakness (myopathies, etc.) may produce a weak suck.

- Respiratory and endurance problems may contribute to a weak suck. The suck may be strong initially but become weaker as the feeding progresses. While the techniques below may be helpful in the latter portion of the feeding, feeding modifications related to the problems of respiratory compromise and endurance (see page 257) should also be considered.

Treatment Techniques

Facilitating a stronger sucking pattern: In some infants, providing oral stability will allow oral structures to produce stronger, more effective movement. Maximal stability is provided by optimal positioning and using firm cheek and jaw support (see figure 5-12). A small bottle may make it easier for the feeder to place the fingers to provide these three points of stability. Small bottles such as a Volu-feed® are available in hospital nurseries. Slight traction on the nipple by gently trying to pull it out of the mouth also may promote stronger sucking.

Increasing the flow of liquid: Manipulating the flow of liquid allows the infant to get a larger bolus in response to a weak suck. Many babies with a weak suck can coordinate swallowing and breathing with a much larger bolus than their weak suck can produce. Increasing the bolus size, however, must be done with caution. When the bolus becomes too large it may cause coughing or choking and can result in less active, weaker sucking as the infant attempts to reduce the bolus size by modifying the sucking pattern. Techniques to increase the flow of liquid are discussed in chapter 7.

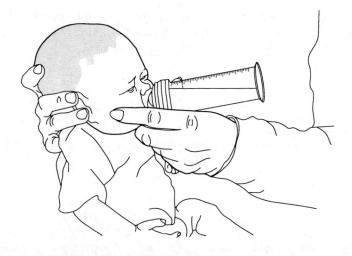

Figure 5-12 Feeder provides jaw and cheek support during feeding. (Note feeder's hand position and use of small-sized bottle.)

Problem: Excessive Jaw Movement

When the jaw moves excessively during sucking, it does not provide a stable base for tongue movements. This can result in abnormal tongue movements and inefficient feeding. Lip seal may also be compromised by marked jaw depression if the lower lip or corners of lips are not able to maintain contact with the nipple.

Causes and Contributing Factors

- Jaw instability is the primary cause of excessive jaw movement. In the term newborn, positional jaw stability is the result of appropriate tone and the physical approximation of the oral-facial muscles and structures. Adequate development of the neck flexor musculature provides a stable base for appropriate jaw movement. This is supported by a slightly tucked chin position. In older infants, postural stability provides the primary jaw stability and is the result of the balanced active control of the muscles of the jaw.

- Premature infants often show jaw instability. Maturationally, they have poorly developed tone and bulk in the oral-facial muscles and structures, as well as minimal active neck flexion. Neck hyperextension is also common, further reducing positional stability to the jaw.

- Low oral-facial tone or facial weakness may result in poor jaw stability and therefore excessive jaw movement.

- Neurologically based hypertonicity may result in poorly balanced control between the muscles opening and closing the jaw. This may lead to strong downward "thrusting" of the jaw.

- Neck hyperextension, whether the result of immature development of neck flexion, abnormal muscle tone, or some ongoing stress to the infant, is generally associated with excessive jaw movement.

- Abnormal tongue movement can also contribute to excessive jaw movement as the infant attempts to use marked jaw depression to create negative pressure suction.

Treatment Techniques

Postural support: Head and neck alignment is a key in treating excessive jaw movement. A position allowing neck hyperextension will contribute to this problem as described above. Using a position with the head in neutral alignment, or in slight flexion, will provide additional positional stability to the jaw, improving the effectiveness of other treatments.

External support: External support is provided by firm pressure of the feeding specialist's finger under the jaw. This will allow the clinician to grade the range of movement of the jaw. The bottle is held between the thumb and index fingers while upward pressure is provided to the mandible by the third or fourth finger (figure 5-13). Care must be taken to keep the pressure distal and under the mandible, as pressure proximally will be under the base of the tongue and could interfere with sucking. The amount of upward force needed to reduce jaw excursion will vary among babies. Although substantial pressure is often needed for organized and graded jaw movement, use as little external support as possible to allow development of maximal internal stability. The amount of pressure needed may vary throughout the feeding session. The feeder should periodically remove the support and "test" whether it is still required.

Increased neck flexion: At times an infant will not respond well to the external support technique described above, or a feeder will have difficulty carrying it out. An alternative method of providing additional jaw stability is to bring the head into strong neck flexion. The chin should be close to the chest, with the chest then providing pressure and helping to grade jaw movement. To be effective, the head must be held very stable so that excessive jaw movement is not possible by increasing neck extension. To maintain this position, an angled-neck bottle may be useful (see figure 5-8, page 226). The baby's respiratory pattern must be continually monitored, especially in preterm infants, since marked neck flexion may produce airway obstruction.

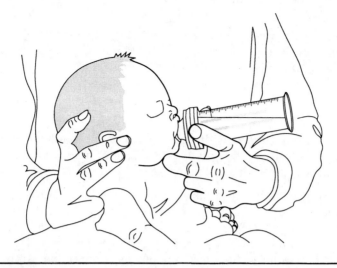

Figure 5-13 When jaw control is provided during feeding, firm pressure is applied to the mandible.

Neuromotor preparation: In addition to the techniques described above, handling techniques prior to feeding, with the goal of reducing overall muscle tone, may benefit the infant with jaw thrusting resulting from increased muscle tone.

Facilitating appropriate tongue movement: As jaw instability often results in abnormal tongue movements, poorly coordinated tongue movement may lead to excessive jaw movement. Specific treatments to the tongue may be needed. Techniques beginning on page 235 should be considered, based on the type of tongue movement noted.

Problem: Poor Lip Seal

When lip seal is poor, negative pressure suction may be reduced if the seal on the nipple is broken intermittently. A smacking or kissing sound will accompany this intermittent loss of suction. Excessive fluid loss, with a steady stream of formula from the corners or lower lip, may also be noted when the lip seal is weak. Both reduced suction and excessive fluid loss lead to inefficient feeding.

Causes and Contributing Factors
- Low muscle tone or weakness, due to prematurity or other conditions, makes maintaining adequate lip seal difficult. Lip seal may be chronically loose, particularly laterally in the corners of the mouth.

- Excessive jaw movement and wide jaw excursions may make it difficult to maintain a consistent lip seal, leading to "smacking" sounds as the suction is broken.

- Abnormal tongue movements with a strong protrusion component may push fluid out of the mouth. Rather than a steady stream, a gush of fluid during each suck is often seen. Although this may look like a problem of lip seal, often the lip seal is adequate, and the abnormal tongue movements require treatment.

Treatment Techniques

Treat underlying problems: If poor lip seal is the result of facial weakness/hypotonia or excessive jaw excursion, treatment should begin with these underlying problems (see pages 233 and 241).

External support: Direct external support to the cheeks and lips may help increase lip approximation around the nipple. Place the thumb and index or middle finger on the sucking pads and provide pressure to purse the lips laterally (figure 5-14). For some infants it may be appropriate to use this technique simultaneous with external support to the jaw (see figure 5-12, page 241). This may be easier with a small bottle such as a Volu-feed® (available in hospital nurseries). This small bottle can be supported between the thumb and the index finger, leaving the other fingers free for jaw and lip/cheek support.

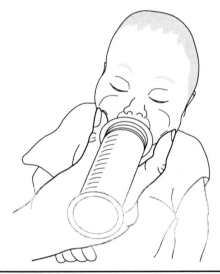

Figure 5-14 Feeder provides cheek control during feeding.

Problem: Poor Cheek Stability

Cheek instability can lead to poor lip seal, as appropriate lip movement is dependent on stable cheek movement. Maintenance of stable cheeks is important in allowing the size of the oral cavity to increase during sucking to produce suction. When the cheeks are unstable, the lateral borders of the oral chamber may not hold firmly during sucking. Excessive jaw excursion may then result as the infant attempts to increase the size of the oral cavity to produce suction.

Causes and Contributing Factors

- Facial hypotonia and weakness may lead to poor cheek stability.

- Since the fat pads are the primary contributor to cheek stability in young infants, if they are small or diminished, cheek instability may result.

Treatment Techniques

Increase facial tone: Techniques described on page 233 should be considered.

External cheek support: Direct external support to the cheeks may help improve cheek stability during sucking. Place the thumb and index or middle finger on the sucking pads and provide pressure (see figure 5-14). For some infants it may be appropriate to use this technique simultaneously with external support to the jaw (see figure 5-12, page 241). This may be easier with a small bottle such as a Volu-feed® (available in hospital nurseries). The bottle can be supported between the thumb and the index finger, leaving the other fingers free for jaw and lip/cheek support.

Problem: Poor Initiation of Sucking

Difficulty in eliciting sucking at feeding time can be very frustrating to the feeder. A hungry baby will also become increasingly frustrated if not able to initiate sucking. This may lead to crying, fussing, and/or "tuning-out." These signals are unclear, leading the feeder to think the baby is not hungry, when in fact the baby is hungry but not able to initiate sucking.

Causes and Contributing Factors

- An infant may root excessively to the stimulus of the nipple and not be able to inhibit this reflexive response to initiate sucking. The baby's head will turn wildly, keeping it from latching onto the nipple.

- Some babies orient to the nipple with extreme mouth opening and are unable to close the mouth to begin sucking. This may be due to increased tone or marked extensor patterns of movement.

- Ineffective tongue protrusion or a lapping pattern may be the infant's initial attempt at sucking. This may be part of a mildly hypersensitive response or the result of poorly developed sucking patterns.

- Poor state and organizational abilities, as well as hunger, may contribute to the infant's problems initiating sucking.

Treatment Techniques

Treatment of underlying problems: If poor state and organizational abilities appear to contribute to this problem, treatment techniques beginning on page 211 should be considered. If oral tactile hypersensitivity is present, the techniques starting on page 247 may be helpful. If neurologically based increased tone is contributing, preparatory neurodevelopmental handling may be appropriate (see page 218).

Controlling excessive rooting: To control excessive rooting, provide firm stabilization and control of the head through positioning. This will make it difficult for the baby to quickly shake the head from side to side. Stabilize the front of the head with jaw control as needed. Place the nipple firmly on the midline of the baby's tongue, with slight downward pressure to give a central point of stabilization. Cheek support may also be needed to provide the baby with a central reference point.

Assisting with mouth closure: For the infant who has difficulty closing the mouth due to increased tone, firm jaw control may be needed to assist in physically closing the mouth, as well as in grading subsequent mouth opening. Vibration to the jaw may be necessary to relax jaw tension and assist in mouth closure.

Facilitating appropriate tongue movements: For a baby using ineffective tongue movement due to poorly established sucking patterns, techniques to facilitate normal tongue movement may be necessary. Techniques beginning on page 235 may be appropriate.

Problem: Poor Palatal Movement

A baby with poor palatal movement may have difficulty producing appropriate oral and pharyngeal pressures. If the soft palate does not adequately seal against the tongue, oral suction will be interrupted prematurely. The volume of fluid per suck may then be reduced and feeding becomes inefficient. During sucking a "click" is often heard as this seal is broken.

Decreased velar elevation may also lead to nasopharyngeal reflux. If nasopharyngeal seal is poor, pharyngeal pressure can be inadequate and the bolus may not clear the pharynx normally during swallowing. This can be visible, with vomiting or formula coming out of the baby's nose during feeding, though it can also be present with no visible sign. In either case, it may lead to irritation of the nasal membranes.

A floppy, poorly controlled soft palate may cause intermittent airway obstruction, resulting in poor air movement, noisy breathing, and an increased risk of apnea with bradycardia.

Causes and Contributing Factors
- Abnormal muscle tone (increased or decreased) may be associated with a floppy, poorly moving palate.

- Submucous clefts can contribute to poor palatal movement.

Treatment Techniques
In general, palatal problems are not easy to treat in infancy. Maturation is frequently needed to change velar function. Palatal elevation may be improved by using a palatal training appliance (see page 227 for more detail) as described by Shelley and Boxall.[21]

Oral-Tactile Hypersensitivity

Infants with feeding dysfunction may demonstrate inappropriately modulated responses to tactile stimuli in and around the face and mouth. Placing a bottle in the mouth or putting toys to the mouth may result in hypersensitive responses (such as grimacing or head turning) or aversive responses (such as gagging, which leads to vomiting). These abnormalities in sensory processing can significantly limit oral feeding abilities and are among the most challenging problems facing feeding specialists who treat infants with complex feeding disorders.

Hypersensitive responses are heightened or exaggerated out of proportion to the magnitude of the stimulus. Babies who have a low threshold for oral-tactile stimuli will frequently demonstrate hypersensitive responses. They may, however, be willing to engage in oral-tactile exploration within their limited range.

Oral-tactile aversive responses are at the extreme end of the continuum of hypersensitive responses. They are more easily elicited, stronger, more negative, and often include a behavioral response to the stimulus. A baby may cry, grimace, wiggle, arch away, or keep the mouth closed when asked to feed. If the feeder persists the baby may begin to gag, and if that warning is not heeded, may vomit. Aversive responses are so strong that they may be observed merely on visual presentation of the spoon or bottle.

Both hypersensitive and aversive responses can be part of a global tactile processing problem or may be localized to the face and mouth. The aversive and hypersensitive responses may be to touch only or may also be to tastes, temperatures, textures, or smells.

The basis for these hypersensitive and aversive responses is multifactorial and includes:

Immaturity and illness: Many infants who show these responses are born prematurely, with immature central nervous systems, and are not equipped to deal with the intensity and multitude of stimuli present in the extrauterine environment. The premature infant, rather than being unable to register and process sensory information, seems to be overly sensitive to these stimuli and unable to buffer or filter the input due to lack of inhibitory controls.[42]

A chronically ill infant may be at the mercy of its physiologic status, with all its resources harnessed toward simple survival. In this state, the slightest increase in sensory stimuli may prove to be overwhelming. With immaturity, lowered threshold, and lack of regulatory filtering mechanisms, a pattern of hypersensitive/aversive responses may develop. The oral area is particularly vulnerable due to the richness of tactile receptors and the relative maturity of these receptors at birth.

Delayed introduction of oral feeding: In the premature or chronically ill infant, introduction of oral feeding is frequently delayed, often substantially. Not only is the introduction of liquids often delayed, but the progression toward solids or cup drinking also lags. Illingworth and Lister, in a classic article, discuss the role of the critical or sensitive period for the acquisition of oral feeding skills.[30] This critical or sensitive period is the time when the infant is most ready to learn a particular skill if the appropriate stimuli are applied. If this critical or sensitive period is missed, learning the skill at a later time will be more difficult, if not impossible. Many infants with complex feeding disorders have not been fed by mouth for long periods of time, and the onset of oral feeding has been significantly delayed. Having missed the critical period, their response to the sensory components of feeding and their acquisition of oral skills is often impaired.

Unpleasant oral-tactile experiences: Babies who develop abnormal responses to oral-tactile stimuli have often undergone many negative and traumatic oral-facial experiences during the course of medical treatment. Many have been intubated repeatedly or for long periods of time. They have had their faces taped and retaped to hold endotracheal tubes and feeding tubes in place. They have been suctioned frequently through the endotracheal tube or directly into the mouth. Pleasurable and comforting oral stimulation may not have been provided or might not have been possible. If the endotracheal tube was placed in the mouth, they may have been unable to engage in simple hand-to-mouth behavior or sucking on a pacifier. These babies, therefore, undergo a period of relative oral deprivation combined with aversive oral stimuli. They learn a pattern of defensiveness to stimulation in and around the oral area, which tends to persist well beyond the end of the medical interventions and is then reflected in oral hypersensitive and aversive responses.

Treatment Techniques

Reduce aversive oral-facial stimuli: As unpleasant or aversive oral-tactile experiences can play a large role in the development of oral hypersensitivity, a logical first step in treatment is to reduce or eliminate such experiences. Care routines should be evaluated to determine which aspects of care may be perceived by the child as unpleasant. They might then be modified by reducing or eliminating oral suctioning, using an indwelling NG tube rather than placing the tube for each feeding, or perhaps moving to a gastrostomy if prolonged tube feeding is anticipated. Taping procedures can also be modified to reduce trauma to facial skin and still hold tubes securely. When unpleasant procedures like suctioning must continue, techniques described by Als for containment and environmental modification can help improve the infant's tolerance of these procedures.[42]

Grading: A key to treatment of oral hypersensitivity and aversion is the provision of *graded* oral/tactile stimuli. This type of treatment may be called "oral-tactile normalization." Treatment must begin in the range where the child is comfortable, slowly build up to the point where it is not tolerated, then step back slightly. The therapist must dance on the edge of the infant's tolerance or the treatment will not be effective in making changes.

An adaptive, well-modulated response to the oral-tactile input is the goal. Therefore, careful monitoring of the baby's response to the stimuli through changes in the autonomic, motoric, and state-related behaviors is crucial. If a positive response is observed, further stimuli may be presented. If a stress behavior surfaces, the intensity of stimuli should be lowered slightly. Sensory input must be advanced slowly in order to increase the infant's tolerance one step at a time.

Tactile stimuli can be graded along several continuums. The first is the area of the body or face. A hypersensitive baby will generally show the most tolerance to tactile stimuli presented furthest from the lips and tongue. For some infants it is necessary to start with input to the hands and arms, then work up to the neck, chin, and cheeks. As the infant tolerates stimuli to these areas, the program can progress to include the lips, then finally move into the mouth to the gums and tongue. Care should be taken to avoid frequent stimulation of the gag response.

The type of tactile stimulation can also be graded. Texture generally falls along a continuum from smooth to soft to unusual or prickly. Pressure falls on a continuum from firm to light. Food textures also

---

form a continuum from liquid to pureed to chunky but uniform (i.e., applesauce or cottage cheese) to crunchy and harder chewing foods. Hypersensitive infants tend to have greater tolerance for smooth textures, firm pressure, and pureed foods. There are individual variations, however, and a particular baby may do well with a texture that is out of sequence. These continuums provide a framework for therapeutic intervention, although controlled experimentation outside the continuum, while carefully monitoring the infant's responses, can provide valuable information for progressing treatment.

A program of graded oral-tactile normalization can use a number of sensory modalities, and these are described below.

Touch/Pressure: Firm touch/pressure is known to have an integrating effect on the central nervous system.[31] This can be provided to the child in various ways.

- Rub the child's face, arms, or body with items of various textures. The therapist's hands, a textured brush, stuffed animals, or textured cloths can be used.

- Firmly rub the gums or stroke the tongue. Mueller and Morris and Dunn describe this technique, which can be effective in decreasing oral hypersensitivity.[4,8,32] The therapist should provide firm pressure on the outer gum ridge starting at the midline and traveling toward the back of the gums. This procedure should be repeated three or four times on each side of the upper and lower gums. Pause between upper and lower gums to allow the child to swallow any saliva produced during the procedure.

- To provide touch/pressure input to the tongue, the therapist places the finger at the front of the tongue and "walks back" on the tongue until just in front of the point of triggering the gag response. In some babies, raised eyebrows or an eye blink indicates this point. Some infants will tolerate only one brief touch or quick swipe on the gums or tongue. If that is the infant's tolerance level, begin there.

- Touch/pressure can be provided throughout the day during the infant's activities of daily living. Bathing and dressing are wonderful forums for providing increased sensory input. After the bath, the parent can spend some extra time rubbing the child's face and body with the towel or massage the child with lotion. While dressing, the parent can provide input to the face, hands, and feet by rubbing them with the child's clothing.

Vibration: Vibration is an excellent modality for use in oral normalization. Vibratory afferents are carried along an entirely different neural pathway than light touch and touch/pressure; therefore they have the potential of being more integrating and less likely to stimulate an aversive response. Mild vibration can be an extremely effective treatment modality even with preterm babies.

In addition to vibratory movements made by the feeding specialist's finger, small, hand-held mini-vibrators (e.g., from North Coast Medical, Inc., 187 Stauffer Boulevard, San Jose, CA 95125), such as those used for chest PT, may also be useful. Although the vibrator can be placed directly on the cheeks or lips, a better method is for the therapist to hold the vibrator in the hand, against the index finger. The vibration is transmitted to the therapist's finger, which can then be placed on the desired structures. This is a particularly effective way to provide vibratory stimuli inside the mouth and on the tongue (see figure 5-10, page 234).

The vibrator can also be placed against a pacifier or nipple so that the baby receives vibration while sucking. This has been an effective technique to encourage babies to suck on nipples or pacifiers when they have previously refused. An electric toothbrush is another means of supplying vibratory input to children of toothbrushing age.

Oral Exploration: Mouthing of toys and hands is a crucial component of oral exploration and oral normalization in the infant. As babies explore the world through the mouth, their ability to tolerate increasing complexity and variety of oral sensations improves. The point at which the gag reflex is elicited in the mouth moves progressively further back, as the child places more objects farther back in the mouth. This normal process of oral exploration may not be part of a baby's experiences if there is a prolonged illness or if the baby is reluctant to engage in self-directed oral exploration due to oral hypersensitivity.

The feeding specialist's role is to reintroduce this crucial stage of normal development in a manner the baby can tolerate. The clinician can assist the baby with mouthing various objects, adjusting frequency and duration to the baby's limits. The clinician's fingers, the baby's fingers or hands, toys, or pacifiers may be used. The ongoing use of a pacifier is particularly important in maintaining sucking abilities in the non-orally fed infant and may assist in maintaining the link between the mouth and the stomach. A NUK® toothbrush trainer is an excellent tool to use for oral exploration. This soft, rubberized, textured brush is easy for babies to hold and is frequently so appealing that babies begin to suck or bite it.

The key to oral exploration is variety. The feeding specialist must guard against the baby becoming "stuck" on sucking or mouthing only one particular item, which is then perceived as safe. When the transition back to oral feeding with a bottle or spoon is desired, the baby may be

---

unwilling to allow anything except that "safe" item in the mouth. This is especially true for pacifiers, as very few are exact matches to the shape of nipples through which liquids can be obtained. An infant that is to be non-orally fed for a lengthy period, with the hope of returning to a bottle, should be encouraged to suck on a variety of things, including a nipple through which liquid can flow (see page 411). The infant should be carefully supervised while sucking on a loose nipple, as nipples are not designed with the safety features of pacifiers.[33]

Integrate treatment into daily care routines: Oral-tactile normalization techniques using touch/pressure, vibration, oral exploration, and other modalities can be done in preparation for a feeding session, or they can be done at nonfeeding times. Integrating these techniques into daily routines has the advantage of increasing the amount and frequency of pleasurable oral experiences. It is often noted clinically that when short, frequent applications of sensory stimulation are used, the amount of sensory input can be increased more quickly. Because much tactile integration is felt to take place at a subconscious level,[31] providing tactile input while the baby is attending to something else may allow the use of stronger stimuli.

Coordination of Sucking, Swallowing, and Breathing

The concept that the individual functions of sucking, swallowing, and breathing are the cornerstones of infant feeding has been emphasized throughout this text. The smooth and timely *coordination* of these three functions is prerequisite for safe and efficient feeding. In addition to being functionally related, sucking, swallowing, and breathing are anatomically related. Feeding and breathing share a common space—the pharynx, which serves as a conduit for air going to and from the lungs and for food going from the mouth to the stomach. This dual role underlies the problems that are seen when sucking, swallowing, and breathing are poorly coordinated. Because of their close functional and anatomic relationship, dysfunction or immaturity in any of these three systems has a profound effect on the other two systems.

The appropriate coordination of sucking, swallowing, and breathing produces the rhythmic pattern that is a hallmark of infant feeding (see figure 5-15a, page 256). Therefore, problems coordinating sucking, swallowing, and breathing often present themselves as abnormalities in the rhythm of nutritive sucking. Three commonly seen abnormal rhythms are described below, and treatment techniques are suggested.

Prolonged Sucking—Feeding-Induced Apnea

During prolonged sucking, the baby has long sucking bursts without interspersing breaths at appropriate intervals (see figure 5-15b, page 256). This leads to a feeding-induced apnea, possibly resulting in oxygen desaturation and bradycardia. A baby with this problem is having difficulty "pacing" sucking and swallowing with breathing. Babies with this pacing difficulty often have strong, rapid sucking and may have difficulty initiating breathing, even after the nipple has been removed from the mouth. Prolonged sucking may be more pronounced at the beginning of the feeding than at other times. By the middle to end of the feeding, sucking and swallowing generally slow, and pacing may improve.

The prolonged sucking pattern is much more common in premature babies and is felt to be related to maturation, although it can also be observed in full-term infants. In the full-term infant, however, it is unclear whether this is an isolated finding or a subtle precursor of future problems. Our experience has been varied—some full-term babies have feeding-induced apnea as an isolated symptom but go on to have apparently normal development in the first one to two years of life. For other infants, patterns of abnormal motor skills and development have emerged during the first year. Thus, a feeding pattern of prolonged sucking without breathing, when seen in the full-term infant, should be considered a "red flag." Careful developmental follow-up should be planned.

Treatment Techniques

External pacing: The feeder assists the infant in appropriately interspersing breaths during sucking bursts. This is done by carefully counting the number of suck/swallows and removing the nipple from the baby's mouth after the third to fifth suck without a spontaneous breath. For some babies it may be sufficient to simply break the suction by inserting a finger into the corner of the mouth while leaving the nipple in place. Keeping the nipple in contact with the baby's lips lets the baby know that it is present and helps eliminate agitation. Tilting the bottle downward to stop the flow of liquid may also be effective. The feeding specialist must be certain, however, that the baby is able to initiate breathing with the nipple in the mouth. Throughout the feeding, the infant's self-pacing should be "tested" by allowing more than five sucks and watching for spontaneous breathing. Babies often show improved regulation later in a feeding. External pacing is an extremely easy, yet very effective technique for treating the sometimes serious problems associated with feeding-induced apnea. As the baby's own control mechanisms mature, this treatment usually becomes unnecessary.

Case example:
Alice was a full-term infant, born after an uncomplicated pregnancy, labor, and delivery. She did well until 7 hours of life, when she became cyanotic while she was given a bottle of glucose water. Oximetry at that time showed normal oxygen saturations at rest, but drops in saturation to 78% to 83% with feeding. An H-type tracheoesophageal fistula was suspected but was ruled out by a barium swallow.

A clinical feeding evaluation was then requested. Alice demonstrated extremely robust, rapid sucking; however, she made no attempt to breathe during 12 continuous suck/swallows. At this point the bottle was removed from her mouth. She *continued* sucking for several seconds before taking a large, gasping breath. No color change or oxygen desaturation was observed during this episode. This sequence was repeated several times.

Alice's problem was obviously feeding-induced apnea without appropriate pacing of breathing. By using external pacing, Alice was able to take her entire feeding without difficulty. Her mother was taught this technique and she was discharged without subsequent problems.

Allow increased maturity: In a very young premature infant who is just beginning oral feeding (i.e., 32 to 35 weeks) and who shows noticeable problems breathing during sucking bursts, it may be prudent to postpone nippling for a week to allow increased maturation. Although external pacing may be tried, it may not be successful. Small, immature babies still may not appropriately pace their breathing, despite external assistance, and may continue to have periods of apnea and desaturation. Often the very young and immature infant will become disorganized. This can lead to increased stress and fatigue, decreased oxygen saturation, and possibly apnea or bradycardia. The increased maturation of only one week can make infants more resilient and able to deal with this stress, as well as bringing them closer to adequate self-pacing.

Decrease the rate of flow: Slowing the rate of liquid flow from the nipple may reduce the frequency of swallowing, allowing the infant more time to organize the swallow/breathe pattern. Using a thicker liquid or slower-flow nipple (smaller hole, firmer consistency; see chapter 7) may be helpful.

Short Sucking Bursts

In this abnormal sucking rhythm, the infant takes only one to three sucks in a burst before pausing for multiple breaths (see figure 5-15c, page 256). The pauses are too frequent and too long compared to the length of the sucking bursts. Swallowing and/or respiratory difficulties may lead to this pattern. If swallowing is delayed, incomplete, or otherwise dysfunctional, the shortened sucking burst may be the infant's adaptive response to the faulty swallowing mechanism; dealing with it by limiting the number of sequential boluses. For a baby with respiratory difficulty, adopting this pattern may be a form of self-pacing that allows frequent pauses to "catch up" on respiration.

Treatment Techniques

For swallowing-related incoordination: VFSS should be done to determine the specific type of swallowing dysfunction. Treatment techniques would then be selected as described on pages 222-232.

For respiratory-related incoordination: After the respiratory status is well understood, consideration should be given to reducing expectations (see page 264) or providing increased respiratory support (see page 261). During feeding, supporting the baby's use of this pattern of short sucking bursts may be appropriate until the respiratory status is improved.

Disorganized Sucking

This is a very disorganized and uneven pattern. The duration of sucking bursts and pauses may vary considerably. Even if burst-and-pause lengths remain somewhat consistent, there is an uneven pattern of breathing and swallowing within the sucking burst (see figure 5-15d, page 256). Coughing and choking are frequently noted. Possible causes include general neurologic disorganization, mild respiratory problems, or a nipple flow rate that is incompatible with the infant's sucking characteristics.

Treatment Techniques

Assisting with external organization: Many external modifications that limit or carefully control environmental input may assist the infant in becoming more organized. These include:

- bundling the infant to decrease excessive movement

- reducing the level of light and extraneous noise

- providing external rhythms through rocking and/or music.

Acknowledging respiratory problems: The respiratory status should be well understood, with expectations and amount of respiratory support modified as necessary. External pacing—removing the bottle after one or two sucks and allowing a long pause—may improve the organization of sucking, swallowing, and breathing.

Reducing the flow rate: Whether the disorganized rhythm stems from respiratory problems or other disorganized features of the infant, reducing the rate of flow from the bottle may produce more rhythmic coordination. Using a thicker liquid or slower-flow nipple (smaller hole, firmer consistency; see chapter 7) can achieve this. To slow the flow more markedly, small or single boluses may be given.

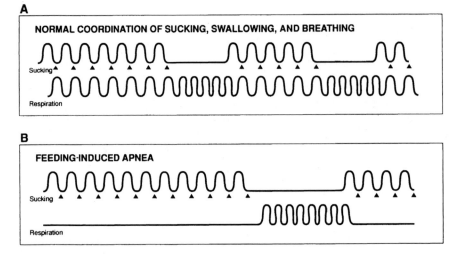

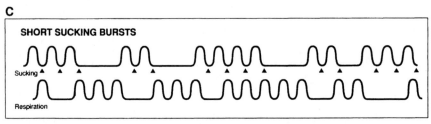

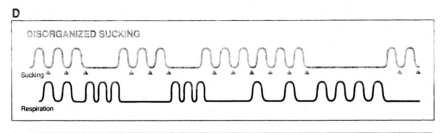

Figure 5-15 Patterns of suck/swallow/breathe organization.

a. Normal, well-coordinated pattern

b. Prolonged sucking (feeding-induced apnea)

c. Short sucking bursts

d. Disorganized sucking

Endurance and Respiratory Compromise

In addition to maintaining homeostasis, feeding is the primary "work" of young infants. "Work" within the body is the process of using oxygen to burn nutrients or calories, to produce a bodily function such as muscle contraction. Thus, any activity (beyond maintaining homeostasis at rest) requires additional oxygen consumption. This can be achieved by increasing cardiac output (higher heart rate and greater stroke volume per beat) and/or through increasing ventilation (higher respiratory rate and greater tidal volume per breath).

In infant feeding, during the initial sucking burst there is slight oxygen desaturation in the bloodstream (although it may still be within acceptable levels), even though there are increased oxygen needs from work of the oral and pharyngeal muscles. During sucking the respiratory rate may decrease, since respirations need to be coordinated with swallowing. Respirations also become more shallow, since the precise timing of the coordination of breathing with swallowing may not allow sufficient time for breaths of larger volume.[40,41] These two factors may lead to less oxygen exchange within the lungs and subsequent desaturation. Respiratory rate and breath size (tidal volume) may then increase during sucking pauses, allowing recovery. Greater cardiac output probably occurs throughout the feeding. The ability to increase ventilation and cardiac output are probably both required to provide the needed increased oxygen for consumption during feeding. In turn, additional cardiac and respiratory work (which may be the *primary* work of feeding) would require further increases in oxygen consumption.

The ability to sustain work is *endurance*, which requires optimal function of numerous physiologic mechanisms. The lungs must exchange oxygen to the blood, oxygen must attach to hemoglobin to be transported by the blood, and it must travel to the heart and be pumped effectively throughout the body. When it reaches a muscle, it must be picked up and properly metabolized. Waste products such as carbon dioxide must reach the venous system, be transported through the heart, exchanged in the lungs, and expelled. In the normally functioning system, the mechanism that generally limits endurance is cardiac output.

If any one of these mechanisms is not functioning optimally, however, "work" will not be able to be sustained—endurance will be limited. In the infant, poor endurance is often manifested during feeding. It results in reduced intake and thus poor weight gain. Should there be any inefficiencies in the system, greater work would be needed to produce the same result. This could also compromise weight gain.

Numerous conditions in the infant can affect the mechanisms described above and can lead to reduced endurance. These include congenital heart disease, muscular weakness from myopathy or other causes, poor nutrition, and a variety of respiratory difficulties, including infant respiratory distress syndrome (IRDS), bronchopulmonary dysplasia, tracheal stenosis, and diaphragmatic hernia. Treatment suggestions for problems of endurance will be discussed below, with a separate focus on problems relating to respiration.

Reduced Endurance

The infant with a primary problem of low endurance will generally have normal oral-motor control and normal coordination of the suck/swallow/breathe mechanism. Initially feeding will go well, but the baby stops early in the feeding (often by falling asleep), before taking an adequate volume. Even for the infant who is still awake and alert, attempting to push the baby to take more food often proves pointless. In other cases, decreased endurance will be manifest by frequent, lengthy pauses in sucking, and feeding sessions can become quite long. This is generally inefficient, as the infant uses more calories staying awake and attempting to feed than are being taken in. Either type of feeding behavior suggests that the baby (1) can no longer sustain the increased physiologic work of feeding, or (2) is no longer willing to sustain this work when its hunger has been temporarily satisfied.

Treatment Techniques

Regulating liquid flow: For some infants, the amount of liquid received at the beginning of the feeding (when the baby is most vigorous) can be increased. A softer nipple with a slightly larger hole will increase flow. Although many infants may be able to adequately coordinate swallowing and breathing with a faster flow, this must be carefully monitored so that respiratory compromise is not induced.

Manipulate feeding schedule: Limiting the length of the feeding session to the period during which the infant feeds most effectively will increase the efficiency of the feeding (i.e., the baby will use the least calories per amount taken). This may be as short as 5 to 10 minutes but should not exceed 30 minutes. The time interval between feedings may then also be reduced, with the added benefit that less volume will be required per feeding. Feedings could become as frequent as every two hours, though care must be taken to allow the infant adequate time to rest between feedings, so that available energy is concentrated on feeding. Two-hour feeding intervals, however, are not appropriate during the night, unless nursing care is available to the family.

Moving to a demand schedule, even in an infant with marginal intake, may increase intake, as the hunger drive can lead to longer or more vigorous feedings. When manipulating feeding schedules, even though the amount taken at each feeding may vary, care must be taken to meet 24-hour intake goals. Changes in feeding schedules must also take into account the family's needs and other demands on their schedule.

Nutritional supplements: An infant who is close to taking the required number of calories may benefit from increased caloric density of the food. Formula can be concentrated or supplements can be added to formula or breast milk to increase the number of calories received per ounce of liquid. Some babies cannot tolerate this increased caloric density or have special needs for fluid balance, so medical supervision and dietary consultation are needed.

Realistic expectations: Endurance problems are frustrating because the infant generally feeds well part of the time. Thus, it is hard to understand why the infant can't feed well all the time, and it is easy to hope that tomorrow will be the day the baby will be able to do it all. Setting realistic expectations may help parents and other caregivers cope with these frustrations and focus on other areas of change. This is a crucial issue in the management of feeding problems in this group of infants and is discussed in depth on page 264.

Respiratory Compromise

When the respiratory system is compromised by structural abnormalities or respiratory disease, there will be increased work of breathing. This "work of breathing" includes two components: activating the muscles that expand the lungs and overcoming resistance in the lung tissue and in the airway.[23] Infant respiratory distress syndrome (IRDS), bronchopulmonary dysplasia (BPD), reactive airway disease (RAD), tracheal stenosis, and musculoskeletal anomalies limiting chest wall expansion are examples of some of the respiratory problems that lead to increased work of breathing.

In a normally functioning individual, the work of breathing represents 5% to 10% of the total work of the body at rest. A similar percentage is maintained even during vigorous activity. In contrast, for the individual with respiratory disease/dysfunction, the work of breathing may be 40% of the total work of the body at rest. In this individual, the percentage of work for breathing may be even greater with activity. While the body may try to compensate by increasing the respiratory rate or heart rate, these mechanisms require additional work. In the infant with respiratory compromise, so much of the available energy for work is utilized by the cardiorespiratory system that there is little reserve for additional activity (such as feeding), with fatigue often resulting.

In addition, some respiratory diseases do not allow adequate gas exchange at the alveolar level. This can result in poorly oxygenated blood and inadequate oxygen supply for any increase in work, even the work of breathing. This compounds the problems of providing adequate resources for the additional work load of feeding. When there is increased work of breathing, other complications may also result. One condition related to feeding is gastroesophageal reflux (GER). A complete discussion of the relationship between respiratory compromise and GER is found in chapter 6.

There is a large range of severity in respiratory dysfunction, from the infant requiring only small amounts of additional oxygen to the infant requiring ongoing mechanical ventilation and possibly tracheostomy. The severity of the respiratory disease, combined with the expected rate of improvement, will affect the selection of treatment techniques. As respiratory problems often result in endurance problems, treatment techniques for endurance should also be considered (see page 258).

Treatment Techniques

Realistic expectations: Even among medical practitioners caring for infants, the high work load of feeding may not be appreciated. Thus, the impact of respiratory problems (particularly mild problems) may be overlooked. In addition, while a baby with respiratory problems may take its whole feeding orally if given adequate time, it can use so many calories in this process that weight gain is compromised. Reduced expectations are often appropriate (see page 264).

Dealing with increased respiratory rate: Infants with respiratory compromise can have a high respiratory rate at rest, or only during work (such as feeding). A very high respiratory rate can lead to disorganization in coordinating sucking and swallowing with breathing. Oxygen saturation may also drop if the infant cannot maintain the necessary rate and depth of respirations while interspersing breaths with swallowing. Aspiration becomes more likely, and apnea or bradycardia may occur, potentially making oral feeding unsafe. While some of the treatment techniques in this section may help to limit increases in respiratory rate, some guidelines are suggested:

- Resting respiratory rate (while awake) should not be above 70 to 75 breaths per minute prior to beginning a feeding session. For an infant who is chronically tachypneic, postponing nutritional oral feeding until the respiratory problems are more fully resolved should be considered. Therapeutic activities with small amounts of fluid may be possible.

- During a feeding session, if the respiratory rate goes beyond 80 to 85 BPM, feeding should be stopped. If the respiratory rate lowers after a brief rest, the feeding could be cautiously continued. If it remains elevated, the feeding should be terminated. Respiratory rate should be monitored during active feeding as well as during sucking pauses and breaks in the feeding. As most cardiorespiratory monitors give an average respiratory rate over 6 to 10 seconds, they may not be sensitive enough to give accurate readings of respiratory rate during brief sucking pauses.

Provide additional respiratory support: This may be done by using supplemental oxygen continuously or only during feeding, and/or providing further medical therapies, such as nebulizer treatments. Feedings may be timed to occur after nebulizer treatments to gain maximum benefit. Regarding the use of supplemental oxygen, three issues deserve discussion:

Ventilation versus perfusion. Providing additional oxygen will be effective only when there is a mismatch between ventilation (the amount of air, and thus oxygen, in the lungs) and perfusion (the ability of the alveoli to exchange gas). Therefore, providing additional oxygen will not be useful in all respiratory problems. Even if the infant has decreased oxygen saturation in the blood, if perfusion is poor, increasing the amount of oxygen will not improve the oxygen saturation in the blood. At the same time, the ventilation-perfusion ratio will change with increased work, so even though additional oxygen is not useful at rest, it may be needed during the increased work of feeding.

Oximetry to determine the need for additional oxygen. In many infants with respiratory dysfunction, the goal is to reduce the amount of supplemental oxygen that is needed. This process is often monitored by using continuous or intermittent oximetry readings (see chapter 2). The oxygen saturation in the blood is used as an indicator of the infant's need for additional oxygen and of the response when it is provided. Intermittent monitoring is often carried out when the baby is at rest, even sleeping, when oxygen needs are least. If supplemental oxygen is reduced following monitoring at those inactive times, when the infant is asked to do additional work, such as oral feeding, fatigue and decreased intake may result. Therefore, oximetry should also occur during times of "work" (such as feeding) to determine the infant's overall need for supplemental oxygen.

Assessment of response to supplemental oxygen. Measuring oxygen saturation via oximetry is only one method by which to judge the need to provide supplemental oxygen. In some cases, a baby with acceptable oxygen saturations may benefit from additional oxygen. The demands of feeding might also be reflected in an increased heart rate, respiratory rate, tidal volume, or stroke volume. A baby, therefore, could be experiencing considerable stress to the respiratory system during feeding, but the parameter affected would not be oxygen saturation; oximetry values could be normal. For this reason, changes in heart rate and subjective assessment of the infant's work of breathing during feeding (including nasal flaring, retractions, and the quantity of respiratory sounds) should be used as additional criteria when making decisions regarding the efficacy of supplemental oxygen.

Case example:
Robert was a former 27-week premature infant with severe chronic lung disease. At 11 months of age, he had just been discharged from the hospital, requiring 1 liter of oxygen by nasal canula and multiple medications. He was nippling all feeds, though weight gain was poor. Prior to feeding, respiratory rate was 50 BPM and heart rate was 130-140 BPM. With feeding, respiratory rate moved to 65-70 BPM and heart rate went to 190-195 BPM. Oxygen saturation with feeding, as measured by oximetry, was adequate. Markedly increased respiratory effort with sternal retractions, labored breathing, and fatigue were noted during feeding.

Increasing the amount of supplemental oxygen during feeding over baseline amounts led to the heart rate elevating only to 160 BPM, with less respiratory effort and fatigue noted. This case illustrates the point that infants may benefit from additional oxygen support with feeding, even though oximetry during feeding is "normal."

A study by Groothius and Rosenburg lends support to the concept that prolonged respiratory support through supplemental oxygen leads to greater weight gain in infants with lung disease.[24] Two groups of infants with bronchopulmonary dysplasia (BPD) were studied. Group A was on a conservative, slow regimen to wean oxygen support, both in the hospital and at home. Oximetry occurred during a variety of activities, including feeding, and saturations were maintained at specified values over several days or weeks before weaning. While group B was managed similarly in the hospital, after discharge oxygen support was weaned more aggressively. While group A demonstrated a growth rate similar to full-term newborns, group B showed a slower rate of weight gain.

External pacing: Some babies with respiratory problems automatically use a pattern of short sucking bursts (see page 254) to compensate for respiratory compromise. Other infants may benefit from having this pattern imposed upon them. Even though an infant with respiratory problems may have a "normal" rhythm of sucking, swallowing, and breathing, the respirations during continuous sucking bursts may not be frequent or deep enough to provide adequate oxygenation during feeding.

The feeding specialist can assist the infant by removing the bottle after two to three sucks, thus imposing a breathing pause. The infant should take several deep breaths before returning to feeding. For some babies it may be sufficient to simply break the suction by inserting a finger into the corner of the mouth while leaving the nipple in place. Tilting the bottle downward to stop the flow of liquid may also be effective. Throughout the feeding, the feeding specialist may want to "test" the infant's self-pacing by leaving the bottle in the infant's mouth longer. Note whether the baby pauses frequently to breathe; the coordination of sucking, swallowing, and breathing; and the baby's overall comfort level. Later in the feeding, when the infant is less eager in its sucking, self-pacing may meet the infant's respiratory needs, and this technique may no longer be necessary.

Case example:
Kramer was a 30-week premature infant who required mechanical ventilation for one week and supplemental oxygen for four more weeks. He was nippling all of his feeds by 7 weeks, when he was discharged from the hospital.

He was referred for outpatient feeding evaluation at 12 weeks of age (2 weeks corrected age) due to prolonged feedings and poor endurance, though weight gain had been adequate. Initially, he was awake and eager to feed, with a respiratory rate of 50-60 BPM. He showed normal oral-motor coordination and strong sucking. He demonstrated the typical pattern of an initial continuous sucking burst, coordinating breathing well. Air swallowing was indicated by the sound of the swallows. He soon looked uncomfortable, with eye widening and slight squirming. He initiated a sucking pause, characterized by a respiratory rate of 80 breaths per minute.

Although Kramer had been breathing regularly during the sucking burst, the rate and depth of respirations were not adequate to meet his needs, leading to a marked increase in respiratory rate during sucking pauses to recover. After giving him a rest period and allowing his respiratory rate to lessen, feeding was resumed. This time external pacing was provided, breaking the suction after two to three sucks and allowing five to six consecutive breaths. The feeding continued with Kramer staying calm, demonstrating considerably less air swallowing, and taking one ounce of formula in five to six minutes. After burping, he initiated a self-pacing pattern of short sucking bursts. The feeding was completed 10 minutes later without obvious fatigue.

When this external pacing technique was used at home, Kramer was calmer during feedings, took his feeding more quickly, was less fatigued, and spit up less frequently. While he had adequate respiratory status at rest, the increased work of feeding (particularly in the early, vigorous portion of the meal) stressed his respiratory and coordination mechanisms, leading to feeding problems. Helping to organize his sucking, swallowing, and breathing in a slightly different manner through external pacing provided better support for oral feeding.

Increased nutritional requirements: As discussed earlier, to perform work the body needs a source of adequate calories and adequate oxygen to burn the calories. When there is increased work of breathing, an infant may need a greater number of calories to support that work and still gain weight appropriately. When developing a nutritional plan to achieve good weight gain, the need for additional calories must be considered. If increased volume is not tolerated, increasing the caloric density of the formula may be possible. Such modifications to the infant's diet should be supervised by a qualified nutritionist or physician.

Establishing Realistic Expectations

When an infant is chronically ill or has a complex feeding disorder, establishing realistic expectations for oral feeding is a difficult task. It requires skill in balancing the medical and nutritional needs of the infant with the parents' needs and expectations, as well as the infant's need to develop or maintain oral feeding skills. This process is difficult regardless of the source of the feeding problem, but it is most frequently an issue with babies who have problems with respiratory support and endurance. Oral feeding skills are generally intact, and it is often unclear how underlying cardiorespiratory problems will progress. This frequently leads to ongoing optimism. In addition, progress in oral feeding and/or reduction in respiratory support are often seen as primary indicators of medical progress. This can lead to enthusiastic pursuit of these goals and the perception of failure on the part of the infant or caregiver if the goals are not readily achieved.

Setting realistic expectations may require changing the way in which progress is measured. We propose that the primary goal for such infants should be good overall growth. This promotes improvement in medical status and supports development. Good growth requires adequate nutritional intake in addition to reasonable caloric expenditure. Improvement in medical status often hinges on growth, particularly in disease processes such as BPD, where overall linear growth is an indicator of growth of healthy lung tissue, or in congenital heart disease, where surgical repair of the defect may not occur until a specified weight is achieved.

Although oral feeding is of great importance and is the first choice in feeding methods, it often comes at a high price to a sick infant. The cost may be fatigue and lack of energy for other activities and/or increased caloric expenditure and poor weight gain. When respiratory support is at borderline levels, endurance for feeding and intake may be further compromised, also leading to poor weight gain. When the cost of feeding an infant orally is high, methods of providing supplemental nutrition should be considered. This decision should be viewed as a *support* for the infant's ongoing growth and medical improvement, rather than the last resort after failure of oral feeding on the part of the infant or caregivers.

In the long run, reducing expectations in the area of oral feeding and supporting the use of supplemental feeding methods or additional respiratory support may be of great service to both parents and babies. As expectations for oral feeding become more realistic (i.e., match the baby's actual abilities), the feeding sessions can focus on the quality of the baby's oral control and on the parent-child interaction. When parents do not have to worry about pushing in every last drop of nutrient, they may be able to relax, enjoy their baby, and renew the bonding process that has been interrupted by the infant's illness or feeding problem. When expectations are reasonably matched to the infant's capacities, parents' feelings of competence are reinforced.

The changing medical status of chronically ill babies is another important consideration in developing appropriate expectations. Babies with respiratory disease or endurance problems frequently have changes in their medical status. There are changes in medication or attempts at weaning from a ventilator or oxygen, in addition to the medical setbacks even a common virus can cause. Any of these changes may impact the level of respiratory support or endurance available for feeding, thereby compromising the baby's intake. If a mechanism for providing supplemental nutritional support is built into an infant's feeding regime, these setbacks will be easier to handle. As the baby's oral intake declines, or effort involved in feeding increases due to a change in medical status, nutrition can be maintained through the support of supplemental non-oral feeding methods. As the baby improves, support can be reduced.

Case example:
Richard was a former 26-week premature infant with severe bronchopulmonary dysplasia. Mechanical ventilation was required for seven months. At 10 months of age, weighing only 10 pounds, he was discharged home with continued severe chronic lung disease. He required oxygen by nasal canula, multiple medications, and extensive home nursing care. He was nippling all of his feedings, which had been one of the goals for discharge.

Richard was rehospitalized at a different hospital one week after discharge due to increasing respiratory problems and poor feeding. As oral feeding was restarted, Richard had difficulty nippling all of his feedings. Clinical feeding evaluation showed that he had adequate oral-motor skills and enthusiastic interest in eating. Respiratory and heart rates were somewhat elevated at rest and showed appropriate increases with feeding. Work of breathing, however, was increased, with sternal retractions and a labored quality to his breathing, both of which were more noticeable during feeding. He took 2 ounces quickly but needed much encouragement to take further amounts.

With this degree of lung disease, the slow rate of improvement, *very poor* growth rate, and increased work of breathing required during feeding, the medical team decided that the expectation for Richard to be a full oral feeder was inappropriate. The cost of full oral feeding was too high and most likely had compromised his weight gain.

Supplemental nutrition by gavage tube was implemented, though limited oral feeding was maintained due to Richard's strong skill and interest. Richard was nippled throughout the day, with continuous-drip feedings given through a nasogastric tube at night. Nippling was limited to 2 ounces at a time, which appeared to be his natural cut-off point. Richard was given a bottle as often as every two hours when he was awake. Two-thirds of his daily intake was by bottle and one-third occurred at night through the tube.

Over one month, Richard's growth in all parameters was described as "outstanding" by the nutritionist. He showed greater gains than in any of the previous months. Modifying the oral feeding expectations for Richard was a key factor in achieving this kind of growth. While the parents had been very resistant to any tube feeding, having been led to believe that Richard could take all of his feedings by bottle, they commented that they felt less stress around feeding time and could enjoy it more when the intake requirements were eliminated.

Non-oral and Supplemental Feeding Methods

Babies should be fed orally to whatever degree is possible for them. Oral feeding in infancy builds the motoric and sensory foundations for more mature oral-feeding skills, as well as oral communication.[4] It also provides comfort and opportunities for bonding with the parent or caregiver. In addition, it builds the connection between oral activity and satiation of hunger. As discussed above, however, for some infants full oral feeding is not possible or is not in their best interest for maintenance of growth and medical improvement. In these cases, non-oral feeding methods are appropriate.

Establishing the Need for Non-oral Feeding

Numerous factors must be considered in making the decision to provide all or some of an infant's nutrition by non-oral means. These include:

Safety of oral feeding: Aspiration poses the greatest risk to the safety of infants during feeding, as food aspirated into the lungs can lead to respiratory disease. When an infant is known to aspirate, is suspected to aspirate, or is at risk for aspiration, non-oral feeding methods may be required (see page 228).

Effectiveness of oral feeding: The ultimate measure of feeding effectiveness is weight gain, which reflects the volume taken in as well as total caloric expenditure. In the face of poor weight gain, and when treatment techniques to facilitate oral feeding have not been fully successful, non-oral feeding methods may be appropriate. Not only can intake often be increased, but the caloric expenditure associated with intake of food is virtually eliminated.

Expectations: While the safety of feeding and weight gain are the primary factors that should be considered in moving to non-oral feeding methods, the expected medical course must also be considered.

An infant with aspiration that appears to be corrected by therapeutic techniques may be allowed to remain a full oral feeder until there is evidence that those techniques are no longer effective in preventing aspiration. On the other hand, an infant who has significant aspiration that does not respond to modifications may immediately become fully fed by non-oral means.

An infant recovering from an acute respiratory infection such as RSV may show poor feeding intake and weight gain. If the baby's weight is adequate and there are no other complicating factors, this pattern may be allowed for a short time, knowing that intake should increase as the respiratory status fully resolves.

In considering the expected medical course, realistic expectations are called for (see page 264). Although medical practitioners often favor optimism in the area of feeding and prefer limited use of non-oral feeding methods, non-oral nutritional support may ultimately be beneficial for both the infant and the parent.

Social factors: Social considerations must also play a role in determining the use of non-oral feeding methods. The parents' skill in orally feeding a difficult baby, as well as their other responsibilities, may limit the time they are able to spend feeding a difficult infant. On the other hand, some parents are not capable of managing the simple care of the tubes used in non-oral feeding.

Options for Non-oral Feedings

There are two basic routes for nourishing the infant or child. The first is *enteral* feeding, where nourishment moves through the digestive tract. The second is to provide *parenteral* nutrition, where nutrient bypasses the alimentary canal and enters the circulatory system directly. Obviously the types of nutrients that are given in these situations will be different.

There are non-oral means of providing nutrition in each of these categories. When total parenteral nutrition (TPN) or hyperalimentation is provided, by definition all nutrition is non-oral as it bypasses the digestive system. Peripheral intravenous lines or central arterial lines may be used to administer parenteral nutrition. Parenteral nutrition can also be provided in conjunction with oral or non-oral enteral feeding.

Enteral nutrition is accomplished through oral feeding and/or non-oral methods using tubes such as nasogastric tube, gastrostomy tube, or jejunal tube. The options for providing non-oral enteral feeding by tube will be discussed in detail below and are summarized in table 5-1.

Nasogastric and Orogastric Gavage Tubes

A slender, flexible gavage tube is passed through either the nose or the mouth into the stomach. It can be removed and replaced for each feeding, or it can be taped in place and left "indwelling" for several days before changing. Most often gavage tubes are threaded through the nose to the stomach (the nasogastric or NG tube). Oral gavage tubes (orogastric or OG tubes) may be used with very small babies or in infants with restrictions of airflow through the nasal passages. Delivery of liquids can be via bolus (the total feeding is delivered over a 15- to 20-minute period) or via continuous drip feedings. In the latter method, liquid is slowly and continuously dripped into the tube via a portable pump set at a specified rate, for example, 30 cc per hour. The pump can be used continuously over 24 hours or for any portion of the day.

Table 5-1 Strengths and Limitations of Various Feeding Tubes

Type of feeding tube	Insertion/Destination	Strengths	Limitations
Nasogastric tube (NG)	Nose/stomach	– No surgical placement required – Oral feeding possible with tube in place	– Insertion and presence in nose/ throat is uncomfortable and may be aversive – May trigger vagally mediated bradycardia – May be cosmetically unacceptable for long-term use
Orogastric tube (OG)	Mouth/stomach	– No surgical placement	– Same as NG, plus difficult to feed orally with tube in place
Duodenal tube	Nose/duodenum	– No surgical placement – Bypasses stomach so decreases risk of GE reflux	– Same as NG, though softer, so may have fewer hypersensitive responses – Must use continuous-drip feeding – Difficult to place and maintain in correct position
Gastrostomy (standard, percutaneous, button)	Surgically placed in stomach	– No aversive oral-facial stimuli – Despite surgical placement, can be removed easily when no longer needed – Sits beneath clothing, cosmetically acceptable	– Requires surgical placement – Site needs daily care and possibly trip to medical facility if tube falls out – Potential risk for increased GE reflux after tube placed
Jejunostomy	Tube surgically placed in jejunum, possibly in association with gastrostomy	– Same as gastrostomy – Bypasses stomach, so reduces risk of GE reflux	– Requires surgical placement – Site needs daily care, requires trip to hospital if tube falls out – Requires continuous-drip feedings

Positive features include:

- Gavage tubes are extremely temporary and require no surgical placement. They are a good choice if supplemental feedings are needed only intermittently or are expected to be needed for a short time.

- Most parents can easily be taught the procedures for placing and caring for these tubes if gavage feedings need to be continued at home.

Negative features include:

- Insertion of a gavage tube can be very uncomfortable for a baby and therefore stressful for the parents. Older babies show particularly strong negative responses as their awareness of the tube increases and their developing memory allows anticipation of the event.

- Insertion can become so aversive to the child that it contributes to hypersensitive and aversive responses to other oral stimuli, sometimes interfering with oral feeding or the development of skills leading to oral feeding. The more often the tube is placed, the more frequent the aversive stimulation.

- An indwelling tube, while placed less frequently, may also be irritating and/or aversive to the oral, nasal, or pharyngeal areas. Taping on the infant's face, which is required to secure the tube in place, can also be aversive to some babies.

- For some babies, the gavage tube can be an ongoing stimulus for the gag reflex, leading to a hyperactive gag response, even when the tube is not present.

- Placement of the tube through the nose or the mouth has the potential to stimulate a vagally mediated bradycardia in some infants.

- The indwelling gavage tube may be cosmetically unacceptable for some parents. Parents may be reluctant to have an obvious symbol of disability when taking their baby out in public. It may be a source of unsolicited embarrassing and/or annoying questions.

While the aversive sensory features of gavage tubes are a primary drawback, our experience is that an indwelling tube generally presents substantially less aversive stimuli than a tube placed at each feeding. This is particularly noticeable in older, more aware babies. The indwelling NG tube is more stable than the indwelling OG tube and does not have as many negative effects on the development of oral-motor control. In addition, the smaller the diameter and the more flexible the tube, the less aversive the stimuli. Bolus feeding may be slower through a smaller tube, but taking a few extra minutes to give a feeding may be a reasonable trade-off for increased comfort. One method of maximizing the positive features of the NG tube and minimizing the negative features is to use the tube only at night, if some oral feeding is possible during the day. It is inserted only one time per day and is in place at night while the child is asleep and least aware of it.

In some centers concern has been raised regarding the impact of indwelling NG tubes on respiratory function. It is believed that the presence of the tube can reduce the size of the nasal airway enough that ventilation might be compromised. Greenspan et al. studied this issue in two groups of infants (<2kg and >2kg).[43] Monitoring respiratory function with a 5 french tube placed either orally or nasally, they found no influence on respiratory status in babies over 2 kg, regardless of tube location. In the smaller infants, however, significant reduction in ventilation was noted with the NG, but not the OG, tube in place. This suggests that the infant's size should be considered when deciding whether a tube should be positioned with each feeding or left indwelling.

Gastrostomy

A gastrostomy (g-tube) is a surgically created fistula through the abdominal wall and into the stomach.[25] A tube is placed through this fistula into the stomach, where it remains to be used for feeding. Common gastrostomy tubes or catheters are the de Pezzer, the Malecot, and the Foley. Their function is essentially the same, although their method of insertion and securing may be different. These tubes are opened for bolus feedings, then sealed with a clamp and secured beneath a child's clothing when the feeding is completed. Gastrostomy tubes can also be kept open and used for continuous drip pump feedings.

Another device, the gastrostomy button, is also available and is increasingly being used with pediatric patients. The "button" is a one-way valve from the stomach to skin level. The closure is similar to that of a snap-top bottle. This is opened for feedings and a longer feeding tube is inserted.[26] After the feeding, this tube is removed and the button is closed, flush with the skin. The gastrostomy button eliminates tubes that may be accidentally pulled out, has less potential to leak, and is easier to conceal under clothing than conventional gastrostomy tubes.

Positive aspects of the gastrostomy include:

- There is no aversive oral or facial stimulus associated with its placement or use. The tube is always available, so there is no aversive procedure prior to using it.

- Despite surgical placement, it is temporary. When supplemental feedings are no longer needed, the gastrostomy tube can be pulled out and the fistula allowed to seal and heal.

- It is cosmetically acceptable to parents, as it can be hidden under clothing.

- While the tube is placed into the stomach, it does not limit the child's positioning or movement in any way. Babies roll over and lie on gastrostomy tubes without problem.

Negative aspects of gastrostomy tubes include:

- For infants, placing a gastrostomy tube generally requires a surgical procedure under general anesthesia. Some babies may not be appropriate surgical candidates due to their underlying medical problems, and thus a gastrostomy is not possible. Some parents are leery of exposing their child to anesthesia and do not want the child to have a scar once the g-tube is removed. A procedure called a percutaneous endoscopic gastrostomy (PEG) does not require a general anesthesia and may circumvent some of these problems.[27] This procedure often has fairly stringent patient selection criteria that may potentially limit its use.

- There is the potential for an increase in gastroesophageal reflux following the placement of the g-tube. Careful evaluation of an infant's GER status before, and monitoring after, g-tube placement are needed.

- The g-tube site needs daily care to prevent infection and insure proper placement.

- A trip to the emergency room may be needed if the tube comes out and the family is not trained in replacement or if the type of g-tube used makes home replacement difficult.

Other Types of Tubes

In addition to nasogastric and gastrostomy tubes, a number of other tubes are increasingly being used to provide nutritional supplementation to infants with complex feeding disorders. These tubes can be inserted to the duodenum (duo tube) or the jejunum (j-tube or jejunostomy), with both destinations lying below the stomach. The tubes can be routed through the nose (similar to an NG tube) or surgically through the skin (similar to a gastrostomy and often in association with a g-tube). These types of tubes are utilized when the baby has significant intolerance to foods being placed in the stomach, resulting in frank emesis or severe gastroesophageal reflux. For some infants, these tubes are the only means of providing adequate and safe nutrition.

When the tubes are placed through the nose, the positive and negative features are similar to NG tubes, though it is generally more difficult to achieve and maintain proper placement. When surgically placed through the abdomen, the positive and negative features are similar to the gastrostomy. As both tubes empty into smaller areas of the digestive tract below the stomach, bolus feeding is not possible, and continuous-drip feedings are required. In addition, these tubes require slightly more daily care than others to cleanse and assure proper functioning.

Decision Making regarding Type of Tube

When tube feeding is required, there is often much discussion regarding the appropriate type of tube, in particular the NG tube versus the gastrostomy. Initially, regardless of the baby's age, supplementation can occur by NG tube. If it appears that the infant's need for supplementation will be brief (less than two to four months) or the need will be extremely intermittent, it is appropriate to use the NG tube. If, however, if appears that supplementation will be required for longer than three to four months, the placement of a gastrostomy is warranted.[28] Additionally, all babies who require tracheostomy for long-term assisted ventilation should receive a gastrostomy. Even if oral function improves dramatically following tracheostomy, respiratory status is obviously significantly compromised when a tracheostomy and ongoing assisted ventilation are required. Babies in these cases generally lack adequate respiratory support for feeding and have a high likelihood of medical setbacks, making it unlikely that they will achieve and maintain full oral feeding within four months after the tracheostomy.

Often the length of time that supplemental feedings will be needed is not apparent at the outset of treatment. The feeding specialist and the rest of the medical team may feel that the baby will progress quickly and soon no longer need tube feedings, so the method of supplementation chosen is the NG. But as time progresses, the feeding problems appear more pervasive or medical problems do not resolve as quickly as anticipated and it becomes apparent that supplemental feeding will be needed for a long time. At this juncture, moving to gastrostomy feeding is appropriate and may have beneficial secondary effects. The g-tube may decrease the amount of oral aversive stimuli, perhaps allowing increased oral skill.

Many parents and professionals, however, find it difficult to make the transition to a g-tube. Since it requires a surgical procedure, it may appear to signal a more permanent and chronic nature to the feeding disorder. Certainly this is a frightening thought for many parents. If, however, the need to move to a gastrostomy is presented as another way to support the child's best feeding performance and an easier method for the parent to manage, the idea may be met with less resistance.

Methods of Utilizing Non-oral Feeding

Making the decision to provide non-oral nutrition is not an all-or-none decision. Various strategies are available for incorporating it into an infant's total nutritional package. These possibilities should be considered during the decision-making process regarding non-oral feeding.

Full non-oral feedings: This is selected for the baby who is not able to feed orally for reasons of motoric deficit, extreme tactile hypersensitivity/aversion, state or arousal problems, medical conditions that preclude oral feeding, or any combination of these factors. This method is also selected when uncorrectable swallowing dysfunction leads to aspiration, compromising health. Even though all feedings are non-oral, a program of oral-motor therapy must be provided. Not only should it address the primary area of dysfunction, but existing oral-motor skills should be maintained for future oral feeding and speech.[44] One simple component of such a program is to routinely encourage use of a pacifier during tube feedings.[34] Oral-tactile responses should also be addressed in an effort to prevent hypersensitivity and oral aversions from developing due to lack of oral input. This will facilitate oral hygiene as well as the possible return to oral feeding (see page 247).

Non-oral nutrition with therapeutic oral feeding: The majority of nutrition is provided non-orally, as some aspect of the oral feeding process is severely limited. Feeding-related functions, however, show adequate competence to allow the infant to complete a small amount of feeding in a safe manner. This oral feeding component generally utilizes therapeutic techniques aimed at improving skills and moving toward larger amounts of oral feeding.

Reduced volume oral feeds with non-oral supplementation: This method is used for the infant who is safe with oral feeding but cannot take full feeds by mouth or does so at great physiologic cost. The infant is generally allowed to feed as much as possible within certain parameters (i.e., length of feeding and frequency of feeding are stipulated), with the balance by non-oral means. Various scheduling combinations are possible, some of which are described below.

Schedules for Non-oral Supplemental Feeding

Once the route for supplemental feeding has been decided, the schedule used for providing supplemental nutrition needs to be established. Many combinations are possible. The one selected will be based on the infant's nutritional needs and the goals of feeding intervention.

Limit nippling at each feeding: Nipple the infant at each feeding using appropriate techniques and staying within the infant's respiratory and endurance limits. Any amount that the baby is not able to nipple at that feeding is given through the feeding tube. This method can be used only when a feeding tube is in place (indwelling gavage tube or gastrostomy). Attempting to place a gavage tube immediately after nippling a feeding often leads to gagging and emesis. When this technique is used, the baby has repeated practice at feeding, with the emphasis on the quality of intake, yet the full caloric needs are backed up by the tube. This is frequently the procedure used when premature babies are beginning to feed.

Alternate nipple feedings with tube feedings: The baby should be close to taking full volume during nippling at a single feeding, since the amount not nippled is then added to the required amount at the next feeding, which is given by tube. This method can be used when there is not a tube in place, as it can be inserted prior to the feeding, when emesis is unlikely. If a tube is in place, the infant may take a smaller amount at the nippled feeding and the balance can be given by tube as described above.

Another variation of this schedule is to allow the baby to nipple feed without supplementation for two consecutive feedings. The amount not taken at each of these feedings is noted, and the baby is gavaged the entire third feeding plus the remainder from the two previous feedings. Again, the baby should be close to taking a full feeding so that the amount remaining plus a full feed is not too large an amount for the baby to handle.

These methods may be appropriate for babies with limited endurance, in which case it is not reasonable to expose them to the demands of oral feeding every few hours. Again, these methods may be used when nipple feeding is introduced to premature babies.

Daytime oral feedings and nighttime tube feedings: In this method, the baby is allowed to nipple as much as possible on demand or a schedule during the day. At night, the balance of the 24-hour caloric needs can be delivered by the tube, using the bolus or the continuous-drip method. Nighttime feeding by continuous drip allows the parents greater opportunity to sleep and supplies the baby with maximal calories for minimal energy expenditure.

The infant is also given maximal opportunity to be an oral feeder. Feeding may improve as the baby becomes progressively more hungry throughout the day. This day/night alternation can be evenly divided into 12-hour segments or any arrangement that meets the child's and the family's needs (for example, 16 hours on the pump and 8 hours nippling).

As with many aspects of infant feeding programs, changes in feeding schedule should be undertaken only in consultation with, and under supervision of, a physician or nutritionist. For additional material regarding nutritional requirements of premature and full-term infants and young children, the reader is referred to Pipes.[29]

Transition from Tube to Oral Feeding

Laying the Groundwork

Ideally, the time to begin the process of moving from tube to oral feeding is the point at which non-oral feeding (including hyperalimentation) is begun. Immediately initiating a comprehensive and relatively aggressive oral-therapy program can improve the speed and success of this transition for some children, particularly infants with normal oral-motor skills who are expected to return to oral feeding within 6 to 12 months. Primary features of this ongoing oral-therapy program should include the following:

- Minimizing negative or aversive oral stimulation.

- Promoting pleasurable oral-tactile experiences and age-appropriate oral exploration.

- Maintaining or building oral-motor skills. For the infant, maintaining sucking skills and interest in sucking may be critical.

- Continuing the association of oral activity with satisfaction of hunger. This can easily be done by having the infant suck on a pacifier during tube feeding. In premature babies, using this procedure has resulted in taking full nipple feedings sooner, better weight gain, and earlier hospital discharge.[34]

- Maintaining *whatever* degree of oral feeding is safe and effective. In our experience, continuing with some degree of limited sucking and swallowing or spoon feeding helps to maintain more effective oral-motor skills, swallowing, and tolerance of tactile and taste input. When it becomes possible, these skills are then *expanded* rather than *introduced.* Following are examples of this principle.

  - An infant struggling with oral feeding due to poor endurance was started on tube feedings. Oral feeding was not maintained, and the infant quickly lost all interest in taking a bottle, even when endurance improved.

- An infant had been fully orally fed but was found to have silent aspiration, so tube feedings were begun. Oral feeding was not allowed, and two months later the infant would not suck on a bottle or allow a spoon in her mouth. It is critical to determine if *some* level of oral feeding is safe, otherwise feeding skills that were present may be lost quickly.

- An infant with micrognathia and apnea with feeding was found to have poor pharyngeal clearance and occasional microaspiration. Tube feedings were begun, but he was allowed to take 15 cc of water by bottle three times per day (in association with tube feedings). Three months later, swallowing had improved, and he was gradually returned to full oral feedings by slowly increasing the amount taken by nipple and changing it to formula.

- An infant with significant bowel loss from necrotizing enterocolitis received total parenteral nutrition. The baby was expected to take months to be able to tolerate more than slow drip feedings through the digestive track. "Sham" oral feedings were initiated and carried out daily. The baby nippled small amounts, which drained out of the stomach through the gastrostomy. Six months later his digestive tract could manage 30-cc bolus feedings, which the infant took by bottle, along with small amounts of semisolids by mouth. Parenteral nutrition was still required for the balance, but as the digestive tract continued to improve, oral-feeding skills were in place and ready for larger volumes.

- Consistency. Whatever program is established needs to be carried out regularly, at least daily, and short programs carried out more often may be the most effective. Just as breast-fed infants who are given a bottle on a regular basis are more likely to continue taking the bottle than those given a bottle only occasionally, babies who consistently utilize adaptive oral-motor skills and tactile responses are more likely to maintain those skills than babies who do not consistently use them.

Unfortunately, many factors may interfere with returning to oral feeding in a timely manner and/or maintaining an aggressive ongoing program focused on this goal. These include the need for *exclusive* tube feedings, prolonged need for tube feeding, oral hypersensitivity and aversion, oral-motor control problems, and developmental delay. For infants and children fed exclusively by NG or gastrostomy tube for long periods, a point may be reached when some member of the team (parent, physician, feeding specialist) would like to take a more aggressive approach toward returning to full oral feeding. At this point, both the child's readiness and the parent or family's readiness must be addressed prior to instituting a program designed to make the transition back to oral feeding.

The transition back to oral feeding is often a lengthy and difficult process. The ill-advised statement "he will eat when he is hungry" does not apply. It is rare that a single event or treatment method is powerful enough to effect the transition from tube to oral feeding. This transition must be seen as a *process* that occurs over time and involves many treatment strategies. Because barriers to this transition include medical, physical, and psychosocial factors, treatments and interventions must address all of these areas.[44]

For both parents and feeding specialists, this transition is usually longer than ever imagined. It sometimes takes years, even when oral therapy has been ongoing. Acknowledging the length of this process at the outset may serve to decrease both therapist and parent frustration over the course of treatment. One way to deal with the frustration that accompanies a lengthy transition process is to set goals that reflect steps in the process rather than the final outcome. For example, the goal may be "playing with or tasting food" rather than eating a meal. If eating is the sole goal, the pressure to meet that goal is great.

Determining the Child's Readiness

Determining a child's readiness to begin the transition to oral feeding involves:

- understanding the original medical condition that resulted in the tube feeding, as well as the child's current medical condition;
- establishing the level and quality of oral-motor skills; and
- determining the status of swallowing abilities.

These factors form the basis of patient selection and can ultimately affect the outcome of the intervention program.

Original Medical Condition Resulting in Tube Feeding

It may seem obvious to state that one needs to know the reason a child was tube fed in the first place. However, the longer the child has been tube fed and the greater the number of facilities where the child has received care, the more likely this original cause will be obscured or unknown. It is essential, however, that one determine whether the original condition that resulted in the tube feeding has been corrected or stabilized. If not, the child is probably not a candidate to begin the transition to full oral feeding. For example, if poor endurance secondary to a congenital heart defect was the factor that led to tube feeding, one needs to determine if the defect has been repaired or the child has developed sufficient endurance to be an oral feeder.

After determining the original reason for the tube feeding, the child's current medical status must be well understood. Not only must information be gathered on function relating to the original feeding problem, but the nutritional status must be evaluated, and the feeding specialist must be aware of any other medical problems that might impact a treatment program focusing on the reintroduction of oral feeding.

Case example:
Sheri was a former 27-week premature infant who required a lengthy course of mechanical ventilation during her initial hospitalization. She was finally weaned from the ventilator to oxygen via nasal cannula. Oral feeding was not begun at this point due to continued and significant respiratory distress. She was discharged home at 7 months of age, still requiring oxygen and being fed primarily through continuous-drip gastrostomy feedings.

She was followed through a community-based therapy program and a pulmonary clinic at a children's hospital. At 20 months of age, mother requested a hospital-based occupational therapy assessment to determine if Sheri might be able to move to oral feeding as her primary means of nutrition. By her mother's report, Sheri was taking some "tastes" of pureed foods, though with much resistance, and her major means of nutrition was continuous-drip feedings at night. She barely tolerated the oral-tactile normalization program developed by her home therapist. Her mother's frustration was obvious as she relayed the history. She was tired of the whole process and wanted Sheri to be eating normally.

As this history was taken, Sheri demonstrated immense respiratory effort. Her breathing was labored with forceful exhalation. When she began to cry, she had immediate color change, despite being on 1 liter of oxygen via nasal cannula. In addition, she still received nebulizer treatments throughout the day.

It was obvious that because Sheri's respiratory disease remained severe, tube feedings were still required. Not only did Sheri lack sufficient respiratory support to meet the demands of a program transitioning to total oral feeding, but she probably also lacked sufficient endurance to take all her needed nutrition by mouth, even if she had been more accepting of oral-feeding activities. Thus, she was not a candidate to begin an aggressive program of eliminating tube feedings, although it was important that her current oral-tactile therapy program continue.

Quality of Oral-Motor Control
Frequently tube feeding is instituted when poor oral-motor control does not allow adequate oral intake. Abnormal oral-motor patterns may result in extremely slow and inefficient feeding, leading to poor nutritional intake and unrealistic time demands on the parent. In this case, prior to beginning

---

the transition to oral feeding, the quality of oral control must be assessed to determine if there has been sufficient change to allow safe feeding in a *reasonable length of time*. If not, then partial or total tube feeding may continue to be in the child's best interest.

Case example:
Candy was a 2-year-old girl with severe mixed spastic/athetoid cerebral palsy. Although she was followed in her public school by occupational, physical, and speech therapy, her mother requested an outside consultation to establish an aggressive program leading to oral feeding. Candy's primary nutrition was by bolus feedings through a gastrostomy tube, although at home she did receive small amounts of many foods by mouth.

On evaluation, Candy had significant motoric abnormalities. It was even difficult for her to sit in her adapted wheelchair because of involuntary, dystonic movements and intermittent extensor thrusts. Her oral control showed a similar level of impairment, with marked tongue and jaw thrust, tonic bite reflex, and stereotyped tongue movements. On videofluoroscopy, she demonstrated aspiration of thin liquids but an adequate pharyngeal swallow with pureed textures. Despite these marked oral and motoric disabilities, she did show an interest in food, seemed to enjoy feeding sessions with her mother, and had food preferences.

The severity of Candy's gross motor and oral-motor impairment, plus the length of time needed to feed her, made it unlikely that she would ever be a totally oral feeder. Therefore the goal of transitioning to greater amounts of oral feeding was not realistic. It appeared more appropriate to focus on "recreational eating." Mother could then focus on the quality of Candy's oral control, allow her to enjoy some of her favorite foods (prepared to create a safe texture for swallowing), and enjoy the social aspects of eating with her daughter.

Swallowing Abilities

Finally, it must be determined whether the child's swallowing ability is adequate to allow safe feeding. The method of choice to evaluate swallowing function is the videofluoroscopic swallowing study (VFSS). Once safe swallowing has been established, parents and feeding specialists can proceed in giving increasingly larger amounts by mouth without fear of compromising the child's health. At times this knowledge may help parents and feeding specialists persevere if the child shows strong behavioral opposition to oral feeding.

Often tube feeding is initiated for reasons unrelated to swallowing ability, possibly before the baby has been fed by mouth. In these cases, the status and safety of swallowing is generally unknown, so swallowing dysfunction is possible. This is somewhat more likely if there are other problems in neuromuscular control or if the baby had a prolonged intubation. Therefore the safety of swallowing should be addressed before proceeding aggressively with an oral-feeding program.

For the child's swallow to be evaluated on VFSS, he or she needs to be able to swallow a small amount of barium. Yet if the child is resistant to swallowing, therapy will be necessary to develop acceptance of swallowing prior to the VFSS. However, if the safety of the child's swallow is unknown, the feeding specialist should be cautious in selecting a substance for therapeutic swallowing activities. In this case, the best substance to use appears to be sterile water (see page 230).

The child may also need an aggressive oral-tactile normalization program in order to tolerate the small amount of liquid or semisolid required to get a meaningful swallowing study. While not all children need a VFSS prior to initiating the transition to oral feeding, if there is any indication of potential swallowing dysfunction this test should be considered. Appropriate activities should then be planned to prepare the child to provide an adequate sampling of swallowing.

Letting Go of Oral-Feeding Goals
When abnormal oral-motor control or other medical conditions have led to tube feeding, ongoing therapy programs generally have a strong focus on maintaining or improving oral-motor skills and other underlying functions in the hope that sufficient change will take place to allow nutritional oral feeding. At some point it may become apparent, however, that moving to oral feeding for primary nutrition is unlikely to ever happen. This could be due to the degree of oral-motor impairment and/or lack of change or the lack of improvement in medical status. This awareness often leads to a shift in the focus and goals of the therapy program. To accomplish this move away from the goal of oral feeding in a manner that supports the child and family, a number of issues must be addressed. These include:

- the quality of the child's life if oral feeding never occurs;
- the parents' desires regarding tube versus oral feeding (and the reasons and feelings underlying these wishes); and
- the parents' level of investment in continuing oral treatment.

Even if the decision is made to give up the goal of moving to nutritional oral feeding, an oral-therapy program should be continued. "Recreational" oral feedings may be possible and desired. In addition, any child needs sufficient tolerance of oral stimulation for ongoing hygiene of the face, mouth, teeth, and gums.

Considering Parent Readiness

In addition to the child being ready, the parents or caretakers must be ready to undertake a program focused on the return to oral feeding. The parents have a key role in the success of programs moving from non-oral to oral feeding. Their support in carryover of the treatment techniques outside of the therapy sessions is extremely important. The more frequently treatment techniques are used, the more likely progress will occur and the faster the changes may be seen. A high degree of *consistency, patience,* and *perseverance* are needed by the people involved in the program. Therefore, communication between the parents and feeding specialist *prior* to initiating aggressive transition programs is essential.

Parents may not be ready or able to follow through with the demands of the intervention program for a variety of reasons. Demands on the parents' time from jobs, other children, or the large amount of care required by the patient may make it difficult for them to follow through on the feeding program as fully as necessary. The parents' individual personality styles may also assist or hinder the program.

The nature of the parent/child relationship is important. The feeding specialist needs to assess the parents' ability to be consistent and firm with the child. The parents' values and their behavioral management style will also impact the treatment process. When the clinician is unaware of the parents' priorities or their ability and willingness to follow through with a particular treatment regime, conflict and misunderstanding can occur, which undermines the goal of transitioning to oral feeding.

Case example:
Alison was a former 32-week premature infant who developed necrotizing enterocolitis. Bowel perforation ensued and she required surgical bowel resection and repair. A gastrostomy was placed at that time. As enteral feeding was introduced, Alison had trouble tolerating the feedings, with frequent periods of loose stools and gastric residuals.

She was hospitalized for three months while feedings were advanced. Alison demonstrated feeding intolerance a number of times during this process, needing to return to total parenteral nutrition at these points. By discharge, she was tolerating full enteral feedings with a special formula and given by a continuous-drip pump through her gastrostomy. She was not able to tolerate bolus feedings. While hospitalized, she also received oral and feeding therapy with the goal of maintaining and building skills in an infant with limited oral-feeding opportunities. At discharge, her feeding pump was turned off two times per day for small oral feedings. While she had normal oral-motor skills and very minimal evidence of oral-tactile hypersensitivity, she was not an enthusiastic oral feeder. Ongoing outpatient follow-up of feeding and developmental status was to be provided by an itinerant therapist in her community.

This family lived in a small semirural community. Alison had three siblings, 3, 6, and 8 years of age. Her father and mother both worked outside of the home, with mother returning to work part-time two months after Alison's discharge. The family felt very protective of Alison because of her medical complications and fragile state as an infant.

Alison returned for occupational therapy follow-up of her general developmental status and oral feeding at 6 months of age (4 months corrected age). Earlier follow-up was not possible due to the family's distance from the hospital. At this visit development was proceeding normally. While Alison was now tolerating bolus feedings, these were all by gastrostomy, with Alison refusing oral feeding.

In recounting the feeding history since discharge, mother described Alison as being somewhat difficult to feed orally. The oral-feeding sessions were not very rewarding for the mother. In addition, she stated that she was very busy, particularly after returning to work, and had little time for oral feeding. The itinerant therapist had also visited infrequently and done little to reinforce the importance of continuing with oral feeding. As Alison was now tolerating bolus feedings, however, mother said that she wanted Alison to become an oral feeder. She expressed interest in working with Alison on this task.

Clinical feeding evaluation revealed no spontaneous sucking (Alison also no longer took a pacifier) and moderate oral-tactile hypersensitivity. When given a bottle, she eventually could comfortably hold it in her mouth, though she chewed and gummed it, rather than sucking.

A program of oral-tactile normalization was developed, incorporating a number of techniques to facilitate sucking. At the same time, activities to provide a background for spoon feeding were introduced. As no further local therapy services were available, the public health nurse was enlisted to assist in encouraging follow-through.

Alison was seen three months later, and there had been no progress toward oral feeding. While mother expressed the desire for Alison to feed orally, she was not able to carry through on any of the necessary activities. She reported that she just couldn't find the time between caring for the other children and working. Alison was well nourished with the tube feedings, and it was convenient for mother to feed her in this manner.

In this case, Alison had lost the oral-feeding skills she had in the hospital due to poor follow-through with the oral-feeding program. When mother did express the desire to return to oral feeding, she did not have the resources to make the time commitment necessary to progress in this area. As she was eager for the results but not ready for the process of attempting to return to oral feeding, an attempt was made to locate other resources in the family and community. An aunt was finally identified who had the time and interest to pursue a regular oral-therapy program with Alison, and slow but steady progress was noted.

Treatment to Make the Transition to Oral Feeding

Nutritional Support
The current pattern of nutritional support needs to be determined, including the feeding schedule, volume, and bolus versus drip feeding. If the child is on continuous-drip feedings, moving to bolus feeding will help normalize the hunger/satiation cycle and insure that the stomach is able to handle a full-size meal. Consultation with a physician, nurse, or nutritionist will be required to make such changes. If the child is not yet able to tolerate bolus feedings, this should become the first goal in the transition process.

Normalizing Hunger/Satiation Cycles
Once the child is on bolus feedings, the hunger/satiation cycle will need to be normalized, and the link between sensations in the mouth and sensations in the stomach must be reestablished. Initially the child's bolus feeding schedule should be arranged so that it approximates the normal eating schedule; that is, three larger bolus "meals" and two smaller bolus "snacks."[35] In this way the child can experience the normal cyclic nature of the stomach being full and then empty. For some children this is a novel experience and can be distressing.

The link between sensations in the mouth and sensations in the stomach needs to be reestablished. For the child still using a pacifier, this can be done by giving the child the pacifier during every tube feeding. The literature gives support to this idea, at least in premature infants. Those infants who sucked on a pacifier during tube feeding discontinued NG feedings earlier, had better weight gain, and were discharged earlier from the hospital.[34] This is an extremely simple procedure that should be implemented with any baby who is able to suck and is receiving some portion of its total intake via a tube.

Once out of the hospital, the child should be included in family meals if at all possible. This gives exposure to the sights, sounds, and smells of the eating process, as well as adults and other children modeling eating behavior. This also allows the child to participate in the important social aspects of eating. Too often, tube feeding becomes totally divorced from the normal eating experience. It may be done in the child's bed or on the run to another activity. Bringing the child to the table while others are eating (and perhaps doing the tube feeding there) is another method that creates more normal eating experiences for the tube-fed child.

Oral-Tactile Normalization

A key feature of any intervention program designed to facilitate the transition to oral feeding from tube feeding is oral-tactile normalization. The rationale and some selected methods of using this technique have been described (see page 247). This can be one of the most challenging areas to deal with when attempting to reintroduce oral feedings. In addition to the non-nutritive methods of oral-tactile normalization, food substances and tastes can be used.

When the child is engaging in normal mouthing of toys, the toys can be dipped into pureed foods. In this way, the pleasurable sensation of toy exploration can be paired with the less familiar and perhaps less enjoyable sensation of taste. Pureed foods can be placed on the tray of a child's high chair, and the child can be allowed to "finger-paint" with the foods. If any hand-to-mouth activity occurs, the child may receive a taste of food. During bathing, the child can be given a wet washcloth to mouth and perhaps extract some liquid. Clear water can be used, progressing to liquids of various flavors. Foods can also be introduced by smells alone. Providing the child with small vials of essences or flavorings to smell may increase the receptivity to oral experiences. All the ways food items can be varied should be considered: texture, taste, temperature, smell. One variation may prove to be a key in making progress in this area. After the child allows food tools (for example, nipples, spoons) and tastes in the mouth, the focus can shift to slowly increasing volume.

Behavioral Management

Any program designed to make the transition to oral feeding from tube feeding needs to have a component of behavioral management; particularly when the child is older and has had prolonged tube feedings. In addition to having sensory processing deficits, many of these children have an overlay of significant oppositional behaviors surrounding eating. Consistent behavioral management strategies are essential. Reinforcers and rewards, whether simple praise or more complicated token systems, are also important to the success of the program.

Recognizing that behavioral opposition to feeding is often a key obstacle in making the transition from tube to oral feeding, some centers have established specific behaviorally oriented programs to deal with this problem. Particularly interesting is one program with the goal of rapid reintroduction of oral feeding in tube-fed patients.[35-37] This multidisciplinary, inpatient program uses firm and consistent behavior management techniques to make the transition from tube to oral feeding in about three weeks, with a high degree of success. Stringent patient selection criteria is

---

a key component of this program, but for some patients this method may be an alternative to a slower, more prolonged approach.

Carryover of Treatment to Other Caregivers

While the feeding specialist plays a leading role in evaluating infant feeding problems, then designing a treatment plan and implementing the treatment, if over long periods of time the feeding specialist is the sole person providing treatment, progress may be extremely slow. Seldom is it possible for a feeding specialist to be present at every feeding, so others must perform some feedings. Thus, involving parents and other caregivers in carrying over the treatment techniques to the feedings they provide becomes an important part of a comprehensive treatment program. It ensures a greater frequency of intervention as well as more feedback on the infant's response to the treatment techniques.

Parents

Parents bring to the treatment milieu not only their own basic personalities and styles but also their mode of response to stress. The birth of a premature infant or an infant with an acute or chronic medical condition not only becomes a stressor for the parent but also places the parent in a state of grief. The parent is grieving for the loss of the expected and dreamed-of perfect child. In dealing with this, parents can go through stages similar to those that the terminally ill may go through—grief, denial, anger, and acceptance. The stage being experienced by the parents will influence their readiness and availability to participate in the treatment. This theme has the potential to reemerge time and time again at critical stages in the treatment process. If a change in treatment is anticipated, such as the placement of a gastrostomy tube, unresolved issues may resurface to complicate the decision-making process.

Feeding a baby is intimately intertwined with the perceived "goodness" of mothering. Feeding a baby is such a primal event that factors interfering with this process potentially undermine the mother's perception of herself as a good mother and her emerging bond with her newborn. Thus, the feeding specialist enters into an already emotionally charged arena. Sensitivity by the feeding specialist is needed to support the mother/baby dyad while providing treatment to the baby for the identified feeding disorder. To do so, feeding specialists must be sensitive to the parents' priorities and goals. These are frequently different from those held by the feeding specialist or other medical staff. Even when the mother is well bonded to the baby and capably following through with all treatment recommendations, the chronicity of the feeding problem combined with the stress of dealing with it many times per day can erode the spirit of even the most invested parent.

It is the clinician's responsibility to choose treatment techniques for carryover to the parent that can be reasonably assured of success. When working with parents, it is easier to train them with smaller components of the treatment, insuring mastery at each level, than to bombard them with the entire picture. The use of return demonstration and written or pictorial materials will foster better and more accurate follow-through outside the treatment session. Videotape, which is becoming increasingly available in homes and hospitals, is another method of parent instruction. This would allow parents to review treatment methods at their own pace and when they are most receptive. The clinician must have a sensitive ear and acknowledge the difficulty of the parents' situation.

Medical Staff

Particularly in the hospital environment, there are potentially numerous staff members involved with an infant. The challenge to obtaining carryover of treatment strategies within that type of setting is gaining consistency with multiple feeders. The various feeders may have different views of the feeding problem and varying skill levels in dealing with these problems. Inconsistencies in management have the potential to compound the baby's original feeding problem.

When the feeding problem is a relatively simple one, the role of the feeding specialist may be to choose the one way the baby should be fed and then help to increase consistency. To determine which is the best way of feeding a particular baby, in addition to conducting a clinical feeding evaluation, the feeding specialist needs to talk to other staff members to gain a consensus of what treatment techniques work the best and under what conditions. Team members will feel much more committed to the treatment plan and therefore more likely to follow through with the program if they have had a role in its creation. Once the feeding techniques are selected, posting written and pictorial instructions at the bedside often is a useful and nonthreatening way to communicate information among caregivers. Writing feeding instructions in the nursing care plan may also improve communication and consistency.

For a more complex feeding problem requiring a high level of skill to treat, lack of consistency in handling could prove dangerous for the infant, particularly if the response to improper feeding techniques is apnea, bradycardia, or oxygen desaturation. The feeding specialist's role may then be to decide which portion of the feeding program will be carried over by other caregivers and which portion will be done solely within the treatment setting. The portions of the treatment regime that would be best suited for carryover outside of therapy sessions would be those that are the easiest to explain, are safest for the baby, and that work consistently. As there is the potential to bruise egos if not all team members are allowed to participate in all aspects of treatment, it may be more readily accepted if the feeding specialist is able to clearly explain the rationale for this division of labor. Exceptions to this division of labor may be made to include the infant's primary nurse, parent, or other special caretaker.

The feeding specialist must constantly communicate with the other caregivers to determine if the program is working well, if follow-through is occurring, or if changes in the program are indicated. Feeding specialists working with infants with complex feeding disorders must be committed to providing continued instruction to other professionals so that all team members working with an infant have a similar skill level. This instruction can occur at the bedside for a specific infant, or through more formal in-servicing. The feeding specialist should attempt to foster an atmosphere of mutual exchange of information and respect among medical staff to best meet the needs of each infant.

Putting It All Together: Developing the Feeding Plan

Throughout this chapter, feeding problems have been broken down into small component parts, with therapeutic treatment and management ideas offered. While this method aids in the organization and presentation of this large amount of material, it does not accurately reflect the way these treatment techniques are used in actual practice. It is uncommon that an infant's feeding problem will be resolved using only one technique or method. The treatment techniques that have been described will be combined and are often used together with medical and surgical treatment or management as part of the total feeding plan.

In addition, selection of techniques or strategies is not a static process but must be fluid, with new treatments and approaches initiated to meet the infant's changing needs. Finally, this list of treatment ideas is not exhaustive. It is meant to provide sound techniques and strategies that may be useful in treating a large variety of infant feeding problems. Background information has been liberally provided to help the clinician understand the feeding problems of the infant and the rationale for various treatments. It is hoped that each feeding specialist will then go on to develop novel and creative treatment solutions for the infant feeding problems seen in practice. Case examples follow to illustrate these three points.

The Use of Multiple Treatment Techniques

Case example:

Quincy was a premature infant, one of twins, born at 32 weeks gestation. He was hospitalized for three weeks with a relatively uncomplicated course. When nippling was introduced, occasional gagging and bradycardia were noted, though these resolved prior to discharge.

At corrected age of term, he was found asleep, blue and limp, 10 minutes after a feeding. Vigorous stimulation was needed to revive him. He was admitted to the hospital for evaluation of apnea. Evaluation revealed Quincy did not have central apnea, but profound acidic gastroesophageal reflux (GER), which at times leads to bradycardia.

Clinical feeding evaluation was also requested. Significant findings included a very strong, rapid sucking pattern and poor integration of breathing with sucking and swallowing, particularly early in the feeding. Later in the feeding a slight noisiness was noted during breathing. In addition, the heart rate was generally in the 180 BPM range, although it dropped 40 beats to 140 BPM several times during the feeding, even after the GER was under better control. While this is not technically a bradycardia, it is certainly a noteworthy drop. It appeared that Quincy's strong suck might be producing such large boluses that coordination of sucking, swallowing, and breathing was compromised and that baroreceptors were stimulated to produce a vagally mediated cardiac response. A VFSS showed normal swallowing in the early part of the feeding but delayed swallowing as the feeding progressed, with no aspiration.

Quincy's feeding plan incorporated a number of components:

- An upright position was used during feeding. This minimized the possibility of GER.

- The formula was thickened with rice cereal. Not only did this help to manage GER, but it provided smaller boluses and slowed the flow of the bolus during sucking.

- A firm nipple with no enlargement of the nipple hole was used. Since Quincy had a very strong suck, he was able to draw the rice cereal through the nipple hole. Keeping the hole small and using a firm nipple both reduced the flow of formula. The reduction in flow from these techniques and the thickening of the formula seemed to improve the "pacing" of respirations during sucking and swallowing and eliminated the drops in heart rate.

- External pacing was provided as needed. The coordination of breathing with sucking and swallowing was monitored closely during feeding. While techniques to slow the flow of milk improved this coordination, periodically Quincy was still noted to have a long sucking burst without breathing. At these times, pacing was provided to break the sucking chain after four or five sucks to encourage breathing.

- The formula was chilled. As Quincy's swallowing delay put him at greater risk for aspiration, chilled liquid was found to speed the triggering of swallowing during the VFSS.

Additionally, upright positioning was used rigorously at nonfeeding times to control Quincy's marked GER, and medication was provided to decrease the stomach's acidity.

To fully manage Quincy's obstructive apnea and bradycardia, a number of techniques were necessary during feeding and at other times. If the feeding plan had been limited to one treatment technique, or even one group of techniques, treatment might have been less successful. The determination that each of these techniques was necessary was based on careful multisystem evaluation as well as observation of Quincy's response to each technique.

Ongoing Modification of the Treatment Program

Case example:
Zachary was a full-term baby born after a normal pregnancy, labor, and delivery. He was cyanotic in the newborn period and soon diagnosed with a complex congenital heart defect. It was immediately surgically repaired, but Zachary had difficulty weaning from the ventilator. Final extubation was at 4 weeks, but oral feeding was delayed due to tachypnea.

He was referred for clinical feeding evaluation at 6 weeks, when oral feeding was medically advisable. Prior to this time, nutrition was bolus feedings gavaged through an indwelling nasogastric tube. Findings included a markedly hyperactive gag and extreme difficulty initiating and maintaining a non-nutritive sucking pattern. He would not initiate any sucking on a bottle, and he showed gagging and poorly coordinated swallowing when given small amounts of fluid.

An oral-therapy program was begun that eventually had three phases, based on Zachary's changing skills and therapy needs.

Phase One: Building oral-motor skills for sucking
- The gag was desensitized by presenting all oral stimuli at the front of the tongue and slowly moving back on the tongue.

- Sucking was facilitated through firm pressure and stroking proximal to distal on the midline of the tongue.

- Carryover was promoted by training parents and encouraging use of the pacifier.

In three days, Zachary was easily initiating strong non-nutritive sucking without gagging. He continued to gag when fluid was introduced.

Phase Two: Building skills to coordinate swallowing with sucking

- During non-nutritive sucking, small amounts of fluid were introduced by dropper, encouraging controlled swallowing with sucking.

- The bottle was given, but was removed after only one suck, giving time to coordinate the swallow. As Zachary had a very strong suck, however, he still had a very large bolus quickly entering the mouth, which produced some gagging.

- A technique was needed to slow the flow of the liquid from the bottle. Therefore, the formula was thickened slightly to allow more time to organize the bolus for swallowing. The bottle could now be kept in his mouth for multiple sucks but was still removed frequently.

On day 8 of treatment, Zachary took 30 cc of thickened liquid without gagging. This took about 10 minutes, and it was noted that the strength of the suck diminished and respiratory rate increased over the time he was nippling. Respiratory rate was in the 80s by the end of the feeding.

Phase Three: Balancing respiratory needs with the need to nipple

- Nippling was attempted at most feedings, with intake of 10 cc to 20 cc over 10 minutes. Nippling was generally stopped due to fatigue or increased respiratory rate.

- Gradually Zachary improved and was taking 30 cc to 40 cc per feeding. His nutritional requirement, however, was 60 cc per feeding. Medically he was ready for discharge from the hospital.

- A home feeding program was developed, with Zachary nippling thickened formula for a maximum of 20 minutes at each daytime feeding, and the balance given through an indwelling NG tube. Parents were trained in gavage feeding techniques and in the signs and symptoms of increased respiratory effort.

Discharge was two and a half weeks after the oral-therapy program began (Zachary was 9 weeks old). At home he steadily increased the amount he nippled. He had less need for the NG feedings, which were discontinued by 4 months of age. Weight gain was good on full oral feedings. Improvement in oral intake during this phase was not due to

---

specific therapeutic techniques but to improved cardiorespiratory status. Feeding management only supported needs in this area to minimize stress to Zachary and encourage weight gain.

Developing Creative Treatment Techniques

Case example:
Allen was a former 36-week premature infant who had apnea, bradycardia, and cyanosis with feedings. Following an interdisciplinary assessment, it was found that he required supplemental oxygen via nasal cannula to maintain appropriate oxygen saturation, he had poor pacing of his swallowing and breathing, and he had atypical gastroesophageal reflux (GER) observed immediately after feeding. If his position was changed from the normal semirecumbent feeding position to more upright for burping, GER to the oropharynx occurred, which triggered an apneic or bradycardic episode. In addition, he had somewhat slow esophageal motility which contributed to the problem. His treatment therefore needed to be designed to strictly limit movement during and after feeding. For further details on the assessment process for this infant, see chapter 4, page 176.

Initially, Allen was fed in an infant seat with a customized seat insert that promoted an erect posture with good trunk support and 90-degree hip flexion to assist with the downward movement of his formula. He remained in the infant seat for 20 minutes after feeding and then could be placed in any position without problem. The time in the infant seat post-feeding was quickly weaned to 10 minutes without difficulty. He was fed thin formula, since his GER was atypical and the thickened formula might have increased his already slow esophageal motility.

Allen's mother, however, had wanted to breast-feed her baby and the feeding specialist felt it was important to attempt to achieve this goal. Modifications to the standard nearly horizontal breast-feeding position were attempted. Allen was fed in a modification of the "football hold" whereby he sat on his mother's leg or next to her on a pillow in an erect position directly facing his mother's breast. When finished with one side, he was lifted straight up to the shoulder on the same side, horizontally transferred to the shoulder on the opposite side, then lowered vertically to the sitting position to nurse again. In this way, the relative movement of his trunk was eliminated and he did not reflux. Following nursing, his mother lifted him vertically to the shoulder on the side just completed and held him there for 10 minutes. With this procedure, Allen no longer had apneic or bradycardic episodes with feedings. Most importantly, the mother was able to have the feeding experience she desired, while simultaneously providing her baby with a safe feeding experience.

While these are not "standard" treatment techniques and are not described specifically in this chapter, they follow the lines of positioning modifications that are frequently a part of feeding therapy. A complete understanding of the specific problems this infant was having allowed the feeding specialist to create an effective, though atypical treatment strategy.

References

1. Case-Smith, J. 1988. An efficacy study of occupational therapy with high-risk neonates. *American Journal of Occupational Therapy* 42:499-506.

2. Trykowski, L. E., B. V. Kirkpatrick, and E. L. Leonard. 1981. Enhancement of nutritive sucking in premature infants. *Physical and Occupational Therapy in Pediatrics* 1:27-33.

3. Brazelton, B. T. 1984. *Neonatal behavioral assessment scale.* Philadelphia: J. B. Lippincott Co.

4. Morris, S. E., and M. D. Klein. 1987. *Pre-feeding skills.* Tucson, AZ: Therapy Skill Builders.

5. White-Traut, R. C., and C. M. Hutchens. 1987. Modulating infant state in premature infants. *Journal of Pediatric Nursing* 2:96-101.

6. Bosma, J. F. 1988. Functional anatomy of the upper airway during development. In *Respiratory function of the upper airway*, edited by O. P. Mathew and G. Sant'Ambrogio, 47-86. New York: Marcel Dekker, Inc.

7. Thach, B. T., and Stark, A. R. 1979. Spontaneous neck flexion in and airway obstruction during apneic spells in preterm infants. *The Journal of Pediatrics* 94:275-81.

8. Finnie, N. R. 1974. *Handling the young cerebral palsied child at home.* New York: E. P. Dutton.

9. Morris, S. E. 1982. *The normal acquisition of oral-feeding skills: Implications for assessment and treatment.* New York: Therapeutic Media.

10. Wilson, J. M. 1978. *Oral-motor function and dysfunction in children.* Chapel Hill, NC: University of North Carolina, Division of Physical Therapy.

11. Bly, L. 1983. *The components of normal movement during the first year of life.* Birmingham, AL: Pathway Press.

12. Connor, F. P., G. G. Williamson, and J. M. Siepp. 1978. *Program guide for infants and toddlers with neuromotor and other developmental disabilities.* New York: Teachers College Press.

13. Logemann, J. 1983. *Evaluation and treatment of swallowing disorders.* Boston: College Press Publication.

14. Logemann, J. A. 1986. Treatment for aspiration related to dysphagia: An overview. *Dysphagia* 1:34-38.

15. Lazzara, G. D. L., C. Lazarus, and J. Logemann. 1986. Impact of thermal stimulation on the triggering of the swallowing reflex. *Dysphagia* 1:73-77.

16. Kirsch, C. M., and A. Sanders. 1988. Aspiration pneumonia: Medical management. *Otolaryngologic Clinics of North America* 21:677-89.

17. Johnson, P., and D. M. Salisbury. 1975. Breathing and sucking during feeding in the newborn. *Ciba Foundation Symposiums* 33:119-35.

18. Bartlett, D. 1985. Ventilatory and protective mechanisms of the infant larynx. *American Review of Respiratory Disease* 131:S49-S50.

19. Mathew, O. P., and F. B. Sant'Ambrogio. 1988. Laryngeal reflexes. In *Respiratory function of the upper airway,* edited by O. P. Mathew and G. Sant'Ambrogio, 259-302. New York: Marcel Dekker, Inc.

20. Mortola, J. P., and J. T. Fisher. 1988. Upper airway reflexes in newborns. In *Respiratory function of the upper airway,* edited by O. P. Mathew and G. Sant'Ambrogio, 303-57. New York: Marcel Dekker, Inc.

21. Shelley, W. G., and J. Boxall. 1986. A new way to treat sucking and swallowing difficulties in babies. *The Lancet* 1 (24 May 1991):1182-84.

22. Leonard, E. L., L. E. Trykowski, and B. V. Kirkpatrick. 1980. Nutritive sucking in high-risk neonates after perioral stimulation. *Physical Therapy.* 60:299-302.

23. Guyton, A. C. 1991. *Textbook of medical physiology.* Philadelphia: W. B. Saunders Company.

24. Groothuis, J. R., and A. A. Rosenberg. 1987. Home oxygen promotes weight gain in infants with bronchopulmonary dysplasia. *American Journal of Diseases in Children* 141:992-95.

25. Nelson, C. L. A., and R. A. Hallgren. 1989. Gastrostomies: Indications, management, and weaning. *Infants and Young Children* 2:66-74.

26. Gauderer, M. W. L., G. J. Picha, and R. J. Izant. 1984. The gastrostomy "button": A simple, skin-level non-refluxing device for long-term enteral feedings. *Journal of Pediatric Surgery* 19:803-5.

27. Larson, D. E., D. D. Burton, and K. W. Schroeder. 1987. Percutaneous endoscopic gastrostomy: Indication, success, complications, and mortality in 314 consecutive patients. *Gastroenterology* 93:48-52.

28. Moore, M. C., and H. L. Greene. 1985. Tube feeding of infants and children. *Pediatric Clinics of North America* 32:401-17.

29. Pipes, P. 1985. *Nutrition in infancy and childhood.* St. Louis, MO: Time Mirror/Mosby.

30. Illingworth, R. S., and Lister, M. B. 1964. The critical or sensitive period, with special reference to certain feeding problems in infants and children. *Journal of Pediatrics* 65:839-48.

31. Ayres, A. J. 1979. *Sensory integration and the child.* Los Angeles: Western Psychological Services.

32. Mueller, H. 1972. Facilitating feeding and prespeech. In *Physical therapy services in the developmental disabilities,* edited by P. H. Pearson and C. E. Williams. Springfield, IL: Charles C. Thomas.

33. Millunchick, E. W., and R. D. Mcartor. 1986. Fatal aspiration of a makeshift pacifier. *Pediatrics* 77:369-70.

34. Measel, C. P., and G. C. Anderson. 1979. Non-nutritive sucking during tube feedings: Effect on clinical course in premature infants. *Journal of Obstetrical, Gynecologic and Neonatal Nursing.* 8:265-72.

35. Blackman, J. A., and C. L. A. Nelson. 1985. Reinstituting oral feedings in children fed by gastrostomy. *Clinical Pediatrics* 8:434-38.

36. Blackman, J. A., and C. L. A. Nelson. 1987. Rapid introduction of oral feedings to tube-fed patients. *Journal of Developmental and Behavioral Pediatrics* 8:63-66.

37. *Management of the child fed via gastrostomy: An oral-feeding approach.* Media Services, Division of Developmental Disabilities, Department of Pediatrics, University of Iowa, Iowa City, IA 52242.

38. Blitzer, A., Y. P. Krespi, R. W. Oppenheimer, and T. M. Levine. 1988. Surgical management of aspiration. *Otolaryngologic Clinics of North America* 21:743-50.

39. Cumming, W. A., and B. J. Reilly. 1972. Fatigue aspiration. *Radiology* 105:387-90.

40. Mathew, O. P., M. L. Clark, M. L. Pronske, H. G. Luna-Solarzano, and M. D. Peterson. 1985. Breathing pattern and ventilation during oral feeding in term newborn infants. *The Journal of Pediatrics* 106:810-13.

41. Rosen, C. L., D. G. Glaze, and J. D. Frost. 1984. Hypoxemia associated with feeding in the preterm and full-term neonate. *American Journal of Diseases in Children* 138:623-28.

42. Als, H. 1986. A synactive model of neonatal behavioral organization: Framework for the assessment of neurobehavioral development in the premature infant and for support of infants and parents in the neonatal intensive care environment. *Physical and Occupational Therapy in Pediatrics* 6:3-53.

43. Greenspan, J. S., M. R. Wolfson, W. J. Holt, and T. H. Shaffer. 1990. Neonatal gastric intubation: Differential respiratory effects between nasogastric and orogastric tubes. *Pediatric Pulmonology* 8:254-258.

44. Morris, S. E. 1989. Development of oral-motor skills in the neurologically impaired child receiving non-oral feedings. *Dysphagia* 3:135-154.

45. Drehobl, K. F., and M. G. Fuhr. 1991. *Pediatric massage for the child with special needs.* Tucson, AZ: Therapy Skill Builders.

6 *Special Diagnostic Categories*

In chapter 4, problem-driven models for the evaluation of infant feeding difficulties were developed. This method of problem solving has been proposed to focus the feeding specialist on the multisystem, interactional nature of infant feeding. While a specific diagnosis may predispose an infant to a particular type of feeding problem, the diagnosis is not the feeding problem, and merely focusing on the diagnosis may inhibit the feeding specialist from considering alternative sources of the problem. As a rule, it is suggested that the orientation to evaluation and treatment be multidimensional and problem oriented. In this chapter, however, the focus will be on specific diagnoses in an effort to highlight feeding problems or treatment techniques that are unique to specific diagnoses. With this background, the feeding specialist will be able to quickly rule in or out particular features of the initial diagnosis when assessing a feeding problem, or move on to alternative solutions.

The Premature Infant

When an infant is born prematurely, the immature organism is thrust into a foreign environment and must cope with demands it is not prepared to meet. The premature infant also has a greater likelihood of developing medical complications such as intracranial hemorrhage, infant respiratory distress syndrome (IDS) (which may lead to bronchopulmonary dysplasia [BPD]), and necrotizing enterocolitis. While dealing with new environmental demands and possible medical compromise, the premature infant is trying to make normal progress in growth and development. As the infant struggles to accomplish these tasks, feeding difficulties are often encountered.

The variety of gestational ages and medical complications seen in premature infants precludes a single, generalized discussion of feeding considerations in the premature infant. As shown in figure 6-1, the premature infant who is not intubated or is intubated only briefly for respiratory distress will have a markedly different course (and experiences) than the infant who develops BPD and requires prolonged ventilation. The degree of respiratory illness and subsequent medical management is a critical factor in considering potential feeding difficulties. Thus, general issues relating to respiratory status and feeding in premature infants will be discussed in detail. The impact of intracranial hemorrhage, necrotizing enterocolitis, and bronchopulmonary dysplasia will then be addressed separately.

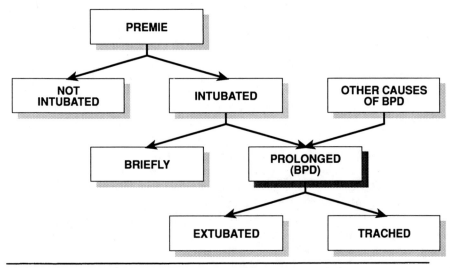

Figure 6-1 The severity of respiratory illness and the subsequent need for intubation will affect the premature infant's medical course.

Respiratory Illness in the Premature Infant

Many infants born before 35 to 36 weeks of gestation develop infant respiratory distress syndrome (IRDS) or hyaline membrane disease (HMD). The primary cause of IRDS in the premature infant is the inability of the immature lungs to produce adequate amounts of surfactant. As production of surfactant is related to maturation, younger premature infants are more likely to have inadequate surfactant and are thus more likely to develop IRDS. Of infants born at 28 to 30 weeks gestation or less, more than 70% will develop IRDS. This proportion decreases with increasing gestational age. Surfactant adequate to prevent the development of IRDS is usually present in infants born at 35 to 36 weeks gestation.[27]

Inadequate amounts of surfactant in the alveoli trigger a "cascade of events" that leads to respiratory insufficiency (figure 6-2). Insufficient surfactant causes alveolar surface tension to increase, resulting in alveolar collapse and atelectasis. This creates an uneven relationship between ventilation and perfusion, as well as reduced lung volume and compliance. Hypoxemia and hypercarbia result, leading to respiratory and metabolic acidosis. This in turn inhibits surfactant production and stimulates pulmonary vasoconstriction, leading to reduced pulmonary blood flow. With reduced pulmonary blood flow, lung tissue becomes ischemic, and blood plasma leaks into the tissue causing the development of fibrin. The presence of fibrin further impairs gas exchange across the capillary alveolar beds, further increasing hypoxia and hypercarbia. A number of "vicious cycles" are created that appear to cause a downward spiral in this disease and impair the production of surfactant, which is needed to reverse the process.[28]

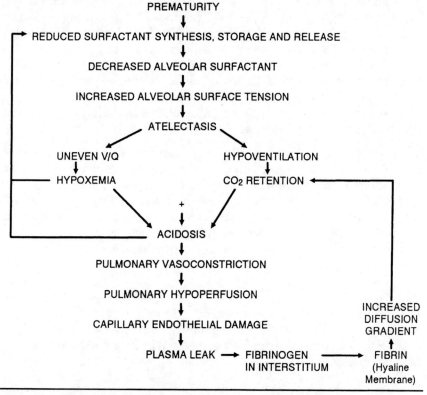

Figure 6-2 The cascade of events leading to respiratory insufficiency in premature infants. Reprinted with permission from: W. Oh, 1983. Respiratory distress syndrome: Diagnosis and management. In *Diagnosis and management of respiratory disorders in the newborn*, edited by L. Stern. Menlo Park, CA: Addison-Wesley Publishing Company.

In the newborn, the clinical manifestations of this process will generally be apparent within the first hours of life. As atelectasis occurs, high pressure is needed for re-expansion of the airways. The infant attempts to produce this by increasing the rate and effort of respiration. This leads to increased oxygen demand and consumption. These deep inspirations tend to collapse the chest wall, which is extremely compliant in the premature infant. Chest wall retraction, rather than lung expansion, is the result. Respiratory distress will be evident as the infant demonstrates tachypnea, grunting respirations, and retractions. Laboratory tests and X-ray findings confirm the diagnosis of IRDS.[27]

Management includes oxygen therapy, correction of acidosis, maintenance of normal arterial blood pressure, temperature control, maintaining fluid and electrolyte balance, and often assisted ventilation. While symptoms may worsen during the first two to three days, noncomplicated IRDS is a self-limiting disease, with recovery generally taking place within a week as surfactant production increases. The process of producing surfactant, however, is sensitive to many systemic factors and can be inhibited by events such as sepsis, intracranial hemorrhage, asphyxia, or persistent patent ductus arteriosus (PDA). Oxygen therapy and mechanical ventilation can also cause epithelial injury in the lung tissue, impairing surfactant production. If surfactant production is not adequate to reverse the disease process within the first week, some degree of bronchopulmonary dysplasia (BPD) is likely to develop[28] (see figure 6-1, page 298).

Those infants recovering from IRDS have experienced a variety of pulmonary changes. While these pulmonary changes may resolve sufficiently to discontinue primary medical therapies, the residual effects are not well understood. As there is variation in rate and degree of recovery, it may be weeks or months before pulmonary mechanisms return to full efficiency in some infants. The work of breathing may be greater, requiring high energy expenditure. Additional oxygen may be needed to support this energy expenditure, and respiratory rate may increase. Respiratory reserve may be minimal, leading to frequent fatigue. Such factors can have a decided impact on feeding. Feeding is the primary "work" of infants (outside of maintaining bodily homeostasis) and therefore requires additional oxygen consumption and respiratory reserve. The potential impact of IRDS therefore must be carefully considered in the premature infant with feeding problems.

Maturation of Feeding-Related Performances

A thorough understanding of the development of feeding-related performances is necessary in considering the feeding problems of premature infants. The progression of feeding skills in this group of infants reflects change in growth, maturation, and experience. These changes will be discussed as they relate to structural maturation, the development of nutritive and non-nutritive sucking, and the development of respiratory control with feeding.

Structural Maturation

The anatomical structures responsible for feeding functions are present well before viability. The development of these structures, however, will not be complete in the young premature infant. Bosma describes several structural features of the immature premature infant that can impact the postural stability that the term infant relies on for successful feeding.[15]

The facial and oral musculature are present in the premature infant, but they are reduced in bulk, and stabilizing tendinous and ligamentous structures are poorly developed. The premature infant also has less body fat and therefore diminished facial fat and sucking pads. Muscle bulk and facial fat play an important role in postural stability during feeding (see page 9). When the infant is poorly developed, stability in feeding is compromised. In addition, the premature infant lacks postural control in the cervical area and thus has difficulty providing adequate stability for competent head and neck motions during feeding, as well as at other times.

The mouth tends to be open in the very young premature infant, providing less opposition of the tongue and lips. With increasing gestational age it begins to close, and the tongue comes into opposition with the hard palate. Finally the lips oppose.[38] When the tongue does not fill the oral cavity, due to its relatively small size in the premature infant or to lack of mouth closure, it moves freely in the mouth, and has less positional stability.[14]

While many aspects of development are felt to proceed in a cephalocaudal direction, Bosma challenges that concept in regard to feeding functions.[15] He points out that pharyngeal functions in the premature infant must be adequate before oral functions mature. The pharyngeal swallow is necessary in a viable infant to clear secretions in the airway. In feeding, therefore, a caudal to cephalo progression may occur. Grybosksi supports this concept, suggesting that an immature suck/swallow pattern may persist until the esophagus is ready to transmit large boluses.[20]

Non-Nutritive Sucking

As illustrated in figure 6-3, there is a developmental progression in establishing non-nutritive sucking rhythms. Non-nutritive sucking (NNS) movements are noted in premature infants at 27 to 28 weeks gestation. This early sucking activity consists of single sucks with long, variable pauses. Between 30 and 33 weeks gestation, non-nutritive sucking becomes more organized and progresses to a burst-pause pattern. The bursts are short but stable in length; however, the pauses are relatively long and irregular. Some single sucks are still noted. Swallowing typically occurs before or after

---

these short sucking bursts. The sucking rate is slower than in infants greater than 33 weeks gestation. During the sucking burst there are 1 to 1.5 sucks per second. Interestingly, esophageal peristalsis has been noted to be poorly coordinated at this age, characterized by lack of smooth peristaltic movement.[19,20] An increase in the respiratory rate during the non-nutritive sucking bursts has also been observed,[8,10] perhaps leading to the increased oxygen saturation during NNS that has been found in some studies.[2]

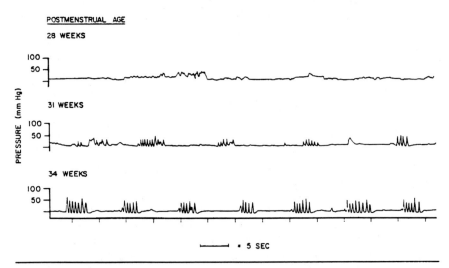

Figure 6-3 The maturation of non-nutritive sucking rhythms in the premature infant. Reprinted with permission from: M. Hack, M. M. Estabrook, and S. R. Robertson. 1985. Development of sucking rhythm in preterm infants. *Early Human Development* 11:133-140.

Around 34 weeks gestation the pace and rhythm of NNS become more stable. There is a greater number of sucking bursts with fewer and shorter pauses. Bursts lengthen, though the number of sucks per burst continues to show stability. The length of the pauses now also stabilizes to produce the smooth rhythm noted in NNS of the term neonate. Swallowing occurs intermittently during sucking bursts, and esophageal peristalsis is smooth and propagative.[20] Differences in the respiratory rate of older premature infants during NNS are noted by some authors[18] but not by others.[10] Interestingly, this is also the time the nursing staff often feels the infant is ready for the introduction of oral feeding.[19]

Nutritive Sucking
A thorough understanding of nutritive sucking (NS) is critical for feeding specialists working with premature infants. It is a complex skill and an early functional representation of neurodevelopmental organization.

Development of adequate nutritive sucking and feeding skills is often crucial to hospital discharge. Daniels, however, clearly demonstrates that there are differences between NS and NNS in premature infants, making the point that nutritive sucking skills cannot be inferred from performance of non-nutritive sucking.[8]

Ellison presents a unique perspective on the emergence of NS skills in premature infants by examining them during the first hour of life.[21] Suction and compression responses were measured in 13 premature (31 to 37 weeks), low-birth-weight (1250 to 2438 gr) infants. The primary mode of sucking at 5 minutes of life was by compression (75% of the total pressure generated by compression). Although the total sucking pressure changed little in the first hour, the compression component contributed only 40% by the end of the first hour, with the suction component increasing. Full-term infants also showed this shift toward an increased role of the suction component, and it was even more dramatic than for the premature infants. Overall sucking pressures for premature infants were considerably lower than for term infants. The relationship between these two pressure components in the subsequent development of sucking skills has not been studied. It could be postulated, however, that the inefficient, weak sucking seen during early feedings in some premature infants may be related to difficulty in shifting from the compression component to the suction component.

It is reported that premature infants can coordinate sucking and swallowing at 32 weeks,[49] with the introduction of feeding sometimes suggested between 32 and 34 weeks (although there are reports of younger infants feeding successfully). Most studies, however, report more adequate feeding skills between 34 and 35 weeks.[9,13] Maturation, as measured by gestational age at the time of feeding, appears to play a larger role in this readiness than weight or chronological age.[11,13] Some feel that experience also plays an important role in improving the efficiency of feeding.[9]

By 34 weeks gestational age, NS in the premature infant, as in the term infant, begins with an initial continuous sucking burst of at least 30 seconds (and generally closer to 70 seconds). This appears to be a stable feature of NS for infants over 34 weeks, with up to 30% of the feeding taken during this time. The infant then moves to a pattern of intermittent sucking bursts punctuated by regular pauses.[6,13] The sucking rate during the sucking bursts is about one suck per second, again similar to that of term infants.

Feeding patterns and sucking in the premature infant are often described as being inefficient. Features contributing to this inefficiency appear to be short, poorly organized sucking bursts, or long or variable pauses during sucking, both leading to a lack of rhythm. Weak sucking strength with disorganized jaw and tongue movements, and thus poor intake per suck, is also noted.[4,9,12,16] These factors may result in longer feeding times and/or insufficient intake. Inefficient feeding patterns are frequently seen in infants below 34 weeks gestational age, but they are also observed in older premature infants. Improved efficiency may be seen with greater feeding experience, but it is the interplay of maturation and experience that impact efficiency. Recently it has also been suggested that respiratory compromise or immaturity may be related to inefficient feeding patterns.[16]

Respiratory Control During Feeding

Although the patterns and characteristics of sucking have been studied for many years in both term and preterm infants, detailed evaluation of respiration during feeding has been undertaken only recently. Shivpuri describes changes in respiration during feeding of premature infants.[11] Older premature infants (36 to 38 weeks) demonstrate decreases in respiratory rate and tidal volume (amount of inspired air) during the continuous sucking phase. During the intermittent sucking phase, respiratory rate and tidal volume increase, returning close to baseline values by the end of the feeding. Oxygen saturation also dips during continuous sucking, resuming baseline values before the feeding ends. This is similar to findings in term newborns.[5] In younger premature infants (34 to 35 weeks), findings are similar during the continuous sucking phase, but respiratory rate and oxygen saturation show a low rate of recovery during the intermittent sucking phase. One proposed explanation for the better performance of older premature infants is improved coordination of respiration with sucking and swallowing as a result of maturation and/or experience.[11]

Premature infants of all ages, as well as term infants, show differences in ventilatory patterns during the sucking bursts as compared to the pauses. Ventilation is clearly reduced during sucking bursts. The respirations are shorter, less frequent, and have a lower tidal volume than prior to the feeding or during sucking pauses.[5,6,11] The degree and type of respiratory compensation that may be produced during the sucking pauses is less clear. Some type of compensation does occur in all but the youngest preterm infants, as respiratory values return to baseline levels during this period. There is evidence, however, that after feeding and after respiratory parameters return to baseline, there may be a subsequent decline in ventilation. In preterm infants, by 4 to 10 minutes after feeding, oxygen saturation and other measures of ventilation have been noted to be lower than baseline or immediate postfeed values.[11,36] Whether this reflects a late response to the decreases in ventilation that occur during feeding or is related to changing needs caused by digestion is not currently understood.

Hypothesizing that decreases in ventilation might lead to hypoxia, hyper-carbia, and acidosis, which might be manifest as apnea or bradycardia, Mathew pursued further study of the respiratory control of premature infants during feeding.[6] Of 24 premature infants (mean age 35 weeks) who were studied once during their first week of feeding, 15 infants demon-strated 39 episodes of apnea. These were primarily short episodes (10 to 19 seconds duration), which occurred during both continuous and intermit-tent sucking. Oxygen saturation consistently decreased during sucking and then rose during the pauses. It fell below 80% only during apneic episodes lasting longer than 20 seconds. Seven infants also demonstrated 11 episodes of bradycardia, all several seconds after the onset of apnea.

Others have also reported apnea during feeding in premature infants, often in babies felt to be feeding adequately prior to detailed study. Rosen et al. and Guilleminault and Coons studied infants not suspected of having feeding problems and reported apnea during feeding in a large number of these subjects.[3,4] For those babies, respiratory airflow typically ceased for longer than 10 seconds, then oxygen saturation fell, at times leading to bradycardia. Coughing and choking were *not* typically noted, and cyanosis was infrequent. The mechanism that triggered these bradycardic events may have been chemoreceptor stimulation during the apnea, by hypoxia and/or hypercarbia.[6] As normal respiration resumed, the infant typically recovered spontaneously, though this was generally after the bottle had been removed from the mouth.

The mechanisms responsible for this type of apnea during feeding are unclear. Possible explanations include an incoordination between breath-ing and swallowing, as discussed in chapters 1, 3, and 5, or a response to stimulation of laryngeal chemoreceptors.[6,50] In Mathew's study, infants showed a greater incidence of short apnea with feeding than during sleep, suggesting that the neurons involved in integration of breathing and swallowing may mature more slowly than those involved only in regula-tion of respiration.[6]

Although it has been assumed that feeding and respiration are well coor-dinated in term infants, there are recent reports of similar apneic episodes in full-term and older infants.[3,7] It is therefore suggested that feeding-re-lated apnea in the preterm infant approaching the postconceptual age of term does not necessarily represent a delay in the development of respira-tory control or feeding skill in the infant. Rather, respiratory control during feeding may not be complete even for term infants in the neonatal period, and thus such findings in a "term-age" premature infant may not be unusual.[22] For the term infant, however, short apneas always occurred at the beginning of the feeding during continuous sucking, oxygen saturation was less likely to lead to bradycardia, and the infant tended to recover while continuing to feed.[3,7]

The incidence of apnea, oxygen desaturation, and bradycardia in premature infants felt to be feeding adequately is clinically relevant. Although most events were self-limiting, or easily limited by removing the bottle, the effects of ongoing intermittent hypoxia during feeding must be considered. It can be hypothesized that these events could contribute to the poor endurance and intake noted with feeding in some premature infants. It also suggests that careful clinical monitoring of respiratory pattern and color, in addition to cardiorespiratory monitoring, may be appropriate during feeding even for the "healthy" growing premature infant.

Progression from Non-oral to Oral Feeding

Non-nutritive sucking: As adequate oral-feeding skills are not present in many young preterm infants, nutrition by non-oral methods is often necessary. These include gavage feeding through nasogastric and orogastric tubes and, in some cases, parenteral nutrition through peripheral or central lines (see page 268). When the infant is not able to suck nutritively, providing non-nutritive sucking opportunities has many benefits.

Studies have found that NNS in premature infants is associated with accelerated maturation of sucking responses, earlier bottle-feeding, better weight gain, improved oxygen saturation and gastrointestinal function, and earlier hospital discharge.[2,23,31-33] Anderson also describes NNS as facilitating self-regulatory state modulation and improvement in muscle tone and coordination.[1] Therefore, in premature infants who are fully or partially non-orally fed, providing NNS opportunities should always be stressed, particularly in association with non-oral feeding.

Readiness factors: Four factors should be considered in determining if a premature infant is ready to attempt oral feeding.

1. Gestational age: The infant should be at least 32 weeks, although success is more likely if the baby is closer to 34 weeks gestation.

2. Medical condition: The baby's condition should be relatively stable, particularly the respiratory status. The infant should be tolerating gavage feedings, the resting respiratory rate should be below 70, and breathing at rest should not be labored. The assessment of this "work of breathing" includes not only respiratory rate but also heart rate, retractions, and audible sounds of effort such as grunting.

3. State: The infant should be able to maintain, at least briefly, a wakeful state.

4. Non-nutritive sucking: A rhythmic pattern should be present and easily maintained.

Meeting all of these criteria provides the infant with the best chance to make a smooth transition to oral feeding. If an infant does not meet some of these criteria, oral-feeding trials should not automatically be precluded, but the baby should be monitored closely and expectations should be reduced accordingly. For example, occasional oral feedings may be possible. An infant who meets only one or two of these criteria, however, is not likely to be successful at oral feeding. Feeding may be more successful if it is postponed one to two weeks, at which time the infant will probably meet more criteria.

Maturational versus medical factors: If an infant does not make a smooth transition from tube to oral feeding, determining the level of concern and subsequent action requires careful consideration of the balance between maturational factors and medical condition.

In regard to maturational factors, it is often expected that all premature infants will be nippling well by 37 to 38 weeks.[17] Drawing a parallel to motor development, however, it is not expected that all babies will roll at 6 months or will walk at 12 months. There is a wide age range for normal acquisition of these skills. Most likely, this concept also applies to early feeding skills. As discussed above, recent literature suggests that even full-term infants do not always show fully coordinated sucking, swallowing, and breathing during feeding.[3,7] As premature birth and subsequent medical complications may interrupt the normal maturational progression, some premature infants may be slower to progress in the maturation of the coordination required during feeding yet still acquire skills within a "normal" time range.[22]

Medical factors must also be considered. In particular, even mild ongoing respiratory problems or the residual effects of "resolved" respiratory distress can compromise the transition to nipple feeding. In addition, neurologic insults that may be associated with prematurity are known to interfere with oral-feeding function. As failure to progress to oral feeding can be an early sign of long-term neurodevelopmental dysfunction, it must be identified in a timely manner for the infant to receive appropriate intervention.

Based on the gestational age of the infant, some guidelines are suggested to aid in determining the level of concern warranted when a premature infant has difficulty making the transition to oral feeding.

- **35 weeks or less:** In an infant this age, maturational factors often explain feeding difficulties. Waiting at least a week and reintroducing oral feeding may be useful. Non-nutritive sucking opportunities should continue to be stressed. If some level of oral feeding is present and not taxing the infant, but further progress is not noted, remaining at that level of oral feeding for 4 to 7 days before increasing the demands may be useful.

- **36 to 39 weeks:** Unless the infant is medically compromised, some oral feeding should be occurring during this period. If no oral feeding has been successful, or if the progress toward full nipple feeding is very limited during weeks 38 and 39, the level of concern increases and potential causes should be explored. Factors related to oral feeding should be carefully evaluated. This would include clinical evaluation of feeding focusing on the development of sucking mechanisms and rhythm, as well as careful assessment of respiratory factors (at rest and with feeding), including respiratory rate, heart rate, oxygen saturation, and work of breathing (see chapter 3). While maturational factors may still influence progress, medical and neurodevelopmental factors should be considered.

- **40 weeks and older:** A premature infant who has achieved a stable and relatively healthy medical status by this age but, who was born quite prematurely or who had a complicated medical course, may not be taking full oral feedings by 40 weeks gestation. Most infants should be approaching this goal, though endurance may be a limiting factor. The pattern and coordination of the oral portion of the feeding should be smooth and well organized, though occasional oxygen desaturation or bradycardia may still be present.

The relatively healthy premature infant at postconceptual age of term who is not approaching taking full oral feedings deserves additional concern and evaluation. If respiratory problems are not resolving, or they show a pattern of improvement and then rapid decline, microaspiration may be present. Microaspiration occurring during feeding *or* during episodes of gastroesophageal reflux could be compromising respiratory improvement and should be considered for assessment. If significant problems persist in coordinating sucking, swallowing, and breathing, it becomes more likely that central nervous system factors, rather than maturational lags, may be involved. If medical or neurodevelopmental factors are specifically identified that suggest the transition to nipple feeding will be prolonged, the potential need for a gastrostomy tube should begin to be considered.

Feeding specialists may take exception to these guidelines, which find it acceptable for older premature infants to continue to receive some feeding by tube. With the dual pressures to minimize the length of hospital admissions and to have infants fully nipple feeding prior to their discharge, there is considerable pressure on hospital staff *and* on the premature infant in the area of feeding. Not only is nipple feeding often being introduced earlier and with expectations for rapid progress, but respiratory support is often being decreased simultaneously. Frequently the goal is an expedient discharge with the infant weaned from respiratory support and with the infant taking all feedings by nipple.

While these are useful long-term goals and may work as hospital discharge goals for some infants, in our experience they may be counterproductive for other infants and thus result in longer hospitalizations. The progression to nipple feeding must be completely individualized to be the most successful. Each infant's response to nippling should be carefully monitored, including respiratory rate, heart rate, color, oxygen saturation, work of breathing, sucking characteristics, and state/behavioral responses.

If weaning from respiratory support (including medications) is occurring simultaneously with increases in oral feeding, this should be reconsidered. Each change should be separated by at least one to two days to allow the infant to adjust to the change and to provide time for careful monitoring of the baby's response. When the infant is continually challenged to increase feeding and to quickly wean from respiratory support, without careful attention to the spectrum of ways the infant is communicating its response to those changes, there may be an increased incidence of complications such as respiratory infection and other pulmonary setbacks, gastroesophageal reflux, or aspiration.

This approach is not meant to prolong hospitalizations unnecessarily and need not prolong the hospital stay for most premature infants. For infants with whom feeding and respiratory support are the only remaining hospital issues, however, providing home oxygen and some level of gavage feeding should be considered. This may expedite discharge without increasing the risk of complications or setbacks that could prolong the hospitalization or lead to rehospitalization. A very individualized approach, along with modifying the expectation that all infants should nipple fully and without respiratory support by discharge, may reduce the incidence of premature infants who require subsequent rehospitalization for feeding-related problems or poor weight gain.

Feeding-Related Problems Commonly Seen in Premature Infants

Problem—The sleepy baby:
The infant may show poor general state modulation, with rare periods of arousal. "Sleepy" babies do not spontaneously wake for feedings and show minimal interest in nippling, quickly returning to sleep.

Basis for the problem: Young premature infants characteristically spend most of their time in sleep states. While brief spontaneous alerting may be noted at 32 weeks, even at 37 weeks alertness may be of poor quality.[26] As feeding is enhanced by an awake state, difficulty achieving or maintaining wakefulness can compromise feeding. While problems in arousal may be strictly maturational for some infants, others appear to utilize sleeping states to "tune out" excessive stimulation. In addition, as the infant does begin to demonstrate increased differentiation of states at about 36 weeks,[26] nursery routines based on time schedules do not enhance this emerging behavior. Instead, the infant is expected to wake for a feeding or a treatment, then sleep at other times.

Treatment strategies:

- Environmental modifications may be needed. If sleep appears to be utilized as a defense behavior to tune out environmental stimuli, feeding should not begin until appropriate modifications have been made to the environment (see page 210).

- Arousal may be necessary. Some premature infants may appear to awake as they are lifted out of bed and positioned for feeding. However, this arousal may not be adequately sustained for feeding. More complete arousal may be accomplished by using the techniques suggested on page 212.

- Demand feeding schedules may take advantage of the infant's emerging periods of awake alertness. Several authors describe the use of demand feeding in premature infants who are beginning to demonstrate state differentiation independently.[24,25,51] They describe achieving adequate intake in a majority of infants. Also reported are fewer gavage feedings prior to full nipple feeding, as well as earlier hospital discharge.

- Evaluation of oxygen saturation should be considered. Intermittent hypoxemia has been noted during feeding in preterm infants, without obvious signs of its presence.[3,4,6,11] As this could result in lethargy, drowsiness, and difficulty maintaining adequate arousal to complete a feeding, evaluation of oxygen saturation during feeding may be useful.

Problem—Difficulty with sucking mechanics:
While premature infants are generally able to produce a coordinated sucking response, wide jaw excursion and inefficient tongue movements may compromise sucking strength. In addition, tongue-tip elevation is often noted, which makes nipple insertion difficult.

Basis of problem: As described earlier, when compared to the term infant the premature infant shows differences in oral size and structural relationships that can compromise stability during feeding. In particular, the premature infant often has difficulty developing adequate stability in the tongue and jaw. Since the tongue does not fully fill the oral cavity, it does not receive positional stability through continual opposition to other oral structures. It is therefore hypothesized that the baby elevates the tongue tip to oppose the hard palate and achieve a degree of stability in this manner. With the tip elevated, the development of normal tongue movement is inhibited.

Wide jaw movements may also be the result of poor positional stability. The facial "exoskeleton" (composed of subcutaneous fat, thick skin, and sucking pads) provides stability for mandibular movement in the term infant.[15] In the preterm infant, it is poorly developed and therefore not able to stabilize jaw movement adequately. Postural maintenance of a neutral neck position also provides stability to mandibular movement. Poor muscle bulk and limited control of the craniocervical musculature in the premature infant preclude developing adequate neck stability and thus impact jaw movement.

Treatment strategies: Specific treatment techniques for these problems in oral control, as well as others that may be seen less frequently in premature infants, are described in chapter 5. While efficacy of most techniques is based solely on clinical judgment, Leonard et al. have studied the effectiveness of one particular treatment technique on improving the sucking mechanics in premature infants.[30] The infants studied had difficulty feeding, with many described as having a weak suck, though specific problems of oral control were not identified. When the infants were given repetitive pressure over the cheek area during prolonged sucking pauses, increased sucking rate and intake resulted. Similar study of other intervention techniques is warranted.

Problem—Difficulty coordinating sucking, swallowing, and breathing:
Rhythm patterns reflecting the coordination of sucking, swallowing, and breathing are often abnormal in the premature infant. In particular, it is common for premature infants to have prolonged bursts of sucking and swallowing without interspersing breaths—also referred to as feeding-induced apnea (see page 253). This often leads to oxygen desaturation but may or may not lead to bradycardia. Coughing and choking or color change

may or may not be seen. In other infants a dysrhythmic sucking pattern may be noted, consisting of short, irregular sucking bursts.

Basis for the problem: Recent literature suggests that the task of coordinating respiration with sucking and swallowing during feeding is a more complex task than has been appreciated. Even term infants demonstrate undetected feeding-related apnea in the first weeks of life, potentially due to incomplete maturation in the coordination of sucking, swallowing, and breathing.[3,7] Premature infants, who have less mature respiratory control, appear to be even more susceptible to problems in this area.[4,6,11,22]

Treatment strategies:

- Careful monitoring of respiratory rate, heart rate, and oxygen saturation is called for in premature infants, particularly in those who show clinical signs of possible difficulty coordinating sucking, swallowing, and breathing. Such monitoring can help determine the physiological impact of immature coordination of these components. In the presence of marked compromise during feeding, oral feeding can be postponed briefly until there is further maturation.

- Treatment techniques to provide external pacing of sucking, swallowing, and breathing rhythms may also be very useful in the premature infant (see page 253).

- Mathew and Pierantoni suggest that some feeding-related apnea may be related to high milk flow.[29,22] Changing nipples or using other methods of limiting milk flow may be useful (see chapter 7).

- There is some evidence that premature infants coordinate sucking, swallowing, and breathing more effectively at the breast than on the bottle.[34-36] If breast-feeding is planned and if early bottle-feeding trials are not fully successful, breast-feeding may be tried (see chapter 8).

Problem—Reduced endurance:
Frequently the premature infant stops nippling before taking an adequate amount of nourishment. Although the baby may fall asleep part way through the feeding and be difficult to arouse for continued feeding, initially the infant is generally easy to arouse and eager to feed, unlike the truly sleepy baby. Some infants do not fall asleep but simply stop feeding before taking the required amount. Such behavior is often an indication of problems of endurance.

Basis of the problem: The primary contributor to reduced endurance may be respiratory compromise resulting from infant respiratory distress syndrome (IRDS). It appears that even when IRDS seems to be resolved, subtle differences in respiratory performance persist. While oxygen therapy may not be required at rest, if the work to maintain homeostasis is greater than in an infant with a fully competent respiratory system, the infant may not be capable of the increased respiratory work required in feeding. This is consistently a problem in infants with bronchopulmonary dysplasia (BPD) and is discussed further in that section. In infants who meet the criteria for BPD but fall into the mild category, the potential for decreased endurance may be overlooked.

Treatment strategies: Treatment strategies and techniques are discussed on page 257. Possibilities include providing additional oxygen, manipulating feeding schedules, providing nutritional supplements, modifying the flow of liquid, and adjusting expectations.

Necrotizing Enterocolitis

Necrotizing enterocolitis (NEC) is a gastrointestinal disease typically seen in premature infants but also occurring in term infants. In one report, the mean gestational age at onset was 31 weeks gestation, and mean birth weight was 1460 grams.[39] The incidence approaches 12% in infants with birth weights below 1500 grams.[42] It typically develops between day 3 and day 10 of life, though wide variation is possible. Risk factors have been identified, with prematurity being the most significant. Other risk factors include neonatal complications, many of which are implicated in reducing gastrointestinal blood flow.[41] Of interest is the fact that 95% of patients with NEC have been fed formula, breast milk, or both prior to acquiring the disease.[40]

Feeding intolerance, abdominal distention, and gastric retention of feedings are early diagnostic signs. The disease may remain in this mild and benign form or progress to moderate or severe levels involving cellulitis, peritonitis, and intestinal necrosis which may lead to bowel perforation. Progression from the mild form to a severe form can occur very rapidly, with mortality reported in 20% to 40% of those with severe NEC.[39]

While the cause of NEC is not well understood, the process seems to involve an enteric bacteria reacting with a substrate (probably milk) and producing excessive amounts of abdominal gas, which then causes or adds to mucosal injury. Several mechanisms have been implicated in the pathogenesis of NEC, though most likely a combination of these mechanisms is actually involved. These include gastrointestinal and immunologic immaturity, ischemic injury, the presence of pathogenic enteric bacteria, and enteral feeding practices.[39,53] While the immature gastrointestinal system is particularly vulnerable, the specific factors leading to this vulnerability are also not well understood.[53]

Treatment includes antibiotics, nasogastric tube decompression, and bowel rest. Fluid replacement and other medical management appropriate to the patient's condition may be instituted. However, if bowel perforation is recognized, surgery is indicated. Short necrotic bowel segments may be resected, with continuity of the remaining bowel segments established immediately by primary anastomosis. More typical is bowel resection and enterostomy or ileostomy, with anastomosis at a later date.[39]

Any premature infant developing NEC experiences a significant setback in overall medical progress. This setback can impact other problems, such as respiratory distress syndrome. Deterioration in medical condition, as well as the subsequent recovery, places additional stresses on the infant and may interfere with neurodevelopmental and behavioral progress. Enteral feeding is stopped and when restarted must proceed very slowly. At times infants demonstrate difficulty tolerating the return to enteral feeding, slowing the process of moving toward oral feeding.

Impact of NEC on oral feeding: The impact of NEC on feeding in the premature infant is greatest when surgery has been necessary. If large portions of the bowel have been removed, enteral feeding may not be possible, as nutrient absorption will be inadequate to sustain life. Total parenteral nutrition (TPN) may be required (see page 268). Even when smaller bowel segments are resected, recovery is prolonged. Intestinal adaptation is gradual, occurring over months to years.[39] A primary problem during this recovery process and intestinal adaptation is malabsorption, which often persists even after anastomosis.

When malabsorption is present, the process of introducing enteral feeding can be remarkably slow and thus may interfere with the development of oral-feeding skills. The process of moving toward enteral feeding will always include periods of parenteral nutrition. If the need for TPN persists, a catheter or line may be surgically placed directly into a central vein (central line).

As the infant becomes stable with parenteral nutrition, small amounts of enteral feeding are introduced. This is often done using a continuous drip feeding pump. Large boluses of food, which are more difficult for the intestine to manage, are avoided, and the amount of enteral feeding can be advanced in very small increments. Initially only one to two cc/hour may be introduced into the stomach, with similar increments of advancement possible. The use of a continuous drip feeding pump, however, necessitates the use of a feeding tube such as a nasogastric or gastrostomy tube.

When reasonable feeding volumes are tolerated by continuous drip, small bolus feeds are introduced. At this point small nipple feedings may be allowed. Further advances in the volume of bolus feedings and formula strength will, it is hoped, bring the infant to the point of obtaining all nourishment from enteral methods, allowing parenteral nutrition to be discontinued.

Despite slow and gradual advancement of enteral feedings, this process is characterized by frequent setbacks. The infant may reach a level at which the bowel is no longer able to handle the work of nutrient absorption. Gastric retention or excessive stooling may result. Contracting viral and bacterial illnesses common to the hospital nursery can also interfere with this process. When feeding intolerance becomes apparent, the bowel is allowed to rest, using parenteral nutrition only, and the process must begin again.

Although at times this process progresses fairly rapidly, occurring over a few weeks, for some infants it takes months to years and is characterized by numerous periods with little to no enteral feeding. Not only are the oral-feeding opportunities severely limited, but long-term tube feeding may be required. During periods of TPN or continuous drip feeding, hunger patterns become distorted. In addition, when infants are deprived of normal oral-feeding experiences, they may adopt abnormal patterns of oral movement and develop resistance to oral-tactile experiences and exploration.

Initially these infants may have "normal" oral-feeding skills; however, the factors just described suggest the need for a feeding specialist to assist in managing an ongoing program of oral activity. The focus of intervention should be maintaining and facilitating the development of the oral skills that will be necessary for returning to oral feeding when medically feasible. Various treatment strategies and considerations are outlined below. While appropriate for infants with NEC, they should also be considered for any infant who has a "short-gut" syndrome or gastrointestinal malabsorption, as the clinical course and feeding related problems are similar. When prolonged tube feeding has been necessary, following the recommendations on transitioning from tube feeding to oral feeding in chapter 5 would be appropriate.

Treatment strategies and considerations:

Non-nutritive sucking (NNS): Since oral feeding may be restricted for long periods, encouraging NNS becomes very important. Although NNS should accompany tube feedings, many times feeding may be entirely by TPN, or by continuous drip methods. This precludes accompanying "feeding" with NNS, so liberal use of the pacifier should be encouraged at all times. Many benefits of NNS for the non-orally fed premature infant have been described in the section on prematurity. The following benefits are particularly pertinent to the infant with NEC:

- Enhanced maturation of the sucking reflex and increase in strength and rhythm of sucking are noted with NNS.[2,23] This could aid in the transition to oral feeding.

- Improved gastrointestinal motility has been reported in association with NNS.[31] Although these responses are noted in premature infants without NEC, it would be of interest to study the effect of NNS on absorption and feeding tolerance in patients with NEC.

- Improved ability to modulate behavioral state is also associated with NNS.[1] This ability is particularly desired in a premature infant additionally stressed with the disease process of and recovery from NEC.

- Interest in sucking is maintained. Lepecq[52] evaluated eight infants 11 to 13 months old who had no nutritive or non-nutritive sucking experience and found no differences when he compared their NNS patterns to those of normally feeding infants. Our experience, however, has been quite different. In infants who have had no previous nutritive or non-nutritive sucking experiences by the time they reach 4 or 5 months, it is difficult if not impossible to elicit a sucking response.

It appears that as reflexive sucking diminishes, if sucking has not been reinforced through nutritive or non-nutritive sucking experience, this motor pattern is no longer easily elicited. A related observation can be made regarding healthy infants. Although a pacifier may be used in the newborn period, if this practice is not continued, by 4 or 5 months of age most infants will mouth or chew a pacifier but will not suck on it. This occurs despite the fact that a bottle is taken easily.

It is felt that these responses are reflective of the fact that the older infant becomes extremely aware of the tactile qualities of objects in the mouth. Sucking is used only on objects that have very specific and familiar tactile qualities. Other oral patterns are used for other objects. For this reason, it is suggested that the infant with NEC be exposed to a variety of nipple shapes for NNS. At least one should be shaped *exactly* like a bottle nipple. We have seen infants who have very strong NNS skills on only one type of pacifier who have had considerable difficulty transitioning to the bottle. By the time oral feeding could finally be introduced, they were reluctant to suck on a bottle nipple (with or without fluid) that was a different shape from their preferred pacifier (see chapter 7).

Minimize negative or aversive oral stimulation: Although the medical course of the infant with NEC may have included the types of negative oral stimulation to which every premature infant is exposed, the infant with NEC is more likely to require prolonged tube feeding and the associated aversive oral stimulation. As discussed in chapter 5, nasogastric or orogastric tubes will produce significantly more negative oral stimulation than gastrostomy tubes. Since the need for long-term tube feeding is so routine in infants after bowel resection, particularly when large amounts of the bowel are removed, in some centers gastrostomies are placed during the initial surgery. In some instances an infant uses it for only a short period, but typically it is necessary for several months. During that time it provides many benefits to the infant, including a reduction in aversive oral stimulation.

Encourage pleasurable oral experiences: This includes non-nutritive sucking, as well as other pleasant tactile stimulation to the face, lips, and mouth. Developmentally appropriate oral exploration of hands and toys should be encouraged.

Integrate oral-feeding experiences into the enteral or parenteral nutrition program: Two approaches have been used with some success; both are based on the hypothesis that providing some amount of experience coordinating sucking, swallowing, and breathing will help the infant maintain greater interest and skill in the nutritive aspects of sucking.

When a continuous drip enteral feeding regimen is used, nippling is often not considered until boluses of a reasonable size are tolerated in tube feedings. This may deprive the infant of many weeks of nutritive sucking experience. Introduction of some nipple feeding could be considered during periods of continuous drip feedings. When drip rates reach 10 cc per hour, two or three times per day the pump can be turned off for one hour and the infant then nipple-fed 10 cc. This amount does come as a bolus, but it is recognized that even during continuous drip feedings volumes such as this accumulate in the stomach, forming a bolus that the infant is already capable of digesting.

Another way to integrate oral feeding into an enteral or parenteral feeding program is through "sham feedings." These have been used in our center, with some positive effects. This technique requires a gastrostomy tube in place. The infant nipples a small amount (10 cc to 20 cc) of fluid with the gastrostomy lowered and draining to gravity. The fluid then exits the stomach via the gastrostomy. Gentle aspiration of the stomach contents with a syringe may be necessary if the fluid does not drain well. The appropriate fluid to use for each infant must be determined in conjunction with the medical team and can vary from sterile water to specialized formulas.

Intracranial Hemorrhage

Intracranial hemorrhage (ICH) is a frequent complication in premature infants. It occurs in one-third to one-half of infants with birth weight below 1500 grams and is typically noted in the neonatal period. Lower birth weight and gestational age put an infant at greater risk.[43] Detailed discussions of ICH are found elsewhere,[43-45,48] though several points merit inclusion here as they are salient to a discussion of the relationship of ICH to feeding.

Intracranial hemorrhage is a broad term, describing a wide variety of lesions to the brain. These can vary from cortical, cerebellar, and brain-stem bleeds to subependymal or intraventricular bleeds. The latter are particularly common in premature infants. The extent of bleeding can also vary, influencing the amount of damage to the brain. Severe ICH can lead to hydrocephalus.[47]

As would be expected with a condition having a wide range of presentations, there is also wide variation in outcome. A full understanding of outcome is only now emerging, as follow-up studies are completed using sensitive brain-imaging techniques that have recently become available. Adding to the difficulty in formulating a complete picture of outcome, studies vary tremendously in regard to study group, definition of terms, and outcome measures. Deficits that have been identified are in motor skills (sometimes associated with cerebral palsy), speech, and cognitive skills. Seizures and visual problems are also noted. Individual outcomes, however, range from profound damage to apparently normal functioning.[43]

While less favorable outcomes are generally associated with more severe ICH, to date no method exists to predict accurately whether an individual infant will do well or poorly. Additionally, the specific type of problems an infant might develop as a result of ICH are elusive. During infancy it is particularly difficult to determine what, if any, consequences might occur. Outcome becomes more apparent during development over the first year, though some outcome studies still identify subtle deficits at 3 years of age that are possibly linked to neonatal ICH.[46]

This information has several implications in terms of feeding in the premature infant with ICH:

1. ICH itself does not put a premature infant at higher risk for feeding problems. Many infants will have no sequelae from their bleeds. If deficits do result, only some of these might have an impact on feeding performances.

2. While careful observation of neurodevelopmental parameters (including feeding skills) is warranted in infants with severe ICH, even in this group feeding difficulties may not arise.

3. Based on knowledge of the types of deficits reported in outcome studies, infants with feeding problems related to ICH might be expected to show dysfunction in the motoric aspects of feeding. Deficits may be found in oral-motor control as well as in the general postural control needed for feeding. Abnormal motor control in the pharyngeal area might result in swallowing dysfunction. Therefore, these particular areas should be carefully evaluated in the infant with feeding dysfunction who has also experienced ICH.

4. It has been noted that children diagnosed with cerebral palsy have often experienced feeding difficulties in infancy. As cerebral palsy is a frequently reported outcome in infants with ICH, when early feeding problems are present, their significance as an early marker of long-term motor impairment should be considered. Very close neurodevelopmental follow-up is suggested. Alternate explanations for early feeding problems in this group, however, are also possible.

Bronchopulmonary Dysplasia

Bronchopulmonary dysplasia (BPD) is a chronic pulmonary disease process generally seen in neonates after treatment with positive pressure ventilation. The vast majority of infants developing BPD are premature infants being treated for infant respiratory distress syndrome (IRDS). Instead of recovering from IRDS in the first one to two weeks of life, they follow a course of prolonged pulmonary compromise leading to BPD. Full-term infants treated for meconium aspiration, pneumonia, or other respiratory disorders can also develop BPD[1-4] (see figure 6-1, page 298). The criteria for diagnosis of BPD include:[7]

- Positive pressure ventilation for at least three days during the first weeks of life.

- Clinical signs of abnormal respiratory function, that persist beyond 28 days of life.

- Supplemental oxygen required longer than 28 days of life.

- Diffuse abnormal findings characteristic of BPD on chest X-ray.

It appears that BPD develops as a consequence of both the initial lung injury *and* of the treatment to repair it.[3] Not all infants with a primary respiratory insult develop BPD; however, a number of factors have been associated with an increased risk of developing BPD.

Prematurity: There is an inverse relationship between BPD and gestational age and weight. Smaller, more premature infants show a greater incidence. Bancalari reports that BPD develops in 50% to 85% of infants with birth weights below 1000 grams, but in only 5% to 16% of infants who weigh over 1000 grams at birth.[1] Obviously these smaller birth weight infants are also at higher risk for respiratory distress syndrome due to structural or functional immaturity of the lungs. This provides a larger pool of infants with congenitally dysfunctional lungs and the potential to develop BPD.

Oxygen toxicity: Prolonged, continuous inhalation of high concentrations of oxygen can lead to endothelial damage and bronchiolar changes. This increases the risk for subsequent compromise in pulmonary dynamics. Although short courses of intense oxygen therapy may not add to the incidence of BPD, when oxygen is used over longer periods, high concentrations may act synergistically with other factors to play a role in the development of BPD.[4,23]

Positive pressure ventilation: To maintain adequate expansion of the airways in the damaged lung, positive pressure is required during mechanical ventilation. It is speculated that this pressure may produce trauma to the lung tissues (barotrauma).[23] While not all infants requiring positive-pressure ventilation develop BPD, all infants who develop BPD have undergone positive-pressure ventilation.

Patent ductus arteriosus (PDA): Evidence of PDA is frequently seen in the clinical course of infants with BPD. The mechanism felt to be responsible for this association with BPD is the development of pulmonary edema. When a PDA is present, there is increased pulmonary blood flow, which leads to an increase in interstitial fluid in the lungs. Pulmonary compliance decreases and airway resistance increases, possibly necessitating higher ventilatory pressures and oxygen and/or prolonging the need for ventilation, thus increasing the risk of BPD.[1,2]

Fluid overload in the neonatal period: It has been reported that infants who develop BPD had greater fluid intake during the neonatal period than those not developing BPD. It is felt this difference is related to fluid overload resulting in pulmonary edema, similar to the mechanism seen with PDA.[1,2,4]

Pulmonary Changes

Initial respiratory failure is followed by treatments that produce damage to cellular tissues of the lungs and thus alter pulmonary dynamics. Fluid leaks into interstitial spaces, causing pulmonary edema. Plasma proteins interfere with surfactant production and the functioning of existing surfactant. Surface tension of the alveoli then increases and many alveoli collapse (atelectasis). Remaining functional alveoli may have lost the integrity of their cell walls and coalesce, leading to hyperinflated areas (emphysematous). It is reported that by 2 weeks of age, one-third to two-thirds of the lung tissue is atelectatic and the remaining lung tissue is overinflated.[4]

In addition, cellular damage leads to excessive mucus production while ciliary motility may be impaired. The mucus is not effectively removed, blocking airways and stimulating airway receptors that trigger spasms, thickening of tissue, and reduction in airway diameter. Fibrotic changes are also noted.[3,4]

Complications that might arise in these sick infants during this time (such as intracranial hemorrhage, PDA, pneumothorax, or respiratory infection) may result in the need for higher concentrations of inspired oxygen and increased airway pressure during mechanical ventilation. As shown in figure 6-4, a vicious cycle is created wherein medical treatment and its sequelae aggravate pulmonary damage.

Bozynski describes the injury to the lungs in BPD as "pervasive" and affecting all elements of the lungs and airways.[3] These airway changes result in numerous problems of pulmonary function.

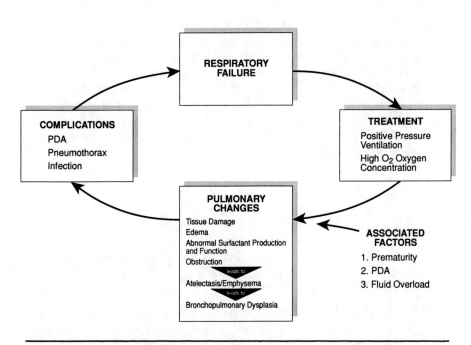

Figure 6-4 In bronchopulmonary dysplasia a vicious cycle is created whereby medical treatment and its sequelae aggravate pulmonary damage. Adapted from Bancalari.[1]

Increased airway resistance: The airways narrow due to pulmonary edema, thickening and spasm, and the presence of mucus. This leads to a reduction in dynamic compliance, which is more noticeable at higher respiratory rates.[1,25]

Decreased pulmonary compliance: Fibrotic tissue, overdistended lung units, and collapsed lung parenchyma lead to reductions in static compliance.[1,4,25]

Increased work of breathing: It is more work to inhale and expand the lungs when lung compliance is poor and airway resistance is high. The work of breathing for an infant with BPD has been likened to a healthy adult breathing through a straw. This activity requires considerably more effort due to the increase in airway resistance created by the comparatively narrow "airway" of the straw. When the work of breathing is great, larger amounts of oxygen and calories are consumed to move a given volume of air. Weinstein reports that oxygen consumption increases 25% in infants with BPD.[6] Wolfson has calculated that the work of breathing in infants with BPD is several times that of healthy term or preterm infants.[5] Intercostal retractions, nasal flaring, and "barrel chest" may be noted during excessive pulmonary work.[3]

Impaired gas exchange: Gas exchange is impaired at the alveolar level due to collapse and overinflation of the alveoli. In addition, there is often a mismatch between ventilation and perfusion. Pulmonary blood flow is still present in areas of alveolar "dead space," leading to a functional reduction of pulmonary blood flow in areas where gas exchange is possible. This results in varying degrees of hypoxia (low oxygen concentration in the blood) and hypercarbia (high concentration of carbon dioxide in the blood). Supplemental oxygen and/or more aggressive mechanical ventilation is then required to maintain an appropriate balance of oxygen and carbon dioxide in the blood.

Increased respiratory rate: To maintain the high level of oxygen needed to support the work of breathing in a system in which impaired gas exchange creates inefficient use of each breath, the respiratory rate often increases substantially. Although increasing the amount of inspired air in each breath could help compensate for these pulmonary compromises, tidal volume is generally decreased, leaving an increase in the respiratory rate as the primary compensatory mechanism.[1]

Increased vulnerability to respiratory fatigue: Infants with BPD seem to be vulnerable to respiratory muscle fatigue. This may be due to an intrinsic difference in the respiratory muscles of the premature infant. It may also result from the high chest wall compliance of the infant. The respiratory muscles are then at a mechanical disadvantage, having a less "stable" base to work from in creating lung expansion.[4]

"Deconditioning" may also play a role in patients who have undergone prolonged mechanical ventilation.[2]

Medical Treatment and Management

Many treatment strategies are used in trying to prevent the development of BPD and in its acute treatment and chronic management. As the mechanisms of BPD are more clearly understood and as technology improves, new treatment strategies are possible. Although some of these therapies are promising, the measure of their effectiveness awaits the completion of conclusive clinical research studies. In general, however, the goals of all medical treatments of BPD are to minimize damage to the lungs, promote growth of new lung tissue, maintain optimal oxygenation, and prevent additional complications.[7]

The risk of oxygen toxicity is reduced by minimizing the concentration of inspired oxygen. Reducing barotrauma to the lungs is also desirable. When an infant is on intermittent positive-pressure ventilation, the lowest possible peak pressure that will still maintain adequate ventilation is used. Pressures are reduced as quickly as possible.[1,26] More recently, high-frequency oscillatory or jet ventilation has been used with some success. Relatively low tidal volumes are provided at supraphysiologic respiratory frequencies, leading to lower intrapulmonary pressures.[20] Diuretics may be used to manage initial pulmonary edema, which contributes to declining pulmonary status.[26] Short-term use of corticosteroids may also produce marked improvement in pulmonary function, though risks associated with long-term use remain a major concern.[29]

Other treatments are used in an attempt to prevent the development of the primary respiratory insult. Tocylitic drugs may be used in some cases to arrest premature labor and allow further lung maturity prior to birth. When it is not possible or advisable to stop preterm labor, acceleration of fetal lung maturation and induction of surfactant production has been attempted by the use of antenatal steroids.[4,18] In small premature infants, surfactant is being provided in the neonatal period, with research studies continuing in this area.[28]

Longer-term therapies become supportive in nature. Once the infant is weaned from the ventilator, supplemental oxygen is required. O'Brodovich and Mellins describe oxygen as being "the most essential medication for the infant with significant BPD."[4] Theoretically, providing oxygen, and thus reducing hypoxia, should decrease minute ventilation and allow calories to be used for growth and repair. Oxygen requirements decrease gradually as the disease process improves, but increases may occur during feeding, physical activity, or episodes of pulmonary infection or edema. In severe BPD, the need for supplemental oxygen may persist for many months or years.[1,21]

Fluid management is important, and water and salt intake may need to be limited. Diuretics may be needed, though complications may arise with long-term diuretic therapy. Bronchodilators may be used to help reduce airway obstruction and decrease airway resistance.[26] Finally, nutrition must be optimal. Although fluid restriction, increased caloric demands, and poor feeding tolerance may interfere with nutrition, good nutritional status plays a key role in the process of pulmonary repair and growth of new lung tissue.[1,24]

Clinical Course and Complications

Although some infants with BPD die from either progressive respiratory failure or other acute complications, most survive. Gradual improvement is seen in pulmonary function and other parameters, though the rate of improvement is dependent on the severity of the disease process.[7] Those with mild to moderate BPD may be free of associated treatments and care by 6 months to 1 year of age. Those with severe lung disease may continue to require related care until 2 to 4 years of age or even longer. The impact of BPD in infancy on pulmonary function in later childhood and in adult life is poorly understood, though deficits may be apparent in some patients.[4] Problems that may complicate the long-term recovery from BPD include:

Prolonged ventilation: The criteria for diagnosis with BPD include mechanical ventilation for at least three days. Unfortunately, many infants with BPD require much longer periods of mechanical ventilation. Although weaning from the ventilator is attempted as quickly as possible without jeopardizing the infant, the degree of lung damage and related complications often lead to the need for prolonged ventilation.[2]

Tracheostomy: When the need for ventilation persists, multiple weaning attempts have failed, and/or significant lung damage is present and resolving slowly, a tracheostomy may be performed. The time line and criteria for placing a tracheostomy vary among centers but are individualized for each infant's situation. The infant with BPD who requires a tracheostomy will have high care needs. Other considerations regarding tracheostomies are discussed on page 333.

Prolonged need for oxygen therapy: As described above, supplemental oxygen therapy may be necessary for days to weeks or even many months after mechanical ventilation is terminated. Long-term, low-flow oxygen therapy is currently possible in home settings and therefore does not necessarily lengthen hospitalizations.[3,4,21]

Prolonged hospitalization: Those infants with more severe forms of BPD, or multiple complications, often require prolonged hospitalization. To a large degree, the length of hospitalization is dependent on the length of time mechanical ventilation is required. While psychosocial and cost motivations are encouraging adaptation of many treatment modalities to the home environment (e.g., low-flow oxygen therapy, gavage feedings, and even ventilators for infants with tracheostomies), the infant must be medically stable. Planning and training for home care is time consuming. Prolonged hospitalization not only adds to a family's financial burdens, but also creates abnormal social relationships between the infant and the parents and interferes with age appropriate developmental opportunities.[3,21]

Infection: The borderline pulmonary status of infants with BPD puts them at increased risk for acquiring respiratory infections and makes recovery from such infections a difficult process. Frequently infants with BPD must be rehospitalized during their first year of life due to respiratory infections, and in some cases an infection may precipitate death.[1,4] Those requiring prolonged hospitalization are at increased risk for acquiring nosocomial infections, such as cytomegalovirus and respiratory syncytial virus. Additionally, the incidence of otitis media is higher in infants who have been mechanically ventilated.[3]

Reactive airway disease: Children with BPD seem to be more prone to problems with reactive airway disease. The compromised lungs of infants recovering from BPD are more susceptible to aggravation from irritants, including air pollution, wood smoke, and cigarette smoke. Microaspiration of oral secretions, or food during swallowing, or from GE reflux also contributes to reactive airway disease. Such reactive airway disease may lead to setbacks in the overall respiratory status.[3]

Heart failure: The chronic hypoxemia common to most infants with BPD can lead to pulmonary hypertension and possibly cor pulmonale leading to heart failure. While attempts are made to manage this progression, heart failure may be the cause of death in an infant with BPD.[2,3]

Acquired tracheobronchial abnormalities: Various abnormalities of the trachea and bronchi may be noted in infants who have been intubated. Tracheal stenosis, tracheomalacia, and bronchomalacia, as well as granulation tissue and narrowing of the bronchi have been reported. Abnormal tissue proliferation may be related to trauma from large endotracheal tubes and their subsequent abrasion, infection, or vigorous suctioning that contacts the trachea and main-stem bronchi. Barotrauma may damage the cartilaginous structures, leading to instability.[8,9,10]

Osteopenia: Premature infants typically have poor calcium deposits in their bones at birth. Parenteral nutrition solutions are low in calcium, and diuretics cause excretion of existing calcium. Therefore an infant with BPD, particularly undergoing these treatments, is at risk for developing osteopenia, or fragile, poorly mineralized bones. The risk of subsequently developing fractures of the ribs and long bones is high.[2,3]

Gastroesophageal reflux (GER): As described in detail starting on page 336, there is a close association between respiratory dynamics and the development of GER. Increased respiratory effort can influence intra-abdominal pressure gradients, increasing the likelihood of GER. In addition, the presence of GER can compromise respiratory status, secondary either to microaspiration or reflex responses in bronchial tissue when receptors in the esophagus are stimulated.[2,3]

Growth failure: Infants with BPD are often noted to demonstrate poor weight gain and growth, even when given "adequate" calories for age. It is hypothesized that their higher energy expenditure for breathing may actually increase their caloric needs. Unfortunately, many other factors interfere with consuming the required calories. Oral-feeding ability is often limited due to respiratory compromise or poorly developed oral-motor skills. Fluid restrictions may necessitate concentrated formulas that may not be tolerated, and GER may lead to loss of some calories previously consumed.[1,11,12]

Developmental delay: While developmental delay is seen frequently in infants with BPD, perinatal and neonatal events may be the primary contributing factors, rather than the presence or absence of BPD.[21,22] More severe BPD, longer hospitalization, and prolonged need for oxygen have been associated, however, with less optimal developmental outcome, even when accounting for the degree of prematurity.[30] The degree of developmental delay during the first two years of life, when medical status is most compromised, may not correlate well with later developmental performance as health status improves.[21,22]

Feeding-Related Problems Commonly Seen in BPD

Feeding problems are *common* in infants with BPD. Rare is the infant with moderate to severe BPD who escapes feeding difficulties throughout the course of recovery. Even infants with mild BPD frequently have feeding problems, often exacerbated by the expectation that because their lung disease is so mild feeding should not be affected. Difficulties in feeding primarily stem from ongoing respiratory problems as well as motor, tactile, and behaviorally based problems resulting from medical interventions.

While oral feeding is an important goal for the infant with BPD, the crucial goal is providing optimal nutrition. It is becoming increasingly apparent that adequate nutrition is a key to facilitating lung repair and growth, both of which aid in the recovery from BPD.[1,12,24] If oral feeding leads to marginal nutrition or excessive energy expenditure, nutrition should take precedence over oral feeding. In this case, providing supplementary non-oral nutrition should be seen as aiding the infant's overall recovery from BPD, and maintenance of oral skills should still be addressed (see chapter 5).

Problem—Decreased endurance:
It is common for infants with BPD to have difficulty taking the required volume by nipple. Reduced endurance is often a key factor. Poor coordination of sucking, swallowing, and breathing, as well as abnormal oral-motor patterns that lead to feeding inefficiency, can also contribute.

Basis of the problem: For infants with BPD, the percentage of total work needed for respiration is several times greater than in infants with healthy lungs.[5] In healthy persons this percentage remains constant, even with additional work. In those with chronic obstructive pulmonary disease such as BPD, however, the percentage of energy used in breathing *increases* during further activity. For infants, the activity of feeding requires additional work, thus adding stress to an already limited respiratory system with minimal reserve. Fatigue develops and the infant may stop feeding prior to taking adequate calories. Factors that make oral feeding inefficient will magnify limitations in endurance.

Treatment Strategies:

- Decrease the work of breathing. Medical treatment that supports increasing pulmonary compliance and lowering airway resistance will help decrease the work of breathing. In particular, if inhaled bronchodilators are prescribed, administering them prior to a feeding may be useful.

- When the workload is increased, such as during feeding, oxygen consumption is also increased. Providing additional oxygen at feeding time is recommended, even after it has been eliminated during rest.[1] When long-term, low-flow oxygen has been provided, substantial improvement in weight gain has been reported.[12] Supporting the increased work of breathing during feeding may minimize the impact of reduced endurance.

- Feeding schedules can be manipulated and nutritional supplements used to assist the infant with poor endurance. These are described further on page 258.

- Expectations may need to be adjusted and supplemental non-oral-feeding methods utilized to provide adequate nutrition and support optimal growth (see page 264).

Problem—Poor coordination of sucking, swallowing, and breathing:
Although the young premature infant may present with feeding-related apnea secondary to immature neuromotor coordination of these functions, the infant with BPD is likely to be somewhat older when oral feedings are initiated. Maturational factors should be considered, depending on the age of the infant; however, it is more common that respiratory factors will limit the coordination of sucking, swallowing, and breathing. Decreased respiratory control may lead to an abnormal sucking pattern consisting of short, irregular sucking bursts with long pauses.

Basis of the problem: When oral feeding is initiated in the infant with BPD, significant compromise of respiratory function is present. In particular, the respiratory rate is often quite elevated and little respiratory reserve is present. Coelho suggests that in this case the reciprocity between swallowing and respiration may be disrupted.[13] If the infant with BPD has a tracheostomy and is on mechanical ventilation (see page 335), coordination of sucking and swallowing with the pre-set respiratory rate of the ventilator may be difficult.

Airflow is interrupted for approximately one second with each swallow, thus reducing the amount of time available for breathing. Repeated swallowing is a key aspect of infant feeding; however, if an infant swallows 30 times per minute, the time available for respiratory activity is cut in half.[32] Knowing that the work of feeding actually increases respiratory demands, one can see how the infant struggling to breathe at rest, and with minimal respiratory reserve, could become compromised with feeding. Choking or coughing may result as the infant gasps for air. Some infants may learn to compensate by utilizing extremely short sucking bursts. Thus, fewer swallows are necessary and there is less interruption of breathing. Feeding, however, becomes quite inefficient.

Treatment strategies:

- Careful monitoring of physiologic parameters, particularly respiratory rate, is necessary. Feedings may need to be limited or postponed if the infant remains tachypneic (see pages 142 and 260 for guidelines).

- Use of the short sucking burst pattern should be encouraged or facilitated as an adaptive response to high respiratory demands (see page 254).

- Expectations may need to be adjusted and perhaps supplemental non-oral feeding methods utilized if the infant's feeding pattern is adaptive yet inefficient (see pages 264-276).

Problem—Abnormal oral-motor patterns:
Although some infants with BPD have well-organized, strong sucking, abnormal oral-motor patterns are frequently noted during sucking. Jaw excursion may be wide and tongue movements poorly coordinated. In particular, central grooving may be minimal, the tongue may be bunched or humped, and protrusion may be noted. The degree of dysfunction may range from mild, producing inefficient sucking patterns, to severe, whereby the infant is not able to initiate or maintain any functional sucking. Related to these oral-motor problems, posture during feeding may reflect strong neck extension.

Basis of the problem: Numerous factors may impact oral-motor control in the infant with BPD. Primary may be the lack of normal sucking experiences, though neuromotor control problems due to central nervous system damage must also be considered. An orally intubated infant may have completely missed sucking experience during the period of intubation. Depending on the length of intubation, reflexive sucking responses may not have been facilitated to build a basis for the volitional responses of the older infant. If sucking was present during oral intubation, abnormal patterns may have been utilized. The shape and position of the endotracheal tube may have encouraged tongue protrusion and limited development of central grooving.

Additionally, head and neck posture can alter oral-motor patterns during sucking. The infant struggling to breathe, on or off a ventilator, often adopts a strongly extended neck position. It is presumed that this posture is adopted as an attempt to more fully open the airway and ease respiration or to minimize the discomfort of the endotracheal tube.[33] Stress responses may also exaggerate this posture. An extended position provides little positional stability for sucking and leads to wide jaw excursion and tongue protrusion.

Structural changes to the oral cavity may also be noted. Commonly seen is the high, grooved palate formed by continual pressure of the oral endotracheal tube and lack of contact between the tongue and the hard palate. This may impact the pressure dynamics during sucking.

Treatment strategies:
- Normalization of total body posture and alignment should be emphasized during feeding (see page 215), as well as at other times. Ideally, marked neck extension should be reduced to aid oral-motor control; although even a neutral alignment may not be tolerated by these infants. Changes to the habitual posture of the infant with BPD

---

may cause the infant to be stressed. This may be more detrimental to oral feeding than the abnormal oral patterns associated with neck extension. Not only may a new position be uncomfortable, but it may make respiration more difficult, thus interfering with feeding. Slight neck extension, therefore, may be accepted. The goal of improved neck and head positioning during feeding may need to be addressed slowly.

- After identifying the specific components of abnormal movement in the sucking process, treatment techniques as described in chapter 5 should be utilized.

Problem—Swallowing dysfunction:
When recurrent and unexplained episodes of respiratory deterioration or reactive airway disease are noted in infants with BPD, swallowing function should be questioned. Silent microaspiration can be seen in infants with BPD, leading to cycles of respiratory deterioration. Some types of incoordination between sucking, swallowing, and breathing may also reflect swallowing dysfunction in this group of patients.

Basis of the problem: Intubation for mechanical ventilation may damage structures of the larynx, causing incomplete protection of the airway during swallowing. Moderate to major laryngeal injury has been reported in 44% to 55% of infants who are intubated.[19] In adults with chronic obstructive pulmonary disease, reduced strength in all aspects of swallowing is noted, along with reduced ability to use pulmonary air to clear the larynx and insure airway protection.[13] Such observations may also be made of infants with BPD and suggest further mechanisms for swallowing dysfunction.

Treatment strategies: If swallowing dysfunction is suspected, evaluation with VFSS should be completed. Treatment strategies would depend on the specific findings during the VFSS (see page 222).

Problem—Oral-tactile hypersensitivity:
It is not uncommon to find the infant with BPD pulling back as a nipple is placed on the lips, and becoming agitated or gagging as a nipple is placed in the mouth. These responses indicate oral-tactile hypersensitivity, seen frequently in infants with BPD. Hypersensitivity can significantly interfere with feeding as well as other aspects of the infant's care.[31]

Basis of the problem: Due to the need for mechanical ventilation, the early oral experiences of the infant with BPD are substantially altered. The infant is both deprived of normal, pleasurable oral sensations and experiences aversive oral stimulation during required medical treatment. While the infant is mechanically ventilated via endotracheal tube, oral feeding is not possible. Unless the baby is nasally intubated, even sucking on a pacifier cannot be attempted. Although the infant may develop "sucking" on the endotracheal tube, the size and shape differ markedly from a nipple or pacifier. Pleasurable oral experiences are severely curtailed.

The ongoing presence of an endotracheal tube is an uncomfortable experience, particularly to the oral area, which is rich in tactile receptors. Taping and retaping of these tubes is necessary to hold them securely; yet it is unpleasant. Discomfort is also noted as the tube is suctioned. While the degree of oral-tactile hypersensitivity often appears linked to the length of intubation, even after extubation insertion of feeding tubes and other treatments may prolong aversive oral stimulation.

Treatment strategies:

- Aversive oral input should be minimized. In the infant with BPD there is little choice regarding the presence of an endotracheal tube and the need for care such as taping and suctioning. It is possible, however, to reduce the negative impact of these procedures on the infant through care practices that support the infant's neurobehavioral organization. Als and colleagues have developed a program of intervention that includes attention to the timing, sequencing, and frequency of procedures.[15,16] The infant's behavioral state is prepared for the procedure, postural containment is provided during the procedure, and unhurried reorganization and stabilization are allowed after the procedure. Initial research results suggest that such supportive care may reduce the length of time mechanical ventilation is necessary and therefore reduce the amount of time associated aversive procedures are required.

- Pleasurable oral-tactile input should be maximized. Nasal intubation should be used if possible, as it allows the opportunity for pleasurable non-nutritive sucking experiences. Stroking to the head, face, cheeks, and lips can also be provided. Supporting the infant's neurobehavioral organization may be necessary for these activities to be enjoyable.

- While the previous strategies should help minimize the development of oral-tactile hypersensitivity, for the older infant in whom hypersensitivity is interfering with progress in oral feeding, additional treatment strategies are discussed on page 247.

Problem—"Learned" behaviors that interfere with feeding:
It is clear to most feeding specialists who are experienced with very young infants that associations formed during the first few months of life can be the basis of behavioral responses that may interfere with feeding.[31] Although early behaviors may be simple head turning or extremity flailing to indicate displeasure, these behaviors become more "sophisticated" with advancing development.

Basis of the problem: Erikson describes the task of the infant as developing "trust": trust that the needs for comfort and food will be met.[14] For the infant requiring prolonged intubation and hospitalization, this may prove a difficult task. Although nutrition is provided, non-oral or parenteral methods may separate the feelings of fullness and satiation from the mouth. Comforting measures may be difficult to provide and may be overshadowed by uncomfortable medical procedures. As these procedures are stressful and aversive to the infant, fight-or-flight responses may develop, particularly if appropriate comforting measures are not present to offset this stress. Mildly negative messages may turn into strong behavioral statements if they are not heeded. Pleasurable oral stimuli may be minimal if present at all.

This background gives the infant little reason to participate in oral feeding "when it is time." Interestingly, oral feeding is also the one area in which the infant maintains some sense of control. Caregivers may provide nourishment by tube feeding, but forcing an infant to develop oral feeding is difficult and typically unsuccessful. Negative behaviors may be reinforced as the infant is successful at controlling the feeding situation.

Treatment strategies:

- Techniques described by Als to aid in neurobehavioral organization have the added benefits of helping the infant build trust in the environment and caregivers.[15,16] The consistency and reliability of the care can minimize stress. Als's research also found that infants who had received this regimen of care were completely orally feeding significantly sooner. It is tempting to speculate that in these infants fewer early behaviors resisting oral-motor and oral-tactile experiences will develop.

- While the techniques of Als can help build a general background of trust, specific trusting relationships must be established with those participating in oral-motor and feeding programs.[15,16] Understanding the infant's behavioral communication, and respecting it, can aid in building this trust.

- The infant's control over the feeding process should also be respected. Communicating this to the infant helps build trust and may facilitate the infant's participation in the process.

- If "behavioral" management techniques are utilized, steps should be small and should focus on reinforcement of positive eating behaviors.

Tracheostomy

A subgroup of infants with BPD will require placement of a tracheostomy. Most often a tracheostomy is performed when prolonged ventilatory support is required for infants with the most severe BPD,[17] although infants with diagnoses such as subglottic stenosis or tracheomalacia may also require a tracheostomy despite having reasonable underlying pulmonary function.[8] Tracheostomy eliminates the need for ongoing orotracheal or nasotracheal intubation and the associated discomfort. It also facilitates caregiving and often allows initiation of home-care planning. While this discussion of tracheostomies focuses on the infant with BPD, most points are also applicable to infants with tracheostomies placed for other reasons.

With a tracheostomy in place, varying levels of respiratory support may be provided. A ventilator with intermittent positive pressure may be used to give the infant some or all breaths, along with additional oxygen (figure 6-5). Continuous positive airway pressure (CPAP), without intermittent breaths, may be utilized by some infants on the ventilator. Other infants may not require assisted ventilation; however, moist air (with or without additional oxygen) may be supplied via a "trach collar."

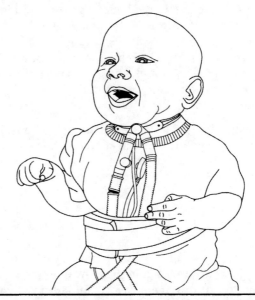

Figure 6-5 Infant with a tracheostomy who requires mechanical ventilation.

Although the presence of a tracheostomy has significant implications for speech and, to a lesser degree, motor development in the head and neck area, this discussion will focus on its relationship to the feeding process. Oral feeding is quite possible with a tracheostomy in place, even during infancy. The safety and functional nature of the feeding, however, must be determined. Such evaluation is based on a clear understanding of the feeding process and the relationship of the tracheostomy to that process.

Relationship of a Tracheostomy to the Feeding Process

Respiratory status: As emphasized throughout this text, compromised respiratory status and pulmonary function will limit oral-feeding skills. If a tracheostomy is placed for supportive care in an infant with severe BPD, the tracheostomy may not improve pulmonary function. The infant will continue to demonstrate problems of limited reserve and poor endurance. The impact of continued respiratory compromise on feeding should be assessed as for other infants with BPD (discussed earlier in this chapter) and will probably limit oral-feeding ability.

If the tracheostomy is placed to manage subglottic stenosis or tracheomalacia, respiratory status may improve, with pulmonary function showing only minimal to moderate impairment. Respiratory factors must still be considered, but it may play a smaller role in feeding.

Oral skills: Although tracheostomy placement should not have a direct impact on oral-motor skills, it is often placed after prolonged intubation. As discussed previously, prolonged intubation and the subsequent lack of normal oral-motor activity and sucking experience can lead to impaired oral function. Removal of the endotracheal tube after tracheostomy allows increased therapeutic activity to facilitate normal oral-motor skills, though changes may be slow. In this case, abnormal oral-motor control can be a limiting factor in feeding infants with a tracheostomy.

Swallowing ability: The presence of the tracheostomy tube in the larynx can lead to impairment in swallowing function. Nash describes several mechanisms whereby the tracheostomy may lead to swallowing dysfunction,[17] though previous damage from endotracheal intubation may also contribute.[8-10] The tube itself may mechanically restrict upward movement of the larynx, limiting the laryngeal elevation necessary for complete epiglottic closure. Chronic air diversion through the tube may lead to desensitization of the larynx and loss of protective reflexes. Upper airway bypass may also contribute to uncoordinated laryngeal closure. Each of these swallowing impairments may lead to aspiration during the swallow. In addition, if a cuffed tracheostomy tube is used, overinflation can easily cause obstruction in the esophagus and overflow of contents into the airway, leading to aspiration after the swallow.

The reported incidence of swallowing dysfunction after tracheostomy varies from 1% to 69%,[17] and little specific information is available for pediatric patients. Some of this wide variation in reported incidence is accounted for by differing methods of evaluation.

Questions confronting the clinician include how rigorous should one be in evaluating swallowing function in tracheostomy patients prior to initiating oral feeding? Also, if evidence of aspiration is noted, how restrictive should management plans be regarding oral feeding?

Some authors describe giving methylene blue dye or a similar substance prior to oral feeding in tracheostomy patients.[17,31] The tracheal aspirate is then screened for evidence of aspiration. VFSS can be used for more definitive evaluation of swallowing dysfunction. Another option is close clinical observation during initiation of oral feeding. Evidence of swallowing dysfunction during feeding or subsequent respiratory deterioration would then indicate the need for detailed swallowing studies.

Maintaining some level of therapeutic oral feeding is often desirable, even in the patient with evidence of aspiration, as long as it is not compromising pulmonary status (see page 228). It is often patients with tenuous respiratory status, such as those with BPD, however, who are not able to tolerate even minimal amounts of aspiration. As discussed previously, microaspiration during feeding or from gastroesophageal reflux can lead to reactive airway disease and deterioration of respiratory status.

Coordination of sucking, swallowing, and breathing: In infants with tracheostomies, the coordination of sucking, swallowing, and breathing is altered, though this is not well understood. Neither ventilated nor spontaneous breaths flow through the pharynx, essentially separating the air and food channels. As the infant is weaned from the tracheostomy, or develops air leaks around the tube and begins moving air through the larynx, coordination of breathing with sucking and swallowing is necessary. If the infant has not had to rely on precise timing and coordination of swallowing and breathing to protect the airway, dysfunction may now become apparent. In non-ventilated infants, monitoring the rhythm of feeding and the coordination of sucking, swallowing, and breathing should be ongoing. External pacing should be provided as necessary to help the infant develop an adequate pattern of coordination. In the ventilated patient this may not be possible, but appropriate pacing of sucking, swallowing, and breathing should be encouraged, incorporating the ventilator rate.

Gastroesophageal Reflux

Gastroesophageal reflux (GE reflux or GER) is the spontaneous return of gastric contents into the esophagus. Symptomatic gastroesophageal reflux is an important clinical problem in infants. Any parent will confirm that reflux with emesis occurs all too frequently in healthy infants. On the other hand, some babies who never demonstrate vomiting as a symptom of their reflux have significant GER that may cause numerous and significant sequelae. The distinction, therefore, between babies considered symptomatic or asymptomatic does not depend upon all-or-none phenomena but rather on the frequency and extent of the reflux-related symptomology.

Many factors result in reflux, including (1) transient and inappropriate relaxation of the lower esophageal sphincter, (2) transient increase in intra-abdominal pressure,[1] and/or (3) spontaneous free reflux from abnormally decreased lower esophageal sphincter tone. Morbidity from reflux includes emesis (vomiting), which can lead to failure to thrive, esophagitis or heartburn,[2] stricture formation, aspiration, reactive airway disease,[3,4] and/or apnea and bradycardia.[5]

The natural clinical course of reflux shows that by 18 months, 60% to 80% of infants will be free of symptoms, with the greatest improvements occurring around 8 to 10 months as the child begins to sit up and solid foods are added to the child's diet. Another 30% will have symptoms until at least age 4.[6,7] It is generally accepted that GER gradually resolves with maturation.[8]

The detection of gastroesophageal reflux in babies with feeding difficulties is important secondary to its association with respiratory disease, its ability to influence a baby's willingness to feed, its effect on weight gain, and its ability to alter respiration and heart rate. There is an interrelationship and interdependency between GER and respiratory disease in children—there are several mechanisms by which reflux can cause respiratory disease and, conversely, many ways that respiratory disease can cause reflux.[9,10] A vicious cycle can occur, with reflux producing respiratory disease and the respiratory disease or its treatment further aggravating the reflux. A complete understanding of this interrelationship is needed for effective evaluation and management. Orenstein and Orenstein provide an excellent review of this relationship.[10]

GE Reflux as a Causal Factor in Respiratory Disease

The most obvious mechanism by which GE reflux can cause respiratory disease is through aspiration of the refluxed material. Several other factors related to GE reflux, however, have more recently been identified as contributors to respiratory disease. These include reflex bronchospasm, reflex laryngospasm, and reflex central apnea or bradycardia. Through complex interactive processes, the presence of acid reflux in the esophagus has been postulated to increase the amount of mucus secreted in the lungs and possibly change the dynamics of the upper and lower airways. Often one of the only presenting symptoms of GE reflux is the presence of respiratory disease that is not explained by a thorough pulmonary evaluation or is not responsive to traditional pulmonary treatment.[4,11]

Aspiration

Aspiration of refluxed food has long been thought to cause reactive airway disease; however, this type of aspiration is extremely difficult to document. Generally, it is hard to differentiate aspiration of ascending refluxed material from descending aspiration that occurs during swallowing. Procedures to sample the lungs for the presence of stomach contents are invasive and often insensitive to the detection of microaspiration. A diagnosis of reflux-related aspiration can only be suggested, but not confirmed, by a compatible history of coughing or choking after feedings, emesis, and an abnormal chest X-ray. It can also be inferred if pulmonary symptoms abate when GER treatment is instituted.[3]

Reflex Bronchospasm

An association between reflux and reactive airway disease through a vagally mediated reflex mechanism has been postulated. It is suggested that refluxed acid causes bronchoconstriction or heightened bronchial reactivity. Human and animal studies show that the infusion of acid into the esophagus causes bronchospasm. This response is obliterated if the vagus nerve, the afferent mediator of this response, is cut.[10] In a baby such as a former premature baby with some residual component of lung disease, this reflux-driven pulmonary response of bronchospasm will only further exacerbate airway problems and thus affect the ability to feed.

Reflex Laryngospasm

Partial or total closure of the airway can be secondary to laryngospasm induced by gastroesophageal reflux. Acid reflux or mixed gastric contents can reflexively trigger laryngeal adduction. Total closure will result in obstructive apnea, which will impede the flow of air to the lungs even if respiratory efforts continue. Partial airway closure will allow the continuation of airflow, but the resistance to airflow from the narrowed larynx may be audible as stridor. To parents observing this type of reflux-triggered laryngospastic event, it is a frightening experience. They may find their baby, about an hour after eating, either awake or asleep, possibly having just regurgitated, rigid, staring, opisthotonic, ruddy or cyanotic, and struggling to breathe.

Central Apnea and Bradycardia

Laryngeal stimulation with a variety of liquids can result in a centrally mediated apnea and subsequent bradycardia, possibly via the superior laryngeal nerve afferents. The application of cow's milk, water, or other solutions to the larynx can produce apnea in immature animals or humans.[12] Therefore, if refluxed material enters the larynx, whether it is aspirated or not, apnea or bradycardia can result.

Respiratory Disease as a Causal Factor in GER

Respiratory symptoms or disease can trigger or exacerbate reflux if they alter any of the infant's natural antireflux barriers. The primary antireflux barrier is the lower esophageal sphincter (LES). This is not a definitive muscular sphincter at the distal end of the esophagus. Rather, there is a zone of increased intraluminal pressure in approximately the distal one to three cm of the esophagus. Anatomically, the esophagus passes through the diaphragm and enters the stomach at an angle, causing the lower esophageal sphincter to be positioned partially in the thorax and partially in the abdomen[13] (figure 6-6). In this angled position, the baseline positive pressure within the abdominal cavity assists with closure of the LES. Changes in abdominal or thoracic pressure gradients, therefore, will influence the competence of the LES and its ability to maintain the gastric contents within the stomach.

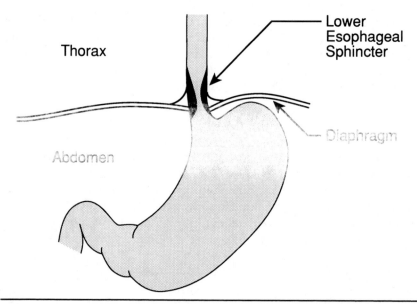

Figure 6-6 Anatomic relationships of the esophagus, stomach, and LES are shown.

Thus, if respiratory disease changes the pressure dynamics within the abdomen or thorax, or its treatment alters the resting pressure of the lower esophageal sphincter, the likelihood of reflux is increased. Respiratory disorders may increase positive abdominal pressure or increase negative intrathoracic pressure over baseline values. Certain drugs used to treat respiratory disease may decrease the lower esophageal sphincter tone or increase gastric acid production. Any of these conditions may produce or intensify GER. In addition, the efficiency of the pharynx and esophagus in clearing the refluxed material and protecting against aspiration plays a critical role in modulating the severity of the respiratory symptoms.[5]

Positive Abdominal Pressure

Pressure within the abdominal cavity can be increased over baseline by forced expiration, as seen during coughing or wheezing. These types of respiratory symptoms are frequently seen in bronchopulmonary dysplasia (BPD), cystic fibrosis, or respiratory infections such as respiratory syncytial virus (RSV). The frequency of GER is increased in all of these conditions. When positive abdominal pressure is increased over baseline, the gastric contents may be pushed back up the esophagus. The force can be such that the LES is unable to oppose it and GE reflux results.

An example of this process is seen in infants with BPD, especially when their respiratory disease worsens. At this time, work of breathing and respiratory effort may temporarily increase, leading to higher abdominal pressure. GE reflux then worsens during this acute respiratory compromise. For some babies with BPD, even their baseline respiratory effort can produce reflux. This GER can then further exacerbate the lung disease by the mechanisms described above. Frequently, the only sign of GER in a baby with BPD is a worsening of respiratory symptoms not explained by other causes.[14]

Negative Intrathoracic Pressure

The baseline normal negative pressure within the thorax can be increased by the forced inspiration that is seen with stridor, tracheomalacia, or hiccups. In this case, the stomach may be somewhat pulled up into the thorax. If the esophagus is shortened in this way (or in the case of a hiatal hernia), the total LES can be elevated above the diaphragm and surrounded by the negative intrathoracic pressure. Since there is positive abdominal pressure on the stomach, the gastric contents flow in the direction of the lowest pressure; that is, they will flow up the esophagus if the pressure gradient overcomes the resting pressure of the LES. Treatment of the underlying respiratory difficulty may decrease the elevated negative pressure and thereby diminish the reflux.

Lower Esophageal Sphincter/Gastric Acid Production

The LES is a zone of increased intraluminal pressure lying between the stomach (with its positive resting pressure) and the esophagus (with its negative resting pressure). It therefore creates a pressure barrier over which the stomach contents need to "climb" to enter the esophagus.[15] Anything that alters or lowers the LES tone will affect its ability to keep the gastric contents within the stomach and will thereby increase the likelihood of GER.

It has been suggested that GER results from an immaturity in the LES. Actually, LES pressures of infants with and without GER appear to be comparable; however, infants who have symptomatic GER tend to have more periods of transient, spontaneous relaxation of LES tone at inappropriate times, which allows gastric material to enter the esophagus.[16] In addition, babies with GER tend to have more frequent transient increases of intra-abdominal pressure than babies without GER. Why some infants have more periods of LES relaxation, and thus more reflux, is not clear.[15]

Several medications commonly used in the treatment of respiratory disease have the side effect of decreasing lower esophageal sphincter tone. Theophylline and caffeine are two medications frequently used for the treatment of central apnea. They can, however, alter LES tone and thereby increase gastroesophageal reflux. In addition to lowering LES tone, theophylline can increase gastric acid production. With more gastric acid there is a higher probability of acid reflux, which can trigger increased mucus production, bronchospasm, or laryngospasm.

The use of indwelling nasogastric tubes for nutritional support can also decrease LES function and possibly cause reflux. The outside of the NG tube itself may act as a conduit for the reflux, further aggravating the problem.

Management of Gastroesophageal Reflux

Once the diagnosis of GER has been made (see chapter 2 for diagnostic tests), management of the problem can begin. Treatment for GER is usually aimed at *managing* the resulting problems and/or treating any of the underlying causal factors described above. The most common cure for reflux, however, is time and maturation. Management is aimed at alleviation of the symptomology so that the infant can thrive. There is a progression in the treatment of reflux. Most conservatively, positional and dietary management is used, with antacids and other medications added as necessary. Surgery reserved for those cases with the most severe sequelae that have not responded to more conservative management. Many infants with GER can be managed well with conservative treatment.[17]

Positional Management
Upright positioning is one of the most commonly used techniques for the management of gastroesophageal reflux and is the foundation upon which other therapies are added. Some disagreement continues to exist regarding the effectiveness of all upright positions in treating reflux, though it is

widely felt that the 30-degree prone elevated position is the most effective for decreasing the frequency of GER when compared to supine, seated, or prone horizontal.[18-20] The prone elevated position does not appear to increase the pressure of the lower esophageal sphincter; therefore its effects are more likely related to the effects of gravity on the stomach contents.[21] Regardless of position, reflux tends to occur more frequently when the child is awake and active than when asleep.[19] Therefore, to be most effective, upright positioning needs to occur throughout the child's entire day and during all activities, whether awake or asleep. This becomes a challenge with infants who have limited postural control due to their young age or those who are mobile in bed. Interestingly, Orenstein found that NNS affected the incidence of GER depending on the infant's position. NNS increased the frequency of reflux episodes slightly in prone, but slightly decreased the frequency of reflux episodes in sitting.[30]

The use of a foam wedge that is angled at 30 degrees and is the width of a standard crib is an inexpensive, comfortable, and effective means of maintaining the upright position during sleeping[17] (figure 6-7). The infant can be positioned in prone or in sidelying and is restrained on the wedge by means of a blanket sling. Other slings for positioning infants in an upright position are commercially available, or a sling can be fabricated.[17, 22] The wedge is generally used for sleeping only, as it is too restrictive an environment for most infants while awake.

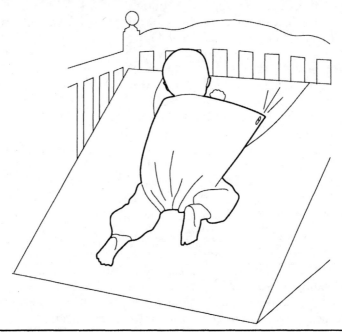

Figure 6-7 Using a foam wedge for upright positioning.

When the infant is awake, upright positioning can be done in a variety of ways. For the small infant, the front carrier pack provides an excellent means for providing erect positioning while allowing movement stimulation and physical proximity to the caregiver. The straight, upright posture combined with the physical containment and vestibular stimulation often proves extremely soothing and organizing to infants with reflux.

Sitting is another means of providing upright positioning. Questions have been raised regarding whether the seated position of an infant actually increases reflux rather than improving it. Orenstein et al. found an increase in the number of reflux episodes during the two-hour postprandial period in an infant seat compared to the prone horizontal position.[23] The small infants in that study, however, were placed in the infant seat with no adjustments to the fit to the infant seat. Thus, they assumed an extremely slouched position, with the hips posteriorly tilted. Orenstein et al. felt that the increase in the number of reflux episodes observed in the infant seat was secondary to this slouched position, which placed the entry of the esophagus into the stomach below the level of the stomach and increased the intra-abdominal pressure.[23] Both factors would tend to bias the infant toward more reflux. A later study has suggested that positioning in the upright slouched position in an infant seat resulted in more awake crying time when compared to awake time in the prone elevated position.[24]

These findings suggest that when upright seating is used, adaptations should be made to optimize posture; the infant's trunk should be erect and symmetrical with nearly 90 degrees of hip and knee flexion. A customized foam infant seat insert can be fabricated to meet this goal (figure 6-8). Such an insert provides lateral trunk support for upright positioning. The base of the insert provides a ledge to allow the baby's knees to flex, resulting in a more neutral position of 90-degrees hip flexion. This, combined with a strap that holds the infant's hips back in the seat, improves alignment between the esophagus and stomach and eliminates abdominal compression. Adaptations to the child's stroller, swing, or walker can be made to mirror this position. An effort should be made to provide the infant with a variety of seating options to minimize boredom and frustration due to the positioning requirements and to encourage the development of motor control in a variety of positions.[25]

Positioning techniques should also be employed while feeding, whether by breast or bottle. The infant should be held at no less than a 45-degree incline and preferably at a 60-degree incline. Attention to positioning while breast-feeding is especially important, as many babies are fed in a nearly horizontal position or while lying down. Even in the conventional breast-feeding position, it is possible to place the baby at roughly a 45-degree angle.

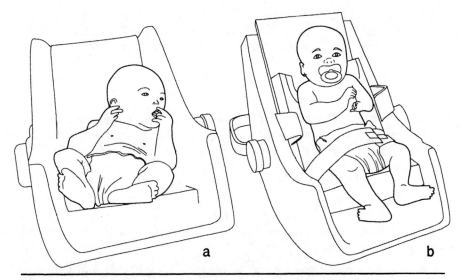

Figure 6-8 An infant seat can be used for upright positioning.
(a) Without modification of the seat, the infant is slouched and the abdomen is compressed. (b) With a foam insert, the trunk position is improved and abdominal compressed is reduced.

For some babies with particularly severe reflux, upright positioning needs to occur even during diaper changes, especially those that occur immediately after feeding. A pillow can be placed on the infant's changing table to allow the infant's trunk to be elevated while the diaper is changed. As the marked hip flexion typical when the legs are raised during diapering can also increase abdominal pressure, rolling the baby's hips to the side should be encouraged. For some parents, changing a diaper with these modifications can be awkward in the beginning; however, most parents quickly become adept at this procedure.

Dietary Management
The use of thickened feedings is probably one of the oldest and most widely used treatments for gastroesophageal reflux. Even so, there is controversy over whether this procedure improves reflux or not.[26] Although the rationale for the use of thickened formula has been that with increased bulk the formula would tend to stay in the stomach and not rise into the esophagus, some feel that thickened feeding causes a delay in gastric emptying, which could increase reflux.[27] Orenstein et al. found that thickening formula with 15 ml of rice cereal per 30 ml of formula produced a decrease in the number of episodes of emesis, did not alter the frequency of reflux episodes measured by technetium scan, and slightly increased gastric emptying time.[28] Most important, these researchers studied the effect of thickened formula on a number of behavioral parameters. They found that with thickened

formula, infants slept longer and were significantly less fussy when awake. With the increased caloric density from the thickened formula combined with less food loss from emesis, these infants probably would have better weight gain. This confirms the observations of Vandenplas and Sacre, who found improvement in the number of reflux episodes with thickened feedings.[29]

While there is conflicting research data on the efficacy of thickening feeding to manage GER, many clinicians and parents report that it is effective. This clinical response to treatment may be the best way to determine if thickened feedings should be used. Ulshen remarks that thickened feeding may be an example of successfully treating GER despite lack of apparent improvement in the laboratory measures used to quantify outcome.[26] The improvement in the behavioral parameters demonstrated by Orenstein et al. may be the crucial factors in determining a parent's ability to deal with a child's reflux until maturation occurs.[28]

Our clinical management protocol for gastroesophageal reflux includes thickening feedings with one tablespoon of standard infant dry rice cereal per two ounces of formula. The rice cereal is added to the bottle of formula or expressed breast milk and is shaken to mix well, and the nipple hole is *slightly* enlarged. Rice cereal is added to every feeding. When the baby is old enough to take solids by spoon but still needs reflux management, unthickened formula can be given in conjunction with thicker pureed foods by spoon.

Thickened feedings can be used even with a baby who is breast-feeding. The mother is instructed to give the baby a very thick mixture of one to two tablespoons of rice cereal in a bottle or by spoon before nursing or between breasts. As many babies fall asleep after nursing, and thus refuse further feeding, the cereal should not be given after breast-feeding.

Some infants experience difficulty with constipation when feedings are thickened with rice cereal. If constipation should become a problem, strained fruits can be given to the baby by spoon or added to the bottle. Dietary manipulations, such as adding cereal or fruit to an infant's diet on a regular basis, should be carried out with nutritional and/or medical guidance.

A large volume of food can distend the stomach, increasing the possibility of transient spontaneous LES relaxation and thereby increasing the potential for GE reflux.[15] Therefore, small, frequent feedings can be useful in managing reflux, as they do not overly expand the stomach. Feeding a baby three to four ounces every three to four hours rather than eight ounces every six to eight hours is preferable. Babies who are overfed, particularly babies who take large volumes because they are calmed with a bottle, can have frequent emesis and appear to have GER.

In severe cases of GER, or those leading to respiratory symptoms, changing to a continuous drip feeding regime either through an NG tube or gastrostomy may be necessary. With the fluid dripped in slowly over a 24-hour period, there is less in the stomach to reflux. When using a continuous drip feeding method it is not possible to thicken feedings, as the rice cereal tends to precipitate out of suspension and clog the feeding pump. Many infants with GER also have a delay in gastric emptying when compared to infants without GER.[15] Thus, as food remains in the stomach for a longer period of time, there is a greater time period during which significant reflux can occur. While medication may improve gastric emptying, it is also minimized when drip feeding is used. The amount of food remaining in the stomach is smaller than during bolus feedings and therefore there is less available to be refluxed.

If these methods of feeding still do not alleviate the reflux symptoms, continuous drip jejunal or duodenal feedings may be necessary. These methods supply nutrition below the stomach, in either the duodenum or jejunum, further reducing the chance of GER.

Medications
Medications are another aspect of treatment in the management of GER. They are often used in conjunction with positional and dietary management and always under medical supervision. The purpose of these medications is to neutralize the stomach acid, decrease acid production, or to increase gastric motility.

Medications may be prescribed to neutralize stomach acid in infants with reflux. Low sodium antacids such as Maalox® or Riopan® are often used to alleviate the pain and discomfort from acid reflux. In babies, this pain is manifested in irritability, crying, and/or pulling the legs up. The neutralizing effect of formula may lead the baby to feed frequently or "snack." Saliva also is able to neutralize 15% to 30% of the acid in the esophagus, so many infants with GER seek out non-nutritive sucking (NNS). In a small series, NNS on a pacifier altered the frequency of reflux, depending on the infant's position.[30] In addition, the sucking and swallowing may increase peristalsis, which may assist in further clearance of the acid reflux.

The effectiveness of antacids is often improved when given after each feeding rather than between feedings.[31] Medications such as cimetadine (Tagamet®) or ranitadine (Zantac®) may be used alone, or in combination with antacids, to decrease acid production and mitigate the development of esophagitis.

Delayed gastric emptying is one of the numerous contributors to GER. Medications such as metoclopramide (Reglan®)[32] or bethanechol[33] may be prescribed to increase gastric motility, stimulate gastric emptying, or elevate the tone of the lower esophageal sphincter.

Surgical Management

If a child's reflux symptomology does not respond to a period of intensive medical management, surgical intervention may be considered.[13] Surgery is usually reserved for the most severe and intractable cases of reflux, in which the effects of the reflux are significant respiratory disease, severe esophagitis, anemia, failure to thrive, or persistent apnea and cyanosis, and where medical management has failed. In these cases, the risk of further recurrent aspiration, respiratory compromise, or prolonged malnutrition is greater than the surgical risk. When surgery is considered, GE reflux should always be confirmed by tests such as those discussed in chapter 2. Antireflux surgery is designed to tighten the LES so that the stomach contents cannot escape up the esophagus. There are several types of surgical procedures that accomplish this; commonly known are the Nissen fundoplication and the gastropexy. A pyloroplasty may be added to help accelerate gastric emptying.

A child's response to surgery is related to the presence of other associated disorders. Giuffre et al. report increase in weight gain and growth and decrease in oxygen requirement in seven of nine infants with BPD following Nissen fundoplication and gastrostomy.[34] The presence of other central nervous system disorders, however, significantly decreases the likelihood that there will be complete resolution of respiratory symptoms following surgery.[35] The long-term effectiveness of these procedures is not clear. There are some indications that they will lose their effectiveness over time. Thus, every effort should be made to control reflux and its related disorders medically before contemplating surgery.

Management of Feeding-Related Problems Associated with GE Reflux

Problem—Feeding Aversion

There may be a small subpopulation of infants with gastroesophageal reflux who develop feeding aversion and refuse to eat or severely limit their intake.

Basis for the problem: Pain from esophagitis is a sequelae of GER.[3,5,13] This pain is like heartburn because gastric acid or acidified gastric contents are escaping the stomach and bathing the delicate esophageal mucosa. Some babies, therefore, may begin to associate feeding with pain and may attempt to eliminate the pain by eliminating eating. Other infants attempt to cope with the pain by taking extremely small, frequent feedings, temporarily neutralizing the acidic reflux. "Snacking" in this manner, however, may result in poor overall intake over a 24-hour period.

Treatment strategies: The primary treatment is diagnosis and aggressive medical management of the GER through positional and dietary management and especially with medications designed to limit gastric acid production. If oral aversion becomes entrenched, oral/tactile normalization techniques may be helpful (see chapter 5, page 247). Early introduction of pureed foods by spoon, with medical approval, may improve intake. The baby may not generalize the aversive behaviors to the spoon or the novel taste of pureed foods. The thickness and bulk of the pureed foods may assist with GER control.

Congenital Heart Disease

The incidence of congenital heart disease is 8 per 1,000 live births.[1] In slightly more than 50% of the cases, congenital heart disease occurs as an isolated defect, and in the remaining cases it occurs in conjunction with a malformation, chromosomal defect, syndrome, or association.[2] In congenital heart disease an anatomic defect in the structure of the cardiovascular system results in abnormal blood flow. These cardiovascular defects can include (1) abnormal connections between the systemic and pulmonary vascular systems, (2) obstruction of the normal blood flow through the heart, or (3) a combination of the two. The location of the defect and the type of blood-flow disruption are the basis for the classification system most frequently used to describe congenital heart defects.

Hemodynamic Principles

Pressure and resistance play key roles in determining blood flow, and thus influence the manifestations and consequences of congenital heart disease. Blood normally flows in the path of least resistance. If resistance is low, blood flow will be high. If resistance is higher than normal, blood flow will be low, and/or greater pressure will be needed to maintain the same level of blood flow. If pressure is higher than normal, blood flow will be greater than normal.

The heart is composed of four chambers, each side possessing an atrium and a ventricle (see figure 6-9, page 348). The right side of the heart receives deoxygenated blood from the body via the superior and inferior vena cava and pumps it via the pulmonary arteries to the lungs for reoxygenation. The left side of the heart receives blood from the lungs and pumps it to the body via the aorta. Normally, the pressure on the left side of the heart is greater than the pressure on the right side. Resistance in the aorta, which begins at the left side of the heart (systemic resistance), is greater than the resistance in the pulmonary arteries (pulmonary resistance). Therefore, if there is an abnormal opening between the chambers of the heart, blood will tend to flow from the left side to the right side, moving from an area of higher pressure to an area of lower pressure. This is called a left-to-right shunt or an acyanotic heart defect, since no unoxygenated blood mixes with the systemic blood.[3]

If a defect results in abnormally high blood flow to the pulmonary arteries, over time the walls of the arteries will thicken. This thickening increases the resistance to blood flow, and therefore reduces blood flow.[3] Anatomic crimping or narrowing (stenosis) of the pulmonary arteries can also lead to increased resistance. Whenever resistance in the pulmonary arteries is abnormally high, there is a slowing of blood flow through the right side of the heart. This increases the pressure on the right side relative to the pressure on the left. If there is also an abnormal opening between the two side of the heart, blood will now flow from the right side of the heart to the left side. This is a right-to-left shunt and allows unoxygenated blood to enter the systemic circulation. Heart defects that result in a right-to-left shunt are referred to as cyanotic heart defects.

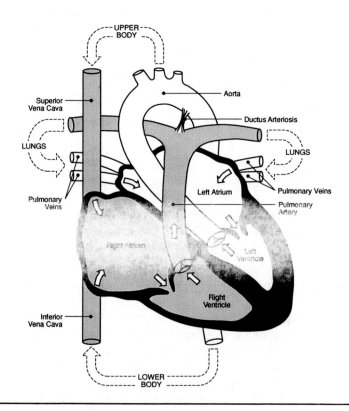

Figure 6-9 Anatomy of the normal heart is shown.

Congestive Heart Failure

Congestive heart failure is a clinical syndrome associated with most congenital heart defects. It is a condition whereby the heart is either unable to supply the body with adequate blood volumes to meet the circulatory or metabolic needs of the body or is unable to adequately dispose of the venous return. Generally, however, it is a combination of the two.[16,26]

In pediatric patients, congestive heart failure frequently results when the original structural defect leads to excessive blood volume flowing to the lungs. This increased blood flow causes the pulmonary arteries to thicken, and therefore resistance to blood flow increases. As the resistance in the pulmonary arteries increases, the heart needs to pump increasingly harder. Pulmonary edema results from the excessive blood flow to the lungs, which causes fluid to seep into the interstitial spaces. The accumulation of fluid causes the lungs to become less compliant, adversely altering pulmonary dynamics and function. Increases in respiratory rate and work of breathing then occur.

When a heart defect is present, the cardiac output may be insufficient to meet the metabolic demands of the body. With increasing insufficiency, the heart may respond with a variety of mechanisms in an attempt to compensate for the inadequate cardiac output. The first mechanism is to increase heart rate. Generally, however, this compensation may not bring cardiac output to adequate levels and requires considerable energy expenditure on the part of the baby. Another, slightly more efficient, compensation mechanism is to increase end-diastolic volume (which increases the stroke volume) and to increase pressure in the ventricles. This continuous increase in end-diastolic volume, however, may result in dilatation of the ventricles first and later in hypertrophy of the heart. Although these compensatory mechanisms—tachycardia, increased diastolic pressure and cardiac hypertrophy—may be somewhat effective in the short run, they extract a toll from the heart and other organs.[26] Progressive congestive heart failure may then result.

Congestive heart failure can occur on the left or right side of the heart depending on the type of heart defect. Some of the features of left-sided heart failure are fatigue, weakness, shortness of breath on exertion, pulmonary edema, pulmonary rales, chronic hacking cough, and cardiac asthma. Right-sided heart failure is characterized by dependent edema, enlargement of the liver, ascites, or oliguria—all a result of increased systemic venous pressure. Infants tend to have left-sided congestive heart failure or a combination of left- and right-sided failure.[26] Cardiac enlargement is present in both left- and right-sided heart failure. Cold extremities may also be a feature of both types of failure. When congestive heart failure is present, some or all of these features may be observed.

Classification of Congenital Heart Disease

Classification of congenital heart disease is generally according to the presence or absence of cyanosis and whether the pulmonary blood flow is normal, increased, or decreased.[4] Although congenital heart disease can be divided into a number of categories, the most common are (1) acyanotic, (2) cyanotic, and (3) obstructive.[1,3] Some of the more common defects will be described.

Acyanotic Heart Disease
In these cardiac defects there is anatomic communication between the chambers of the heart, resulting in a left-to-right shunting of blood. Since no unoxygenated blood reaches the systemic blood flow, no cyanosis is observed. The degree of shunting will depend on the size and placement of the anatomic defect.

Atrial septal defect (ASD): This defect accounts for 5% to 10% of all congenital heart disease.[1,5] A defect is present in the atrial septum that allows shunting of blood from the left atrium to the right atrium. Pulmonary blood flow therefore increases and vessels may begin thickening. Pulmonary resistance then increases slowly, resulting in the development of congestive heart failure. Infants with ASD often present with dyspnea (shortness of breath) or fatigue with exertion.[3] If the left-to-right shunt is large, congestive heart failure may develop quite early.

Ventricular septal defect (VSD): This is the most common form of congenital heart disease and accounts for 20% to 30% of all cases.[1,5] A defect is present in the ventricular septum, and left-to-right shunting occurs. The amount of shunting will depend on the size of the opening, which ranges from tiny to large. Because there is high pressure in the left ventricle, a large VSD can result in increased pulmonary blood flow, again leading to hypertrophy of the vessels and increased pulmonary vascular resistance.

Infants with a small VSD are usually asymptomatic and well developed. Infants with a moderate to large VSD may present, by two to three months of age, with poor weight gain and signs of congestive heart failure such as increased respiratory rate, tachycardia, irritability, or feeding difficulties.[1,3]

Patent ductus arteriosus (PDA): This defect accounts for 7% to 10% of congenital heart disease in term infants.[1,5] It is present in 15% of premature infants with birth weights less than 1750 grams and in 40% to 50% of premature infants with birth weights less than 1500 grams.[1] The ductus arteriosus is a fetal structure that connects the left pulmonary artery with the descending aorta, allowing blood to bypass the collapsed lungs. This connection functionally closes between 24 to 72 hours after birth. Increased oxygen saturation in the systemic circulation stimulates constriction of the ductal smooth muscle. If it does not close, a patent ductus remains and blood is shunted left to right through the ductus. Closure of the ductus may be delayed in preterm infants since the responsiveness of the ductal muscle to oxygen is lower in premature than in term infants.[1]

Infants with a small PDA may be asymptomatic. Those with a moderate to large PDA may present with lower respiratory tract infection and signs of congestive heart failure such as dyspnea, poor feeding, or tachypnea. In premature babies who have infant respiratory distress syndrome (IRDS), the ductus arteriosus may remain open due to the increased pulmonary vascular resistance developed as a consequence of their lung disease. They may develop signs of congestive heart failure as their respiratory disease improves yet the PDA remains open.[1]

Endocardial cushion defect (AV canal): This type of congenital heart disease accounts for 2% of all cases; however, the defect occurs in 30% of babies with Down syndrome.[1] This defect includes a type of atrial septal defect, a ventricular septal defect of the endocardial cushion type, and a cleft in the mitral and tricuspid valve. Failure to thrive, repeated respiratory infections, and signs of congestive heart failure are common in babies with endocardial cushion defect.

Cyanotic Heart Disease
In this category of heart disease there is intermixing of oxygenated and unoxygenated blood in the systemic circulation, resulting in cyanosis. This intermixing may occur due to an anatomic connection between the systemic and pulmonary vascular systems or due to a right-to-left shunting of blood.

There are multiple causes for cyanosis in the newborn, and it is frequently difficult to detect. The etiology of cyanosis can include congenital heart disease, primary lung disease, mechanical interference in lung function such as diaphragmatic hernia, persistent fetal circulation, CNS disease such as intracranial hemorrhage, hypoglycemia, neuromuscular conditions like Werdnig-Hoffman disease, or sepsis.[6] Cyanosis of cardiac origin will not respond to the provision of supplemental oxygen in the same manner as cyanosis from other causes such as lung disease. Clinically, cyanosis usually improves in crying babies with lung disease but will worsen in crying babies with congenital heart disease.[1] Clubbing, a thickening and widening of the tips of the fingers, may result from long-term cyanosis but usually does not appear until the baby is 6 months or older.

Tetralogy of fallot (TOF): This defect comprises approximately 10% of all congenital heart disease and is the most common cyanotic heart defect beyond infancy.[1] This heart defect includes four abnormalities: a ventricular septal defect, right ventricular outflow obstruction from pulmonary stenosis, an overriding of the aorta, and right ventricular hypertrophy. The magnitude of right-to-left shunting of blood will depend on the size of the VSD and the severity of the right ventricular outflow tract obstruction.

Infants with TOF are frequently small for their age, have shortness of breath on exertion, and have hypoxic episodes or "tet spells." These spells occur in young infants, with peak incidence between 2 and 4 months.[1] They typically occur during crying, defecation, or feeding.[3] These hypoxic spells are characterized by rapid and deep respiration, irritability and prolonged crying, increasing cyanosis, and decreased intensity of the heart murmur. A severe spell can result in limpness, convulsions, or even death.[1] The treatment of these spells is aimed at breaking the vicious hemodynamic cycle set up by the defect and includes, but is not limited to, holding the infant over the shoulder in a knee-to-chest position to decrease the systemic return to the heart, as well as the use of medications to correct blood acidosis or to temporarily suppress the respiratory system.

Transposition of the great arteries (TGA): This defect accounts for about 5% of all congenital heart defects and is the most common type of cyanotic heart disease in infants.[1] In this defect, the aorta arises from the right ventricle and the pulmonary artery from the left ventricle. There are two independent and ineffective circulations. Desaturated blood returning to the body goes to the right atrium and, rather than being pumped to the lungs for reoxygenation, is pumped out to the body via the aorta. The tissues comprising the vital organs, such as the brain and the heart, therefore, are perfused by blood with low oxygen saturation. At the same time, well-oxygenated blood returning from the lungs to the left atrium is pumped back to the lungs by the pulmonary artery. This condition is incompatible with life unless there is some communication between the two systems for intermixing of oxygenated and deoxygenated blood. This intermixing can occur through a communicating defect between the atria or the ventricles or at the ductal level, such as a PDA.[1] Early surgical management may include creating such a "communication" between the two systems.

Infants with TGA present with progressive hypoxia and acidosis dependent upon the degree of intracardiac mixing. Congestive heart failure develops early, usually within the first week of life. If the TGA is not identified in the newborn period (usually because there is a great deal of blood intermixing), these infants can also present with frequent respiratory infections, delays in growth and development, or clubbing of the fingers and toes[3]

Hypoplastic left heart syndrome (HLHS): This condition accounts for 1% to 2% of all congenital heart disease and is the most common cause of death from a cardiac defect in the first month of life.[1,7] The primary cardiac defect includes several lesions: a diminutive ascending aorta, aortic and mitral valve atresia or stenosis, and/or hypoplasia of the left atrium and ventricle.[1,7] Several other anomalies are also associated with HLHS, including hypertrophy and dilation of the right side of the heart, dilation of the pulmonary artery, ASD, PDA, or coarctation of the aorta.

Babies with this defect are generally critically ill within the first few hours of life. Their symptoms are usually those of left-sided heart failure: congestive heart failure, sudden onset of cyanosis and progressive respiratory distress, poor feeding and irritability, and tachypnea.[7] In the past, mortality from this lesion was 100%. New surgical procedures (including infant heart transplantation) have improved the prognosis to some degree,[8] although mortality is still 80%.[9]

Obstructive Heart Defects

Interruption and obstruction of appropriate blood flow can occur within the heart or vessels connected to the heart. These types of defects are usually divided into three categories: (1) obstruction of the right or left ventricles (e.g., aortic stenosis, pulmonary stenosis, or coarctation of the aorta), (2) stenosis of the atrioventricular valves (e.g., mitral or tricuspid stenosis), and (3) valvular regurgitation lesions (e.g., mitral, aortic, or pulmonary regurgitation).[1]

Coarctation of the aorta (COA): This defect accounts for 7% to 8% of all cases of congenital heart disease and is present in 30% of individuals with Turner's syndrome.[1,3] A constriction occurs in the aorta at any point from the arch to the bification, but most commonly just below the origin of the left subclavian artery. The location of the coarctation determines the direction of shunting of blood and influences the development of collateral circulation.[1]

Signs of congestive heart failure develop early if the coarctation is severe. In less severe cases, growth and development are normal, but there may be a difference between upper and lower extremity pulses, heart murmur, and changes on the electrocardiogram (ECG).[1,3]

Pulmonary or aortic stenosis: The incidence of pulmonary stenosis is 5% to 8% and aortic stenosis represents 5% of all congenital heart disease.[1] A narrowing occurs in the aorta or pulmonary artery, increasing resistance and decreasing blood flow. Blood does not shunt from one part of the heart to another unless there is also an associated connective defect. The corresponding ventricle generally hypertrophies secondary to the need to generate more pressure to pump blood against the resistance of the stenosis.

Infants with mild pulmonary stenosis may be asymptomatic. Dyspnea and rapid fatigue are present in moderate stenosis, and congestive heart failure may occur in severe cases. In aortic stenosis, most infants are asymptomatic, with occasional exercise intolerance. In both cases, infants are generally acyanotic and well developed.[1]

Treatment of Congenital Heart Disease

Surgical Treatment

Surgery is the primary treatment of congenital heart disease. Surgery can consist of a palliative procedure such as a pulmonary artery banding (PA banding)[10] or Blalock-Taussig shunt,[11] which allows for growth of the heart and vessels to a more favorable size so that total repair of the heart can occur. With advances in cardiopulmonary bypass techniques, postoperative cardiac care, simplification of existing surgical techniques, and the development of new surgical techniques, the majority of patients can undergo primary surgical repair earlier in infancy without a prior palliative procedure.[12-13] Both primary and palliative procedures are occurring at increasingly younger ages (often less than 4 months) with good results.[9]

Adult follow-up studies of patients with surgically repaired congenital heart defects show varying outcomes.[14] For patients with ASD or VSD the prognosis is excellent, with virtually normal exercise tolerance when compared to the general population. Late complications from tetralogy of fallot can include diminished exercise tolerance. Such findings may be related to technical aspects of the original surgical repair, or may be due to pulmonary valve insufficiency. The outlook for patients with left ventricular outflow obstruction is more guarded, with some residual aortic stenosis and/or insufficiency. Successful repair of pulmonary stenosis, especially before 2 years of age, results in a normal life expectancy and exercise tolerance. Long-term follow-up information on infants who underwent an atrial switch procedure for correction of transposition of the great arteries is not available.

Medical Treatment

Medications are also an important component in the treatment of congenital heart disease both before and after surgery. Digitalis or digoxin is frequently used to control congestive heart failure.[1,15] Diuretics, such as Lasix®, Diuril®, or Aldactone®, may be used when hypertension is present, or in conjunction with digitalis for congestive heart failure. These medications act to decrease extracellular and plasma volume and thus reduce stress on the heart.[1,15] Vasodilators, such as captopril, can be used to act directly on vascular smooth muscle to reduce vascular resistance.[1] Irregularities in the cardiac rhythm can be treated with medications such as Inderal®[15] Medical manipulation of the patent ductus arteriosus can occur by administering prostaglandins through the umbilical artery.[1] This is a short-term method of maintaining patency of the ductus until surgery can be performed.

Feeding Problems Commonly Seen with Congenital Heart Disease

Problem—Decreased endurance:
Infants with congenital heart disease may be easily fatigued and may tire before taking in sufficient volume. Depending on the severity of the cardiac lesion and the age of the baby, such an infant may not arouse spontaneously to feed.

Basis for the problem: Tachypnea and poor feeding are classic signs of congestive heart failure.[16] Since the baseline heart rate may be fast, the infant may have limited capacity to increase the heart rate to respond to the energy demands required by feeding. While the baby may be able to respond in the short term, the baby may fatigue quickly. When there is volume overload or pressure overload on the heart, there is little margin to increase the cardiac output and accommodate the demands of the wide variety of organs involved in the act of feeding. The heart may be unable to alter the force or amount of blood that is pumped through the systemic circulation.

Intermixing of oxygenated and deoxygenated blood can result in poor tissue oxygenation as vital organs are perfused with low oxygen content blood.[17] Since oxygen is the fuel for the body's activities, and feeding can be considered a baby's aerobic exercise, the baby with a cardiac defect is at an immediate disadvantage. If the infant's cardiovascular system is not adequate to meet the oxygen debt developed during feeding, rapid fatigue can result. The classic example is a baby with CHD who sucks eagerly for a few minutes, then tires and stops feeding. After a brief rest, the baby may feed again for a short period of time before stopping. Overall intake is less than desired.

With decreased energy stores and decreased delivery of oxygen for work, the baby may have inadequate strength to produce an effective suck. The suck may be weak, although tongue, lip, and jaw movements are usually appropriate. Sucking bursts may be short, with longer than average pauses to rest and recover. This results in an overall decrease in sucking time and intake at each feeding.

Treatment strategies:

- Oral facilitation techniques such as chin or cheek support (see page 240) can be used to increase the strength of suck.

- Switching to a higher flow nipple (see page 406) or slightly enlarging the hole of the nipple may maximize the amount of nutrient the baby receives before tiring. Caution must be exercised when using techniques to increase the flow of liquid, however, so that the increased flow does not alter the baby's ability to coordinate swallowing and breathing and result in apnea during feeding.

- Allowing a 5- to 10-minute break in the middle of feeding may give some babies sufficient recovery time so that they can continue to feed and hopefully ingest adequate volume.

- Altering the feeding schedule may maximize the baby's persistence at feeding. A three- to four-hour interval gives the baby a substantial rest between feedings and potentially greater energy for feeding. This interval between feedings may also increase hunger so the baby is more vigorous at the start of a feeding. When there is a longer interval between feedings, however, higher volume per feeding is required. On the other hand, if the feeding interval is shorter (such as two hours) smaller volumes are needed at each feeding. Thus, less energy may be needed to complete the feeding. A two-hour feeding schedule, however, is not appropriate at night and may be difficult for some families to maintain during the day.

  No matter which interval is selected for the feeding schedule, each feeding (including burping and rests) should not take longer than 20 to 30 minutes. When feeding takes longer, the infant is generally spending much of the time in inefficient sucking activity and resting. This keeps the baby from returning to deeper sleep, which is needed to become well rested for subsequent feedings.

- Supplemental nutritional support through intermittent or continuous gavage feedings may be necessary.[18] It can enhance weight gain and reduce parental anxiety around the issue of feeding intake.

Problem—Early satiety—poor growth and nutritional status:
Failure to thrive is a frequent accompaniment to congenital heart disease.[3] Not only do these infants appear to have suboptimal intake, but often they lack the drive to eat. Many do not wake spontaneously for their feedings. Babies with CHD can appear uninterested in eating and may respond with aversive behaviors, such as gagging, if pressed to eat. The baby who does feed may stop feeding before taking in adequate volume, yet appear satisfied. Weight gain and linear growth are poor.

Basis for the problem: The effects of congestive heart failure may play a part in the poor appetite seen in many infants with congenital heart disease. Congestive heart failure can lead to delayed gastric emptying and gastrointestinal hypomotility, which may blunt the baby's appetite.[19] In addition, the stomach may be compressed by an enlarged liver (hepatomegaly),[20] which can diminish the magnitude of normal feelings of hunger. The infant may also experience a premature sensation of fullness due to reduced gastric capacity or delayed gastric emptying.[19] Thus, the baby may receive inappropriate feedback regarding when to feed or how long to feed.

Delayed gastric emptying and increases in intra-abdominal pressure from increased work of breathing can result in gastroesophageal reflux. The discomfort from GE reflux can provide negative feedback for eating and depress the baby's willingness to feed. Vomiting from GER can further diminish the infant's already meager intake, adversely affecting growth.

Inadequate intake is not the sole reason for growth failure in infants with congenital heart disease. The undernourished state may partly be due to increased metabolic requirements. Oxygen consumption is higher in patients with congenital heart disease. There are increased metabolic demands from the muscles of respiration and the heart muscles.[18] Congestive heart failure may also lead to reduced compliance of the lungs, especially if there is pulmonary edema. Restriction of overall lung capacity can result from cardiomegaly, or elevation of the diaphragm caused by hepatomegaly or ascites.[19] Thus, the baby with congenital heart disease may not only breathe faster but may expend considerably more effort to breathe, which alters its metabolic needs.

With increased metabolic need, greater nutrient intake per day is required for growth. Infants may need at least 150 kcal/kg body weight per day for adequate growth in height and weight, compared to the normal infant who requires 100 kcal/kg per day.[21] The volume required to obtain optimal growth may be beyond the baby's capabilities.

Treatment strategies:

- The caloric density of the baby's formula or breast milk can be increased so that more calories are given per volume of fluid. This approach can increase overall caloric intake and/or reduce the volume the infant is required to take. It is also used frequently with infants who have CHD and are limited in fluid intake secondary to congestive heart failure.

- Supplemental non-oral feeding may be a crucial component of the baby's overall feeding plan. Supplementation can occur through intermittent, nighttime, or continuous drip tube feedings using a

---

nasogastric tube or gastrostomy (see page 266). For some infants 24-hour continuous drip feeding may be the only way to achieve adequate nutrition for appropriate growth.[21] Plans for supplemental feedings must be individualized; they should support optimal nutrition as well as the baby's best oral feeding skills.

- Medical management of congestive heart failure will be important to mitigate its effects on the infant's appetite.

- Implementing positional and feeding management techniques (see page 340) may reduce the amount of food lost through vomiting or improve the baby's willingness to feed. GER can become a problem after surgical procedures even if it was not evident before.

- Increasing the interval between feedings may increase the baby's perceived hunger and allow more time for gastric emptying.

Problem—Associated Problems:

Congenital heart disease often does not occur alone but is present in conjunction with other major defects. Neurologic sequelae that impair central nervous system integrity can occur as a result of cardiac surgery. In these situations, features of the "associated problems" may be the major limitations to oral feeding.

Basis for the problem: In approximately 20%-50% of infants with congenital heart disease the heart defect occurs along with another major extracardiac malformation, a syndrome, or chromosomal defect.[2,22] Defects of the musculoskeletal system such as cleft lip and palate or choanal atresia occur in approximately 7% of cases. Thirteen percent of cases of congenital heart disease occur in conjunction with chromosomal defects such as Trisomy 13 or 21, malformation syndromes of nonchromosomal origins such as Noonan's syndrome, or malformation associations such as CHARGE, VATER, or DiGeorge.[22]

Infants with these types of defects frequently have difficulties in multiple sensory and motoric systems and may demonstrate developmental delay.[23] Feeding problems associated with these other defects are superimposed on the problems already discussed for the infant who has only CHD. For example, oral-motor dysfunction may be present in Trisomy 21, or skills may be hampered by cleft lip and palate or choanal atresia. Swallowing function may be impaired in the VATER or CHARGE association. In each case energy and endurance can also be limited by the heart defect. Developmental delay, if present, will impact the rate of acquisition of normal feeding skills or may influence the baby's persistence at feeding. In addition, the parents' perception of the infant's skill level and their understanding of the impact of the defects on the infant's acquisition of skills may affect the parents' ability to establish realistic expectations for the infant's feeding performance.[24]

Although major advances have occurred in cardiac surgery procedures, morbidity in the form of neurologic sequelae from surgery itself will occur in a small number of cases. Hypothermia and total circulatory arrest during cardiopulmonary bypass can lead to neurologic damage.[25] Cerebral embolism and hypoxic-ischemic encephalopathy can lead to seizures, hemiparesis, cerebral palsy, Horner's syndrome, or developmental delay.[25] Frequently, neurologic sequelae are transient and confined to the immediate postoperative period. If neurological damage continues beyond the postoperative period, the extent of the neurologic damage may affect an infant's oral-motor and feeding abilities to a greater degree than the original heart defect.

Treatment strategies:

- If abnormalities in oral-motor control or postural control are present due to an associated defect or sequelae of surgery, oral and motoric facilitation techniques will be needed to remediate the specific problems identified (see chapter 5).

- The potential for associated defects should be kept in mind during the feeding assessment of any infant with CHD. Observations made during feeding assessment may assist in identifying associated defects. These observations can lead to further evaluation of the musculoskeletal system, neurologic integrity, respiratory control, swallowing, or developmental level.

- Parent education should occur to assist parents in establishing realistic expectations for their infant's feeding. Some parents may see their baby either as more fragile or more sturdy than the actual status indicates.[25] Assisting parents to deal with the sense of loss and grief when a baby is born with a birth defect may ultimately enhance infant feeding by improving the bonding between parent and child. This process is disrupted not only by the initial diagnosis itself but also by the restrictions placed on physical contact and interaction between parent and child due to the baby's illness and pre- or postsurgical care.[20]

Oral-Facial Anomalies

A number of congenital oral-facial anomalies may interfere with infant feeding. Several that are seen relatively frequently and are discussed below include cleft lip, cleft palate, cleft lip and palate, micrognathia, and the Pierre-Robin malformation sequence.

Clefts

A cleft lip results from failure in fusion of the upper lip in the fifth week of embryonic development. A cleft palate results from failure of the palatal shelves to meet and fuse in the midline during the seventh to eighth week of intrauterine development.[24] Cleft lip and cleft palate may occur individually or together.

Clefts may be present unilaterally or bilaterally, and there is great variation in severity. Cleft lip varies from a notch in the upper lip, a relatively minor defect, to a complete cleft lip with an opening through the lip and into the nostril and clefting of the upper alveolar ridge. The most minimal cleft of the palate is the submucous cleft in which the mucosal surface is intact, though the muscles have not closed appropriately across the velum. The uvula is often notched. In the more typical cleft palate, there is a complete opening in the hard and/or soft palate. A number of configurations may be seen, including unilateral, bilateral, and U- or V-shaped openings.[23,19]

The incidence of cleft lip, cleft palate, or cleft lip and palate is one in 600 to 800 live births, with variation based on race and sex. Genetic and environmental factors are implicated in the pathogenesis of these malformations.[23,24,17] In some cases the presence of a cleft is associated with other congenital anomalies, syndromes, and medical complications. One study reports over 40% of infants with clefts having associated malformations.[23] There are a number of management problems that are directly associated with the presence of a cleft. These include feeding problems in infancy, irregularities of the teeth and other dental and orthodontic problems, speech impairments, otitis media, and psychological and emotional problems.[23] Reported feeding problems include poor oral suction, poor intake, lengthy feedings, nasal regurgitation, choking and gagging, and excessive air intake.

Initial treatment focuses on developing a feeding method to insure adequate weight gain, as slow weight gain is often reported in this population. While feeding difficulties may compromise weight gain, nutritional requirements may also differ.[18,21] Potential feeding methods will be discussed in detail below.

The timing of structural repair of these defects is related to the type of defect and the age and weight of the child. Repair of the cleft lip generally occurs when the infant is between 6 weeks and 4 months of age, though some authors advocate immediate closure in the neonatal period.[22,23] Corrective surgery for the cleft palate generally occurs between 12 and 18 months of age, after the rapid craniofacial growth and enlargement of the palatal surfaces during the first 12 months.[17]

Micrognathia and the Pierre-Robin Malformation Sequence

Micrognathia or retrognathia refers to a small or posteriorly positioned mandible (figure 6-10). Externally the chin appears recessed. Internally, the tongue, while generally of normal size, is also posteriorly positioned in relation to the oral cavity. This may lead to glossoptosis, or obstruction of the pharyngeal airway. Micrognathia is often associated with a wide U-shaped cleft of the palate. The triad of micrognathia, upper airway obstruction, and cleft palate is referred to as the Pierre-Robin malformation sequence. Some authors, however, do not consider the presence of a cleft necessary for this diagnostic designation.[2,6]

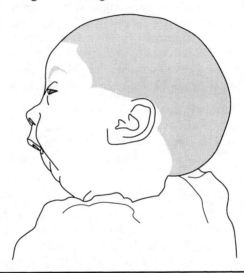

Figure 6-10 An infant with micrognathia.

In utero, an abnormally small mandible can lead to the development of other anomalies. The tongue cannot descend into the oral cavity appropriately, remaining elevated against the base of the cranium and interfering with fusion of the palatal shelves, potentially leading to a cleft palate. Reasons for the initial micrognathia can range from intrinsic mandibular hypoplasia to intrauterine constriction. While micrognathia and the Robin sequence may be isolated findings, they may also be part of multiple anomaly syndromes such as Stickler syndrome.[2]

The most significant neonatal medical complication of the Robin sequence is airway obstruction. The specific mechanism of airway obstruction, however, is not well understood. It may result from one or more of the following factors: (1) mechanical obstruction from the posteriorly placed tongue, (2) ineffective activity of the muscles that protract the tongue, (3) projection of the tongue tip into the cleft, (4) negative pressure of inspiration and swallowing acting to pull the tongue into the pharynx and hinder forward movement, and (5) airway muscle dysfunction.[2,3,6,11-13]

Primary medical treatment is aimed at preventing airway obstruction. The most effective treatment will vary from patient to patient, and a variety of techniques are utilized. The degree of airway obstruction and other associated problems must be considered in determining the medical/surgical treatment. Often simply positioning the infant in prone such that gravity maintains a forward tongue position and a patent airway is successful.[6] Nasopharyngeal tubes (NP tubes) may be used to provide a mechanical opening through the pharynx.[2,26] Surgical procedures are also used. The most commonly described is the tongue-to-lip adhesion. This physically prevents the tongue from moving posteriorly into the pharynx.[4,5] Recently a surgical release of the musculature of the floor of the mouth has also been reported as successful in eliminating airway obstruction.[7] The long-term impact on tongue movements in speech has not been addressed, however. Finally, tracheostomy may be necessary to preserve the infant's life.[2,5]

In infants with Robin sequence, maintenance of nutrition is crucial. Normal growth during the first few months of life will generally bring mandibular enlargement as well as improved tongue position and control. This growth typically eliminates episodes of airway obstruction and other related problems.

Choosing a method of nourishment in this population is complicated. Any condition where there is potential for airway obstruction may limit nipple feeding because of the close association between sucking, swallowing, and breathing. The medical treatment that is selected to manage the airway, as well as the degree of the structural and functional impairment, must be considered in determining the method of feeding. Oral feeding is preferred to maintain and build skills for nippling, other oral feeding activities, and speech; however, it is accomplished more easily when certain treatments are used for airway management (see table 6-1). In some cases oral feeding may be facilitated by altering the medical treatment, though for other infants the severity of problems related to Robin sequence may preclude full or partial oral feeding under any circumstances.

Considerations in Determining Oral Feeding Programs

There is no one feeding method that will be successful for all infants with cleft lip, palate, or Pierre-Robin sequence. A number of factors should be observed during the evaluation of each infant's feeding-related performances and then considered in relation to the feeding methods and medical/surgical treatments available. These factors will be described, then discussed in relation to each of the anomalies described above to provide a framework for selecting appropriate oral feeding techniques (see table 6-2, page 364).

SPECIAL DIAGNOSTIC CATEGORIES

Table 6-1 Comparison of Medical and Surgical Management Strategies for Airway Obstruction Secondary to Micrognathia

	Strengths:	Limitations:
Prone Positioning	• Simple • Low cost	• While oral feeding may be attempted, gavage feeding is generally necessary, particularly if there is a cleft palate • Inconvenient for care and transport of infant • If positioning protocol is not strictly followed, the airway may be compromised
Nasopharyngeal Tube	• Full oral feeding is possible • Feeding can be done in the standard position, using special techniques as appropriate for cleft palate and tongue retraction	• It may be difficult to position the tube correctly and maintain it in this position • Home care is more complex; tube must be changed and suctioned
Tongue-Lip Adhesion	• Full oral feeding is possible • Feeding can be done in the standard position, using special techniques for cleft palate as appropriate	• Surgery is required, with associated risks and costs • Failure rate can be high • Long-term impact on tongue movements for speech is not clear
Soft-Tissue Release in Floor of Mouth	• Full oral feeding is reportedly possible in standard position, with techniques for cleft palate as appropriate	• Surgery is required, with associated risks and costs • This procedure has not been performed on large numbers of patients; therefore, potential complications are not well understood • Long-term impact on tongue movements for speech is not clear

Table 6-2 Comparison of Feeding Components and Feeding Methods for Infants with Oral-Facial Anomalies

	Feeding Components:				Feeding Method:	
	Suction	Compression	Swallow	Respiration	Bottle	Breast
Cleft lip	++/–	+	+	+	Nipple with wide base	Generally possible
Cleft palate	+/– –	+/–	+	+	Small cleft—soft nipple, enlarged hole; Large cleft—assisted milk delivery (squeeze bottle)	Possibly with small cleft or submucous cleft; may need assisted milk delivery
Cleft lip and palate	–	+/–	+	+	Assisted milk delivery (squeeze bottle)	Unlikely
Robin sequence	+/–	+/–	+/–	+/– –	Success depends on degree of airway obstruction and type of management –Long nipple needed –Assisted milk delivery if cleft palate also present	Unlikely

+ = present
– = absent
+/– = may be present, marginally present, or absent

Components of sucking: As discussed in earlier chapters, there are two components of sucking that allow the infant to obtain nourishment by breast or bottle. These are nipple compression and the generation of negative pressure suction. The integrity of each component must be carefully evaluated in infants with oral-facial anomalies.

Suction, which requires the oral cavity to be fully sealed, may not be present. In most cases a cleft produces an air leak that impairs the creation of suction. In addition to suction, the adequacy of tongue and jaw movements to compress the nipple must be assessed in order to determine the most effective oral-feeding method.

Integrity of the swallowing mechanism: The infant must demonstrate airway protection during swallowing to allow safe oral feeding. It is also useful to determine the response of the swallowing mechanism to varying flow rates, as many feeding techniques used for infants with oral-facial anomalies are characterized by rapid rates of fluid flow.

Respiration during feeding: If it appears that respiration is compromised during feeding, the underlying cause must be determined. Etiologies for respiratory difficulties can include: a structural/obstructive phenomenon, a lag in the maturation of coordination, and/or a primary respiratory insufficiency.

Characteristics of breast-feeding: Breast-feeding should never automatically be dismissed in the infant with oral-facial anomalies. Rather, the interface between the infant's feeding strengths and limitations and the breast-feeding process must be understood. The potential for successful breast-feeding can then be considered. See chapter 8 for further discussion of breast-feeding issues.

The antibacterial properties of breast milk may be of particular importance to those infants with oral-facial anomalies, as in some cases there is an increased incidence of otitis media. Compared to commercial infant formulas, breast milk is also a physiologic substance and therefore less likely to trigger coughing and choking responses when in contact with chemoreceptors in the nasal and pharyngeal areas.[20,24] Even if breast-feeding is not pursued, these factors may increase a mother's desire to provide expressed breast milk to her infant.

In breast-feeding, the primary role of the suction component of sucking is to create, position, and maintain an adequate "teat." Once this is accomplished, compression of the nipple may be of primary importance in milk delivery. The flow of milk during breast-feeding is different from that during bottle-feeding. In general it can take up to two minutes of active sucking to elicit the "let-down" reflex and thus strong milk flow. While the flow is rapid following the let-down, it tapers off during the feeding (see chapter 8).

The physical attributes of the mother for breast-feeding must also be considered. There is substantial variation in human nipple shape and size, as well as in rate of milk flow. For the infant with oral-facial anomalies, a "poor fit" between mother and infant characteristics may diminish the prospects of successful breast-feeding. Although initiating breast-feeding in the normal newborn may be challenging, persistence is generally rewarded with success. For the mother of an infant with oral-facial anomalies, however, the process can be time consuming and frustrating, with the possibility of success less clear. Therefore, the mother needs to be strongly motivated to breast-feed before undertaking this feeding method, provided with lots of support, and prepared for possible failure.

Characteristics of bottle-feeding: In bottle-feeding, nipple compression during sucking may play a smaller role in obtaining nutrient. Because of the dynamics of the bottle and nipple, compression of the nipple results in very limited fluid flow. Negative pressure suction plays the major role in efficient fluid flow. During bottle-feeding, suction is not needed to position the nipple in the mouth. The shape and the rigidity of bottle nipples usually insure appropriate positioning when the nipple is fully inserted into the mouth.

Various shapes and qualities are available in artificial nipples. This allows a great deal of flexibility in matching nipple characteristics to sucking characteristics (see chapter 7). A nipple can be selected that matches the particular tongue movements of an infant or that regulates the fluid flow most appropriately.

Feeding Considerations in Cleft Lip

Components of sucking: The mechanical movements of the tongue and jaw are generally appropriate and produce adequate *compression* on the nipple. Depending on the size and exact location of the cleft, the anterior seal may be compromised, reducing the amount of *negative pressure suction* that can be produced.

Swallowing: The swallow typically functions normally and is safe for oral feeding.[8]

Respiration: Respiration is generally normal.

Bottle-feeding: The infant **must** develop full negative pressure suction for effective bottle-feeding. If the amount of suction is reduced or intermittent, feeding will be slow and require greater energy expenditure. If air is leaking through the cleft lip, decreasing suction, this opening must be occluded. A nipple with a wide base that presses against the cleft may produce such occlusion. If it is not possible to occlude the cleft, a system that assists milk delivery will be necessary (see cleft lip and palate, page 369).

Breast-feeding: In the infant with a cleft lip, breast-feeding is often successful with minimal modification. The infant generally has adequate oral mechanics to produce compression of the nipple for milk delivery. Suction to form and position the nipple may be compromised, though the soft tissue of the breast may work better than an artificial nipple to fill the cleft and allow the development of suction for nipple positioning. Mothers nursing infants who do not produce adequate suction for nipple positioning report that manual assistance forming and placing the nipple, as well as feeding when the breast is full and rigid, may be successful.[20,24] The size and shape of the mother's breast may facilitate or limit this process. If the mother's physical shape limits the process, supplementation may be needed.

Feeding Considerations in Cleft Palate

Components of sucking: Mechanical movements of the tongue and jaw are generally adequate to produce nipple *compression.* The effectiveness of the compression will depend on the size and location of the cleft. When a large midline cleft is present, the opposing surface for tongue compression is lacking and will make compression movements ineffective. The degree of *negative pressure suction* achieved by the infant whose palate is intact can never be achieved when a cleft is present. The amount of suction that can be generated and maintained is dependent on the size and location of the cleft. A small cleft may produce a minimal reduction in negative pressure. Posterior clefts may be occluded by the tongue during part of the sucking movement, again minimally reducing negative pressure but leading to inefficient feeding. Submucous clefts limit the development of negative pressure suction to the extent that they impair movement of the soft palate and the glossopalatal seal. Larger clefts completely preclude the development of negative pressure suction. Palatal obturators are used in some centers in an attempt to block the cleft and allow development of suction.

Swallowing: The swallowing mechanism is generally adequate, though the creation of a seal at the proximal end of the pharynx may be achieved in an alternate manner when clefting of the soft palate is substantial.[1] Microaspiration can occur but is not typical.

Respiration: Respiration is generally normal.

Bottle-feeding: Even when the cleft is small and some negative pressure suction is generated, feeding is often inefficient, leading to prolonged feedings and inadequate intake. Providing a soft nipple with an enlarged opening may maximize the effectiveness of these low-pressure sucks and allow greater milk expression from the compression component of sucking. If the cleft is large, it is not possible to generate and sustain negative pressure suction. A system that assists with milk delivery is then usually most effective, though a soft crosscut nipple may also be used (see cleft lip and palate, page 369). Bottle-feeding should always be done in an upright position of at least 60 degrees. This allows gravity assistance in swallowing and minimizes entry of formula into the nasal cavity and eustachian tubes during sucking and swallowing. A bottle with an angled neck may make upright feeding easier (see figure 5-8, page 226).

Breast-feeding: If the palatal cleft is small, the infant may develop adequate suction to form and position the nipple. Once the nipple is positioned, compression should be adequate in the infant with a small cleft. Again, upright positioning is recommended. When the infant cannot produce adequate suction for nipple positioning, the mother can manually assist in nipple creation and positioning. Feeding when the breast is full and rigid, combined with hand expression of milk, may also be successful.[20,24] The size and shape of the mother's breast play a role in this process. If the breast is not a good "match" to the baby's needs, supplementation may be required.

If the cleft is large, not only will inadequate suction make it difficult to achieve proper nipple positioning, but compression may also be compromised by the lack of an adequate opposing surface. When a large cleft palate is present, breast-feeding in the normal manner is generally not successful. The breast-feeding experience may be possible using a feeding tube device, such as the Medela® Supplemental Nursing System (SNS) or Lact-aide (see chapter 8). Usually these devices must be modified to produce milk flow, as the baby creates inadequate suction to operate them in the standard manner.

Feeding Considerations in Cleft Lip and Palate

Components of sucking: When a cleft lip and palate are present, the cleft is generally quite large. Although the mechanical movements of the tongue may be appropriate, when the cleft is large the opposing surface for tongue compression is lacking, making *compression* movements less effective. Due to the large size of the cleft, the development of *negative pressure suction* is not usually possible. Palatal obturators are used by some centers with varying degrees of success. They block the cleft and allow development of compression and possibly suction.

Swallowing: The swallowing mechanism is usually adequate, though the creation of a seal at the proximal end of the pharynx may be achieved in an alternate manner when clefting of the soft palate is substantial.[1] There is some potential for microaspiration.

Respiration: Respiration is generally normal.

Bottle-feeding: When the infant is unable to create negative pressure suction to draw fluid out of a bottle, one of two approaches is generally suggested. A system can be developed whereby the feeder assists in milk delivery, or the nipple may be modified to maximize the amount of milk delivered by the infant's compression forces.

Assisted milk delivery systems include squeeze bottles, ascepto feeders, Brecht feeders, and syringes. Two primary problems arise in using these devices. First, fluid flow is often inappropriately fast and poorly timed with the infant's sucking and swallowing efforts. Second, some of these devices do not stimulate appropriate sucking patterns. Of the assisted milk delivery systems listed, the squeeze bottle with an infant nipple and a regular hole is the best at minimizing these problems.

With any of these milk delivery systems, the flow rate should approximate the normal rate of about .1 to .5 cc per suck. With ascepto feeders and syringes it is difficult to precisely control milk flow, and the flow rate is much greater than normal. Using any system of assisted milk delivery, the feeder must also learn to provide the fluid in rhythm with the infant's sucking movements to facilitate coordinated swallowing.

Whichever milk delivery system is chosen, it should attempt to stimulate normal sucking patterns. The tubing of the ascepto feeder is often put in the side of the infant's mouth, so there is nothing to "suck" on. Syringes may also be positioned to the side of the mouth, but even in the midline, they do not provide an appropriate stimulus for sucking. The squeeze bottle with appropriate nipple (see page 375), therefore, appears to be the best option for assisted milk delivery, as it allows good control of milk-flow rate while facilitating appropriate tongue movements.

A second approach to bottle-feeding the infant with cleft lip and palate is to use a standard bottle but modify the nipple to allow greater fluid flow with compressive tongue movements. This is often done by selecting a long, soft nipple and creating a large crosscut hole. The pressure on the nipple may vary, however, as the opposing surface (palate) is irregular. Both the large hole and varying pressure lead to inconsistent and often rapid milk flow, which can compromise the coordination of normal swallowing and breathing. This may lead to excessive sputtering, coughing, choking, nasal regurgitation, and air swallowing. In our experience, assisted milk delivery with a squeeze bottle is more successful in feeding infants with cleft lip and palate than simply modifying the nipple.

Another approach that deserves attention is the development of a bottle-and-nipple unit designed to deliver milk effectively and consistently using only the compression component of sucking. Developed in England, this unit is known as the Haberman feeder[9,10] (see page 375).

Bottle-feeding should always be done in an upright position (at least 60 degrees) to allow gravity assistance in swallowing and to minimize entry of formula into the nasal cavity and eustachian tubes during sucking and swallowing activity.

Breast-feeding: Breast-feeding is unlikely to be successful in the infant with a cleft lip and palate. There is no suction to form and position the nipple adequately, and compression may be compromised by the lack of an adequate opposing surface. In a study encouraging breast-feeding of infants with cleft lip, Weatherly-White et al. found breast-feeding successful for adequate nourishment in only 1 of 15 infants with cleft lip and palate.[22] The breast-feeding experience may be possible using a feeding tube device such as the Medela® Supplemental Nursing System (SNS) or Lact-aide, though modifications are necessary to provide adequate milk flow. If breast-feeding is attempted, supplementation should be provided initially, and nutritional status should be carefully monitored.

Feeding Considerations in Micrognathia and the Pierre-Robin Sequence

Components of sucking: *Compression* is often compromised by the presence of micrognathia. The tongue is retracted and may not position itself well beneath the nipple to provide compressive forces. The alveolar ridges are not well aligned, so their forces are offset during mandibular elevation. If there is a large cleft palate, there may not be an opposing surface for tongue compression. Infants without a cleft but with micrognathia can typically produce adequate *negative pressure suction*. When a cleft is present, marginal to no *negative pressure* will be generated during sucking activity.

Swallowing: In milder cases of Pierre-Robin malformation sequence, swallowing function is generally intact. For those infants with more airway obstruction and greater difficulty maintaining a stable airway, swallowing dysfunction is more likely.

Respiration: The primary problem in infants with Pierre-Robin malformation sequence is maintaining a patent airway for adequate respiration. Without treatment this problem is exaggerated in supine positions, such as the typical reclined feeding position, as gravity pulls the tongue into the pharynx. If there is airway compromise during feeding, the possibilities for oral feeding will obviously be limited. Therefore oral feeding in these infants is dependent upon the general management of airway obstruction.

Bottle-feeding: Bottle-feeding options are dependent on the type of overall management used for airway maintenance. **A patent and stable airway must be present before oral feeding can be considered.** Oximetry with feeding can help determine if the management of the airway is effective during feeding. Specific feeding techniques will vary based on the presence of a cleft and the degree of tongue retraction.

If airway patency is maintained by prone positioning, the infant's ability to tolerate a semireclined feeding position must be assessed. Although some infants have airway obstruction in supine during sleep, when awake they are able to maintain their airway in this position. For these infants feeding may be attempted in a standard position, though keeping them fairly erect minimizes gravitational pull on the tongue. Another option is to position the baby on its side for feeding. In either case, careful observation of behaviors indicating airway obstruction is necessary. If the infant falls asleep during feeding, repositioning may be necessary. Feeding techniques and devices for cleft palate and tongue retraction should be used as appropriate (see pages 235 and 367).

If the infant must remain prone, feeding may be attempted in that position. In the absence of a cleft palate, some success may be possible using a bottle with an angled neck (such as Corecto® or Degree®) to provide downward flow of milk into the mouth. When the infant also has a cleft palate, feeding in prone is generally not successful. Even if the milk is squeezed into the mouth, the infant lacks adequate suction to move the milk to the back of the mouth and form a bolus for swallowing. Gavage feeding will generally be required unless the overall medical management is changed. If gavage feeding becomes the primary method of nutrition, however, the use of a pacifier should be encouraged and an oral-motor program initiated.

A tongue-lip adhesion may be performed to provide a stable airway. Once the infant is recovered from the procedure and it is established that the surgery is stable, feeding may be able to progress without

---

limitations. Again, techniques appropriate for tongue retraction and cleft palate may be necessary. As breakdown of this repair is commonly reported, its integrity should be monitored carefully and oral feeding reassessed if the repair is no longer functioning appropriately.

A nasopharyngeal (NP) airway may be placed behind the tongue and above the epiglottis. This also allows oral feeding to progress, using techniques for cleft palate and tongue retraction as necessary. Maintaining appropriate positioning of the NP tube, however, is crucial to successful oral feeding. Frequent signs of distress with feeding, or milk regularly coming through the tube, suggest that the tube is not positioned correctly and should be reevaluated.

If a tracheostomy is required, oropharyngeal function is obviously impaired, and complete swallowing evaluation with a VFSS should be considered prior to oral feeding. If swallowing is safe, oral feeding can proceed, considering the factors related to feeding infants with a tracheostomy (see page 333).

Providing the proper nipple can be a key to oral feeding in an infant with a recessed tongue due to micrognathia. The nipple must be long enough to produce adequate contact between the nipple and tongue, or sucking movements will be ineffective, but not so long that it stimulates gagging. To maximize its length, the nipple may need to be fully inserted into the infant's mouth; therefore, a narrow base is suggested. A standard-profile nipple usually works well. A similarly shaped pacifier should also be provided for non-nutritive sucking.

Breast-feeding: For the infant with micrognathia, the possibilities for breast-feeding are again dependent on the degree of impairment and method of airway management, though success is not likely unless the micrognathia is mild and there is no cleft.

Breast-feeding is often difficult for the infant with a recessed jaw and no cleft, even if the airway is never compromised. The malalignment of the alveolar ridges and retracted tongue position may produce inadequate compression of the milk ducts, limiting milk expulsion and leading to reduced milk production. In addition, the retracted tongue may not have adequate contact along the surface of the nipple to support it in the best position. The shape and size of the mother's nipples, along with ease of milk production, may influence breast-feeding success. Supplementing the infant's intake by using a feeding-tube device (see chapter 8) may be necessary to allow breast-feeding to continue in these cases.

If the infant with micrognathia and airway instability must remain prone, breast-feeding is also difficult. While theoretically feeding could be attempted with the mother supine and the infant prone on her chest, establishing an adequate nipple position in the mouth of an infant with micrognathia is unlikely. The additional problem of a cleft palate makes functional nipple positioning and successful breast-feeding very unlikely.

Case example:
Stephen was a healthy, full-term infant born with micrognathia and cleft palate. He developed airway obstruction soon after birth. Although he could be maintained in a prone position, oral feeding was not possible. A nasopharyngeal tube was placed and positioning restrictions were eliminated. Oral feeding progressed well using a squeeze bottle and standard nipple, with full oral feeds by 5 days of age.

Stephen's mother also wished to breast-feed. Stephen could not successfully latch on to the bare breast, but he did suck on the breast when it was covered by a nipple shield. He could not produce suction to draw the nipple into the mouth where the tongue could maintain contact with the breast, but the more rigid shield could be inserted and positioned so that tongue activity could stimulate the let-down reflex. After the initial milk flow, however, Stephen's mechanical sucking was inadequate to maintain milk flow.

The mother enjoyed this breast-feeding activity with her son, then after 10 to 15 minutes gave him expressed breast milk by bottle. She continued this for a number of months, knowing that there was only a small chance it would lead to traditional breast-feeding. In fact, breast-feeding was never successful. Although there are a number of reasons for avoiding the use of breast shields in the infant without feeding problems, in this case it allowed the infant to keep the nipple in his mouth and stimulate some breast-feeding activity, which the mother enjoyed. Milk supply was adequately maintained by pumping.

Feeding Modifications and Devices

New devices, as well as ideas for modifications to existing equipment, for feeding babies with oral-facial anomalies abound. The following section will describe equipment reported in the literature and commonly used in clinical practices. These items are not necessarily recommended but are presented to familiarize clinicians with their function and considerations for their use.

Enlarging nipple holes: While this is done frequently to feed infants with oral-facial anomalies, it must be done with caution. Milk flow can easily be increased to the point that it compromises the coordination of normal swallowing and breathing activity, leading to excessive sputtering, coughing, choking, and nasal regurgitation. In our experience, enlarging the nipple hole is most successful when the infant can develop some suction independently and slight enlargement facilitates nutrient delivery. We have found that the size of hole that must be created for an infant utilizing only the compression component of sucking is generally so large that incoordination of sucking, swallowing, and breathing is frequent.

Slight and predictable enlargement of existing nipple holes can be accomplished by boiling the nipple with a toothpick in the hole, piercing the hole with a hot needle, or creating a 1/8-inch slit. For infants with a cleft palate these techniques rarely result in excessively rapid fluid flow. Using razor blades or scissors to create slits and crosscuts must be done with caution as it can easily lead to excessively large holes. A slit or crosscut works correctly only when the nipple is compressed. For the infant with a cleft palate and poor compression, other methods of enlarging the hole may be more effective.

Lamb's nipple: This long, fat nipple, which is adapted from use with lambs, has historically been recommended for use with the infant with a cleft palate. An enlarged hole, often a crosscut, is generally suggested.[25] This nipple is compressed, often between the lateral alveolar ridges, to release milk. Its large size is felt to allow more milk to enter the infant's mouth with each compression than a standard nipple.

While this system might work for some infants, there are many drawbacks. It is often difficult to correctly size the hole to the infant's compression strength and tolerance for fluid flow. If it is not correctly sized, coughing and choking or inadequate intake will result. The length of the nipple may cause excessive gagging in some infants. In addition, since the infant typically "chews" on this type of nipple, normal sucking movements of the tongue are not encouraged.

Ross® cleft palate assembly: This nipple has been referred to as a "hummingbird" nipple, as it consists of a three to four cm tube flanging out to fit a standard nipple ring. While the long length may cause gagging in some infants, it can be easily shortened to an appropriate length by cutting off the tip. The lumen of the tubing is large compared to standard nipple openings. Therefore, the fluid flow can be very rapid. This nipple does little to encourage normal tongue movements. The tubing is often oriented to the side of the mouth, but even if placed in midline its small diameter may not facilitate normal sucking movements of the tongue.

Obturator nipples: This is a nipple with a flange added across the upper part of the nipple to theoretically occlude the cleft and allow normal suction on the nipple. In practice, however, such nipples may or may not occlude the variety of configurations of palatal clefts, thus leading

---

to marginal success. They are difficult to use and may distort sucking and swallowing patterns.[28] In addition, the infant may not tolerate such a large device in the mouth.

Haberman feeder: This is a new device, developed to eliminate some of the problems associated with modified nipples on conventional bottles that are used for feeding infants with cleft palate. It is designed for effective milk release through nipple compression alone. Valving insures that nipple compression delivers milk into the infant's mouth rather than pushing it back into the bottle. The nipple also has a slit opening. By changing the orientation of the slit in the baby's mouth, flow is controlled during the feeding. Early reports suggest that it can increase amount and efficiency of oral intake and decrease air swallowing in infants with cleft palate.[9,10]

Palatal obturators: These devices may be referred to as oral prostheses, feeding appliances, and feeding obturators. A device is custom fitted to the infant with a cleft palate and inserted into the cleft. This occludes the cleft and allows the infant to develop the negative pressure suction required for breast- and bottle-feeding. Reported benefits include improved intake, along with better feeding skills, increased weight gain, improvements in speech, and easier palatal closure due to guidance of the growth of the dental arches. Disadvantages include the cost and inconvenience of fabricating serial devices as the infant grows, and maintaining proper fit for ease and effectiveness of use.[14-17,27] While some reports suggest that obturators be fabricated routinely for infants with cleft palate,[14,15] restricting their use to infants unable to orally feed by other means may be more appropriate until benefits to the palate repair or speech are substantiated.[16,27]

Ascepto feeders: This is a bulb-type syringe with a piece of soft rubber tubing attached. The tubing is placed in the infant's mouth, often in the cheek area, and milk is delivered by squeezing the syringe. The flow rate of the milk is very difficult to control with this device, often leading to coughing and choking, particularly in the young infant inexperienced at feeding. As no nipple is positioned on the tongue, normal sucking movements are not encouraged.

Squeeze bottles: Several items may work in this way. Disposable nursers can be compressed to push milk out of the nipple, though this may be awkward for the feeder. Standard plastic bottles can be squeezed slightly, though the stiff plastic makes squeezing imprecise.

The Mead-Johnson® cleft lip/palate nurser is a soft bottle that is more easily squeezed and gives the feeder excellent control over the amount of milk delivered to the infant. Although this bottle comes with a crosscut nipple, in our experience the milk flow is more consistent and easier for young infants to handle if a standard nipple with a hole is substituted. In this case, each squeeze of a given pressure will deliver the same amount of milk. With the crosscut nipple, the amount of milk the infant receives with each squeeze varies with the amount of compression on the nipple, and thus the opening in the nipple, at the moment the feeder squeezes. Older infants who are experienced feeders may return to the crosscut nipple to obtain larger volumes of milk and may be better able to cope with the continual variation in fluid flow.

General Considerations

For the large majority of infants with the oral-facial anomalies discussed above, an oral feeding method can be established that works for the infant, works for the parents, and provides adequate nutrition. Analyzing the infant's feeding strengths and limitations and selecting a feeding method are only the first steps in this process. Achieving smooth and consistent oral feeding may take time. Careful evaluation and selection of a feeding method may reduce the time it takes for the infant and feeder to become comfortable and successful at feeding. More complex anomalies and medical complications, however, can prolong the process. Parents must be reassured that early feedings are a learning process and that the feeding should become easier and more successful with practice. Even a parent experienced in feeding must learn how to hold the infant upright, how much to squeeze the bottle, how long to keep the bottle in the infant's mouth, how often to burp, and so on. At the same time, the infant is learning how to coordinate swallowing and breathing when sucking is ineffective and fluid flow may be unpredictable. The infant is also learning how to best communicate its responses to the feeder. Patience and keen observational skills will assist in this process.

For most infants with oral-facial anomalies, oral feeding becomes increasingly easier during the first few months. Not only does the infant gain experience in feeding, but it appears that the normal maturation of the coordination of sucking, swallowing, and breathing allows the infant to handle larger boluses and tolerate more variation in the process of oral intake without coughing and choking. For infants who do not master a system of oral feeding for fluids, the initiation of semisolids by spoon is often welcome. They may be more successful when small boluses of food are delivered into the mouth, and single swallows do not require repetitive coordination of sucking, swallowing, and breathing. Fluid intake, however, must still be maintained.

Common scenarios when problems do arise include the infant who coughs and chokes frequently with oral feeding. While this is reportedly common when feeding infants with oral-facial anomalies, one must ask: How much coughing is too much? In some infants this coughing may indicate abnormal swallowing rather than "typically" increased choking. If swallowing dysfunction is present it may produce such an unpleasant experience that the baby begins to show rejection and avoidance of oral feeding. Coughing and choking can also suggest that fluid flow is too great, but how much can it be reduced and still allow effective feeding? Reduction in fluid flow may reduce caloric intake and further compromise weight gain. Parents may report that feeding takes an hour or more, or that they are feeding the infant every hour. Even if the infant is receiving the required calories, what is the cost to the infant and the family?

The role of supplementary non-oral feedings in this population must be considered. During the initial period of "learning" oral feeding, periodic non-oral supplements may be necessary. For an infant who is coughing or choking excessively or beginning to refuse feeding, the fluid flow may need to be reduced, even if full oral feeding is no longer possible. The short-term use of non-oral supplements is preferable to having oral feeding become so aversive that the infant rejects it. If oral intake is consistently low, or feeding problems marked, non-oral supplements will also be appropriate. When feedings take more than 30 to 40 minutes or they are more frequent than normal for age, modifications to the feeding program should be considered. If the amount of time spent in oral feeding cannot be reduced while nutrition is maintained, non-oral supplements may also be necessary. Guidelines and further information provided in chapter 5 should be useful.

Finally, the impact of surgical repair procedures on oral feeding should be considered. With surgical repair of a cleft lip, there should no longer be an anterior leak in the seal of the oral cavity. When the palate is repaired, or as the cleft becomes smaller with growth, greater suction should be generated, though even with surgical repair of the palate a small anterior opening may be left that is not repaired until 7 to 9 years of age. This information can be integrated into the process of evaluating oral feeding and modifying techniques as the infant's feeding characteristics change. On the other hand, structural repairs do not correct some problems. If neuromuscular incoordination or swallowing dysfunction are present, it is unlikely they will change with surgery. Families should be assisted in developing realistic expectations once surgical repairs are performed.

Tracheoesophageal Fistula/Esophageal Atresia

Tracheoesophageal fistula (TEF) and esophageal atresia (EA) are common congenital anomalies occurring in the neonate. Their incidence is reported to vary between one in 1,500 to one in 4,500 live births, with approximately one-third being born prematurely.[1] Approximately 30% to 40% of these infants have other congenital defects of the oropharynx, gastrointestinal tract, skeletal system, cardiac system, or genitourinary tract.[1] These anomalies often occur together in a complex known as the VATER association, in which vertebral, anal, cardiac, tracheoesophageal, and radial anomalies are present. Advances in surgical management, pediatric anesthesia, neonatal intensive care, and the availability of parenteral nutrition have changed the nearly 100% mortality with TEF/EA to a survival rate of 80%, with survival reaching 100% in those infants weighing more than 2,700 grams at birth.[2,3] Most patients are surviving to adulthood. Mortality is now related more to the associated defects than to the presence of TEF/EA.

Tracheoesophageal fistula and esophageal atresia are classified according to the presence or absence of fistula and the configuration of the esophagus (see figure 6-11). In type A, esophageal atresia without fistula, both segments of the esophagus are blind pouches and neither is connected to the trachea. In type B, tracheoesophageal fistula to the proximal segment, the upper portion of the esophagus is connected to the trachea. Type C, esophageal atresia with fistula to the distal segment, is similar to type A in that the upper portion of the esophagus ends in a blind pouch. The lower portion, however, connects to the trachea. Type D, esophageal atresia with fistula to both segments, has both the upper and lower portions of the esophagus connected to the trachea but not connected to each other.

The last type, type E, is more commonly referred to as H-type or tracheoesophageal fistula without atresia. In this type there is a small fistula or tract connecting the esophagus and the trachea somewhere between the cricoid cartilage and the midesophagus. The size of this fistulous tract can vary, at times being as small as a pinpoint. In contrast to the other four types, which are discovered shortly after birth, the discovery of H-type TEF can be delayed until after the neonatal period. Since both the trachea and esophagus are intact but connected, these babies are able to feed, albeit with frequent coughing. They may come to medical attention secondary to respiratory symptoms.

Surgical repair of the TEF/EA can be accomplished in three ways. First, a primary anastomosis connecting the two portions of the esophagus may be performed very shortly after birth. Although many of these babies will receive a gastrostomy, they frequently do not need it. Second, when the infant has other medical problems or when the distance between the two portions is too great, delayed primary anastomosis may be considered. The baby is generally fed by parenteral feedings or a gastrostomy tube. A replogle tube is placed that removes secretions from the upper blind pouch so they do not spill over into the airway to be aspirated. Many surgeons will try to reduce the long gap between the two esophageal segments by using bougienage, a method of stretching the segments.

In the third method, the staged management of anastomosis, growth is needed prior to repair. In this method, the upper portion of the esophagus is brought out to an opening in the neck called an esophagostomy so that secretions can spill out. This eliminates the need for a replogle tube. The infant receives nutrition via a gastrostomy tube. Sham oral feedings are possible after this procedure, as they should drain out of the esophagostomy. Anastomosis of the esophageal ends occurs at a later time, and may involve reconstruction of the esophagus using other body tissues. Regardless of the type of surgical management, the amount of time that the baby is non-orally fed prior to the anastomosis is one factor that will influence the development of feeding skill and potential difficulties.

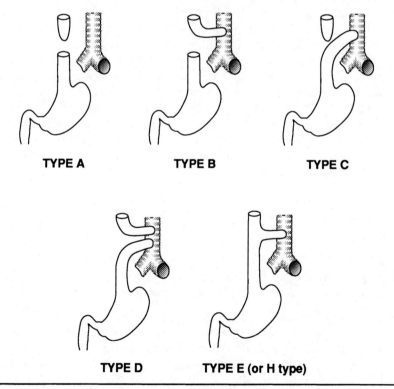

TYPE A   **TYPE B**   **TYPE C**

TYPE D   **TYPE E (or H type)**

Figure 6-11 Types of tracheoesophageal fistulas and atresias.

Long-Term Complications

Long-term complications in infants following repair of TEF/EA will vary according to the type of defect, type of surgical repair, and structural characteristics of the infant. A number of long-term complications are described, including: (1) tracheomalacia, (2) esophageal dysmotility, (3) esophageal stricture formation, (4) foreign-body impaction, (5) gastroesophageal reflux, (6) associated respiratory complications, and (7) nutritional deficits. The occurrence and severity of these known complications will also influence the presence and magnitude of feeding-related problems.

Tracheomalacia: Some degree of tracheomalacia is present in nearly all infants with TEF/EA. This is an inherent structural abnormality of the trachea that causes it to be unstable and prone to collapse. Infants with TEF/EA often have what is described as a "seal-bark" cough, which occurs when the trachea collapses on expiration. Stridor may also be present with tracheomalacia.

Esophageal Dysmotility: Esophageal dysmotility results in fluids and liquids progressing more slowly down the esophagus or in a less organized fashion than normal. Cinefluorographic or videofluoroscopic studies of children with TEF/EA have shown varying degrees of disordered esophageal motility, characterized by a lack of organized propulsive waves. Laks et al.[4] noted that the abnormalities in peristalsis were observed above and below the site of anastomosis, with the entire esophagus involved in abnormal peristalsis. Not only was peristalsis slowed, but the type of peristaltic contraction often led to retrograde flow of the esophageal contents.[4] This could place the child at risk for aspiration. Improvement in esophageal motility is observed over time; however, dysmotility can continue to be present even in asymptomatic patients.

Stricture Formation: Some degree of narrowing at the site where the esophageal ends are joined is expected in all repaired cases of TEF/EA. The formation of a tighter stricture at this site can interfere with the passage of food, particularly solids, into the stomach. Stricture formation can lead to coughing and choking as foods back up in the esophagus and spill over into the airway. If stricture occurs, dilatation, a procedure to widen the narrowed segment, may be necessary.

Foreign-Body Impaction: Esophageal dysmotility, with or without a stricture, can lead to foreign-body impaction. This is especially true in younger children who do not chew well. Inadequately chewed foods may become lodged in the esophagus. Food and saliva can then build up in a functionally obstructed esophagus and overflow into the airway. Endoscopic removal of the impaction is generally required.

Gastroesophageal Reflux: Disordered esophageal motility can contribute to reflux. As mentioned previously, disordered peristalsis can lead to retrograde flow, or reflux of the esophageal contents. If there is typical reflux of the stomach contents into the esophagus, poor motility can impair return of the refluxed material to the stomach. Disordered motility can also result in intraesophageal reflux, whereby the food is refluxed upward prior to reaching the stomach. This can result in aspiration or interfere with the swallowing of subsequent boluses. Lower esophageal sphincter function may be altered as a consequence of mobilizing the distal esophagus to facilitate the anastomosis. The presence of gastrostomy tubes may also worsen GER in TEF/EA patients.

Associated Respiratory Complications: Obstructive and restrictive lung disease can occur in children with repaired TEF/EA.[5] Obstructive lung disease can be secondary to tracheomalacia. Restrictive or reactive airway disease may be secondary to ongoing microaspiration (ascending or descending) or to GE reflux-induced, vagally mediated reflex bronchoconstriction (see section on GE reflux [page 337] for a full discussion of these mechanisms).

Nutritional Deficits: Long-term growth failure of both height and weight have been observed.[4,6] Heights and weights for children with TEF/EA have been reported to be one to two standard deviations below the mean. Growth patterns tended to improve above 13 years of age, and children demonstrated some, but incomplete, catch-up growth. Routine nutritional assessment as part of the child's overall follow-up is strongly suggested.[6]

Feeding-Related Problems Commonly Seen in TEF/EA

The types of feeding problems seen in children with TEF/EA are most frequently due to long-term complications, associated congenital anomalies, or delayed introduction of foods necessitated by delayed surgical repair. If the baby was also born prematurely, the infant may have other feeding problems related directly to the prematurity (see page 297). In the absence of a congenital central nervous system disorder, the majority of babies with TEF/EA have normal oral-motor skills. They have appropriate lip, tongue, and jaw movements for effective sucking. They generally have normal suck/swallow/breathe coordination if no underlying lung disease is present, although swallow/breathe coordination can be influenced by the poor esophageal motility.

Problem—Inability to handle some food types and textures

Infants and children with TEF/EA may have difficulty handling some types of food and/or progressing normally through the various developmentally appropriate food textures.

Basis for the problem: Most parents of children with TEF/EA report some difficulty with feeding, including coughing or choking during feeding, vomiting, or food sticking in the throat. These difficulties are related to the inherent esophageal dysmotility and narrowing at the anastomosis. The most common foods creating feeding difficulties in infancy are junior baby foods, food with lumps, or stringy foods. In adults and older children, fruit, bread, and vegetables are problematic.[7] Inadequate chewing of food (as often seen with toddlers) may result in swallowing pieces that are too large to move easily down the esophagus, or that become stuck at the narrowing or stricture.

Treatment strategies:

- Children are advised to eat in an upright position so gravity can assist the downward movement of foods in the esophagus.

- Parents should be trained in emergency procedures for choking, such as the Heimlick maneuver, so they are prepared to deal effectively with choking episodes should they occur. Food textures should be carefully monitored and thorough chewing encouraged. For a beginning chewer, offer foods that are soft or mashed or that melt in the mouth. Avoid hard or raw fruits and vegetables until the child chews extremely well. Hot dogs and hard candy should not be eaten until the teenage years.[9,10]

- Children are encouraged to drink frequently during meals to "wash down" foods that may be stuck in the esophagus.[8] Liquids and solids should be alternated throughout the meal.

- When there is esophageal dysmotility, more time may be required between swallows to insure adequate clearance of the esophagus. Meals should be eaten slowly. Infants may need external pacing on the bottle or breast. After taking only one or two suck/swallows, the baby is given a pause to allow for esophageal clearance. An infant with dysmotility can show unwillingness to eat, as poor esophageal clearance may make the baby fearful or uncomfortable during rapid sucking and swallowing. External pacing may help minimize such discomfort.

Problem—Gastroesophageal reflux

GE reflux can result in poor weight gain from vomiting, irritability, feeding aversion due to pain, or deteriorating respiratory status from microaspiration.

Basis of the problem: GER can be a significant problem for infants and children with TEF/EA. Foods can progress slowly down the esophagus due to esophageal dysmotility, and they can progress back up the esophagus due to faulty peristalsis. If acid reflux occurs, there is greater risk for esophagitis, since esophageal dysmotility will impair acid clearance. Esophagitis can then contribute to stricture formation at the site of anastomosis. The competence of the lower esophageal sphincter may be impaired because of the surgical repair, or from the inherent defect that created the TEF/EA. Children with TEF/EA are at risk for developing the entire spectrum of consequences of gastroesophageal reflux described in that section of this chapter.

Treatment strategies:

- Following surgery, prophylactic treatment with upright positioning is often prescribed (see page 340). Due to the likelihood of esophageal dysmotility, however, liquids should not be thickened, as this would further slow their progress down the esophagus. Upright positioning is often used for at least two months, with careful monitoring for reflux-related symptoms after discontinuation.

Problem—Prolonged periods of non-oral feeding

Loss of normal oral-motor skills and the development of oral hypersensitivity or aversive feeding behaviors can result from the early and prolonged non-oral feeding methods that may be necessary in some babies with TEF/EA.

Basis of the problem: While TEF/EA repair generally occurs within the newborn period, at times primary repair of the TEF/EA is delayed until medical problems have resolved or there has been sufficient esophageal growth to allow for a tension-free anastomosis. In this case, the baby must be non-orally fed for a significant length of time and may have unpleasant oral experiences, such as prolonged use of a replogle tube for suctioning the esophageal pouch. The baby is thus at risk for developing oral hypersensitivity or aversive responses. If the baby does not have a program of non-nutritive oral stimulation, sucking may not be maintained, and the baby may not develop the prerequisite oral-motor control for more mature skills like spoon feeding or chewing.

Treatment strategies:

- If the baby is undergoing a staged anastomosis and an esophagostomy is present, sham oral feedings can occur. These "feedings" can maintain the baby's oral and swallowing skills during the prolonged period of non-oral feeding. Illingworth and Lister found that the use of sham feedings made the reintroduction of normal oral feeding after repair of the TEF/EA easier and faster.[11]

In our center, the typical progression for an infant who receives sham feedings is as follows:

1. **Early management:** Gastrostomy is placed for nutrition, replogle tube is used to drain secretions from the esophageal pouch, and bougienage may be instituted to stretch the proximal esophageal pouch. During this time non-nutritive sucking on a pacifier is encouraged, particularly at feeding times. NNS is generally possible even with the replogle tube in place.

2. **Staged management approach selected:** Surgery is done to form an esophagostomy, and the stoma is allowed to heal.

3. **Sham oral feedings are instituted:** Nipple-feeding skills are assessed, and techniques for optimal performance are determined. While some infants will need no modifications of standard nippling procedures, some infants may require techniques to slow the rate of flow (see page 406).

As tolerated, nippling is done in conjunction with each daytime gastrostomy feeding. Formula is used for the sham feedings, though to limit waste it is given half-strength. While the infant should take a substantial volume, the goal is for the infant to nipple one-half the volume required for nutritional needs (e.g., if two ounces are given by g-tube, one ounce is given by mouth). Optimally, nippling occurs as the gastrostomy feeding is running into the stomach. If this is not manageable, sham feedings can be followed by g-tube feeding. Cloth diapers are held over the esophagostomy to collect food as it exits the stoma.

Some mothers may be interested in "sham" breast-feeding. This is possible, but the mother's milk supply should be carefully considered. If a mother is pumping breast milk for gastrostomy feedings, using her milk for the infant's nutrition is the first priority. If the mother's supply is abundant, some sham breast-feeding is possible, though the milk will be lost. If milk supply is limited, the mother should be encouraged to put the infant to the breast after pumping, when milk flow and thus milk loss would be minimal. As the goal of sham feeding, however, is for the infant to experience the process and sensations of all aspects of oral feeding, bottle-feeding as described above should also be continued.

4. **Progressive sham feedings:** In many staged repairs, the anastomosis is not done until the infant is 10 to 12 months of age or older. Therefore, it is developmentally appropriate to move beyond nipple feeding. Strained spoon foods should be introduced around 6 months of age and soft finger foods by about 8 months of age. Development of effective chewing skills should be encouraged. Cup drinking can also be introduced. As each new skill is initiated, the baby's responses are carefully monitored, and modifications are made as needed. The ultimate goal of sham feeding is to mirror the oral and feeding experiences of a normally developing child, including variety in food tastes and textures. This is done within the context of providing a *safe* experience for the child.

5. **After anastomosis:** The child who has strong oral and feeding skills will have the easiest time progressing to full oral feeding, though some setbacks and adjustment should be expected. Initial feedings will typically be with liquids or strained foods. Textures must be introduced carefully, as described on page 382. While esophageal dysmotility, GE reflux, and stricture would not have been problems prior to repair, after the repair they can become major problems that affect feeding. Oral feeding techniques may need to be modified if these problems occur.

- Treatment strategies for the non-orally fed baby with TEF/EA where sham feedings are not possible would be the same as for any baby undergoing a lengthy period of non-oral feeding that is superimposed with potentially negative oral experiences. These techniques are described in detail in chapter 5. The general goals would be to: (1) maintain oral sucking abilities and preserve the link between sensations in the mouth and sensations in the stomach through the use of a pacifier during tube feedings as well as at other times; (2) minimize oral hypersensitivity and aversion through graded oral normalization techniques; (3) provide a variety of playful, pleasurable oral experiences; and (4) provide modeling of eating behaviors whenever possible.

References

The Premature Infant

1. Anderson, G. C., and D. Vidyasagar. 1979. Development of sucking in premature infants from 1 to 7 days post birth. *Birth Defects: Original Articles Series* 15:145-71.

2. Measel, C. P., and G. C. Anderson. 1979. Non-nutritive sucking during tube feedings: Effect on clinical course in premature infants. *Journal of Obstetric, Gynecologic and Neonatal Nursing* 8:265-72.

3. Rosen, C. L., D. G. Glaze, and J. D. Frost. 1984. Hypoxemia associated with feeding in the preterm infant and full-term neonate. *American Journal of Diseases of Childhood* 138:623-28.

4. Guilleminault, C., and S. Coons. 1984. Apnea and bradycardia during feeding in infants weighing 2000 gm. *The Journal of Pediatrics* 104:932-35.

5. Mathew, O. P., M. L. Clark, M. L. Pronske, H. G. Luna-Solarzano, and M. D. Peterson. 1985. Breathing pattern and ventilation during oral feeding in term newborn infants. *The Journal of Pediatrics* 106:810-13.

6. Mathew, O. P. 1988. Respiratory control during nipple feeding in preterm infants. *Pediatric Pulmonology* 5:220-24.

7. Mathew, O. P., M. L. Clark, and M. L. Pronske. 1985. Apnea, bradycardia, and cyanosis during oral feeding in term neonates (letter). *The Journal of Pediatrics* 106:857.

8. Daniels, H., H. Devlieger, P. Casaer, and E. Eggermont. 1986. Nutritive and non-nutritive sucking in preterm infants. *Journal of Developmental Physiology* 8:117-21.

9. Casaer, P., H. Daniels, H. Devlieger, P. DeCock, and E. Eggermont. 1982. Feeding behavior in preterm neonates. *Early Human Development* 7:331-46.

10. Paludetto, R., S. S. Robertson, and R. J. Martin. 1986. Interaction between non-nutritive sucking and respiration in preterm infants. *Biology of the Neonate* 49:198-203.

11. Shivpuri, C. R., R. J. Martin, W. A. Carlo, and A. A. Fanaroff. 1983. Decreased ventilation in preterm infants during oral feeding. *The Journal of Pediatrics* 103:285-89.

12. Daniels, H., P. Casaer, H. Devlieger, and E. Eggermont. 1986. Mechanisms of feeding efficiency in preterm infants. *Journal of Pediatric Gastroenterology and Nutrition* 5:593-96.

13. Brake, S., W. P. Fifer, G. Alfasi, and A. Fleischman. 1988. The first nutritive sucking responses of premature newborns. *Infant Behavior and Development* 11:1-9.

14. Bosma, J. F. 1967. Human infant oral function. In *Symposium on oral sensation and perception*, edited by J. F. Bosma, 98-110. Springfield, IL: Charles C. Thomas.

15. Bosma, J. F. 1972. Form and function in the infant's mouth and pharynx. In *Third symposium on oral sensation and perception*, edited by J. F. Bosma, 3-29. Springfield, IL: Charles C. Thomas.

16. Case-Smith, J., P. Cooper, and V. Scala. 1989. Feeding efficiency of premature neonates. *The American Journal of Occupational Therapy* 43:245-50.

17. Shaker, C. S. 1990. Nipple feeding premature infants: A different perspective. *Neonatal Network* 8:9-17.

18. Dreier, T., P. H. Wolff, E. E. Cross, and W. D. Cochran. 1979. Patterns of breath intervals during non-nutritive sucking in full-term and "at-risk" preterm infants with normal neurologic examinations. *Early Human Development* 3:187-99.

19. Hack, M., M. M. Estabrook, and S. S. Robertson. 1985. Development of sucking rhythms in preterm infants. *Early Human Development* 11:133-40.

20. Gryboski, J. D. 1969. Suck and swallow in the premature infant. *Pediatrics* 43:96-102.

21. Ellison, S. L., D. Vidyasagar, G. C. Anderson. 1979. Sucking in the newborn infant during the first hour of life. *Journal of Nurse-Midwifery* 24:18-25.

22. Pierantoni, H. R., L. L. Wright, J. F. Bosma, and K. Bessard. 1986. The development of respiratory control during oral feeding in premature infants. *Pediatric Research* (abstract) 20:382A.

23. Bernbaum, J. C., G. R. Pereira, J. B. Watkins, and G. J. Peckham. 1983. Non-nutritive sucking during gavage feeding enhances growth and maturation in premature infants. *Pediatrics* 71:41-45.

24. Horton, F. H., L. O. Lubchenco, and H. H. Gordon. 1952. Self-regulation feeding in a premature nursery. *Yale Journal of Biology and Medicine* 24:263-72.

25. Collinge, J. M., K. Bradley, C. Perks et al. 1982. Demand vs. scheduled feedings for premature infants. *Journal of Obstetric, Gynecologic and Neonatal Nursing* 90:362-67.

26. Borland, M. 1989. Neuromotor development. In *A guide to care and management of very low birth weight infants*, edited by C. J. Semmler, 216-50. Tucson, AZ: Therapy Skill Builders.

27. Pransky, S. M. 1989. Evaluation of the compromised neonatal airway. *Pediatric Clinics of North America* 36:1571-82.

28. Oh, W. 1983. Respiratory distress syndrome: Diagnosis and management. In *Diagnosis and management of respiratory disorders in the newborn*, edited by L. Stern, 2-13. Menlo Park, CA: Addison-Wesley Publishing Company.

29. Mathew, O. P. 1988. Nipple units for newborn infants: A functional comparison. *Pediatrics* 81:688-91.

30. Leonard, E. L., L. E. Trykowski, and B. V. Kirkpatrick. 1980. Nutritive sucking in high-risk neonates after perioral stimulation. *Physical Therapy* 60:299-302.

31. Widstom, A. M., G. Marchini, A. S. Matthiesen, S. Werner, J. Winberg, and K. Uvnas-Moberg. 1988. Non-nutritive sucking in tube-fed preterm infants: Effects on gastric motility and gastric contents of somatostatin. *Journal of Pediatric Gastroenterology and Nutrition* 7:517-23.

32. Paludetto, R., S. S. Robertson, M. Hack, C. R. Shivpuri, and R. J. Martin. 1984. Transcutaneous oxygen tension during non-nutritive sucking in preterm infants. *Pediatrics* 74:539-42.

33. Burroughs, A. K., U. O. Asonye, G. C. Anderson-Shanklin, and D. Vidyasagar. 1978. The effects of non-nutritive sucking on transcutaneous oxygen tension in noncrying, preterm infants. *Research in Nursing* 1:69-75.

34. Meier, P., and E. J. Pugh. 1985. Breast-feeding behavior of small preterm infants. *MCN* 10:396-401.

35. Meier, P., and G. C. Anderson. 1987. Responses of small preterm infants to bottle- and breast-feeding. *MCN* 12:97-105.

36. Meier, P. 1988. Bottle- and breast-feeding: Effects on transcutaneous oxygen pressure and temperature in preterm infants. *Nursing Research* 37:36-41.

37. Field, T., E. Ignatoff, S. Stringer, J. Brennan, R. Greenberg, S. Widmayer, and G. C. Anderson. 1982. Non-nutritive sucking during tube feedings: Effects on preterm infants in an intensive care unit. *Pediatrics* 70:381-84.

38. Bosma, J. F. 1980. Physiology of the mouth. In *Otolaryngology*, vol. 1, edited by M. M. Paparella and D. A. Shumrick. Philadelphia: W. B. Saunders Company.

39. Walsh, M. C., and R. M. Kliegman. 1986. Necrotizing enterocolitis: Treatment based on staging criteria. *Pediatric Clinics of North America* 33:179-201.

40. Brown, E. G., and A. Y. Sweet. 1982. Neonatal necrotizing enterocolitis. *Pediatric Clinics of North America* 29:1149-70.

41. Yu, V. Y., and D. I. Tudehope. 1977. Neonatal necrotizing enterocolitis II: Perinatal risk factors. *Medical Journal of Australia* 1:688-93.

42. Kliegmen, R. M., W. B. Pittard, and A. A. Fanaroff. 1979. Necrotizing enterocolitis in neonates fed human milk. *The Journal of Pediatrics* 95:450-53.

43. Semmler, C. J. 1989. Intracranial hemorrhage. In *A guide to care and management of very low birth weight infants*, edited by C. J. Semmler, 77-98. Tucson, AZ: Therapy Skill Builders.

44. Pape, K. E., and J. S. Wigglesworth. 1979. *Hemorrhage, ischaemia and the perinatal brain*. Philadelphia: J. B. Lippincott.

45. Tarby, T. J., and J. J. Volpe. 1982. Intraventricular hemorrhage in the premature infant. Symposium on the newborn. *Pediatric Clinics of North America* 29(5): 1077-1104.

46. Weisglas-Kuperus, N., M. Uleman-Vleeschdrager, and W. Baerts. 1987. Ventricular hemorrhages and hypoxic-ischaemic lesions in preterm infants: Neurodevelopmental outcome at 3½ years. *Developmental Medicine and Child Neurology* 29:623-29.

47. Pettett, G. 1986. Medical complications of the premature infant. *Physical and Occupational Therapy in Pediatrics* 6:91-104.

48. Vaucher, Y. E. 1988. Understanding intraventricular hemorrhage and white-matter injury in premature infants. *Infants and Young Children* 1:31-45.

49. Klaus, M., and A. A. Fanaroff. 1978. *Care of the high risk neonate.* Philadelphia: W. B. Saunders.

50. Mathew, O. P. 1988. Regulation of breathing pattern during feeding: Role of suck, swallow, and nutrients. In *Respiratory function of the upper airway,* edited by O. P. Mathew and G. Sant'Ambrogio, 535-60. New York: Marcel Dekker, Inc.

51. Als, H. 1986. A synactive model of neonatal behavioral organization: Framework for the assessment of neurobehavioral development in the premature infant and for support of infants and parents in the neonatal intensive care environment. *Physical and Occupational Therapy in Pediatrics* 6:3-53.

52. Lepecq, J., M. Rigoard, and P. Salzarulo. 1985. Spontaneous non-nutritive sucking in continuously fed infants. *Early Human Development* 12:279-84.

53. Rushton, C. H. 1990. Necrotizing enterocolitis: Part I, parthogenesis and diagnosis. *MCN* 15:296-300.

Bronchopulmonary Dysplasia

1. Bancalari, E., and T. Gerhardt. 1986. Bronchopulmonary dysplasia. *Pediatric Clinics of North America* 33:1-23.

2. Nickerson, B. G. 1985. Bronchopulmonary dysplasia: Chronic pulmonary disease following neonatal respiratory failure. *Chest* 87:528-35.

3. Bozynski, M. A. 1989. Comprehensive management of the infant with bronchopulmonary dysplasia: A growing challenge. *Infants and Young Children* 2:14-24.

4. O'Brodovich, H. M., and R. B. Mellins. 1985. Bronchopulmonary dysplasia: Unresolved neonatal acute lung injury. *American Review of Respiratory Disease* 132:694-709.

5. Wolfson, M. R., V. K. Bhutani, T. H. Shaffer, and F. W. Bowen, Jr. 1984. Mechanics and energetics of breathing helium in infants with bronchopulmonary dysplasia. *The Journal of Pediatrics* 104:752-57.

6. Weinstein, M. R., and W. Oh. 1981. Oxygen consumption in infants with bronchopulmonary dysplasia. *The Journal of Pediatrics* 99:958-61.

7. Guidelines for the care of children with chronic lung disease. 1989. *Pediatric Pulmonology* Supplement 3:3-13.

8. Ratner, I., and J. Whitfield. 1983. Acquired subglottic stenosis in the very-low-birth-weight infant. *American Journal of Diseases in Childhood* 137:40-43.

9. Miller, R. W., P. Woo, R. K. Kellman, and T. S. Slagle. 1987. Tracheobronchial abnormalities in infants with bronchopulmonary dysplasia. *The Journal of Pediatrics* 111:779-82.

10. Jones, R., A. Bodnar, Y. Roan, and D. Johnson. 1981. Subglottic stenosis in newborn intensive care unit graduates. *American Journal of Disease in Childhood* 135: 367-68.

11. Kurzner, S. I., M. Garg, D. B. Bautista, C. W. Sargent, C. M. Bowman, and T. G. Keens. 1988. Growth failure in bronchopulmonary dysplasia: Elevated metabolic rates and pulmonary mechanics. *The Journal of Pediatrics* 112:73-80.

12. Groothius, J. R., and A. A. Rosenberg. 1987. Home oxygen promotes weight gain in infants with bronchopulmonary dysplasia. *American Journal of Diseases in Childhood* 141:992-95.

13. Coelho, C. A. 1987. Preliminary findings on the nature of dysphagia in patients with chronic obstructive pulmonary disease. *Dysphagia* 2:28-31.

14. Erikson, E. H. 1963. *Childhood and society.* New York: Norton.

15. Als, H., G. Lawhon, E. Brown, R. Gibes, F. H. Duffy, G. McAnulty, and J. G. Blickman. 1986. Individualized behavioral and environmental care for the very low birth weight preterm infant at high risk for bronchopulmonary dysplasia: Neonatal intensive care unit and developmental outcome. *Pediatrics* 78:1123-32.

16. Als, H. 1986. A synactive model of neonatal behavioral organization: Framework for the assessment of neurobehavioral development in the premature infant and for support of infants and parents in the neonatal intensive care environment. *Physical and Occupational Therapy in Pediatrics* 6:3-53.

17. Nash, M. 1988. Swallowing problems in the tracheotomized patient. *The Otolaryngologic Clinics of North America* 21:701-10.

18. Oh, W. 1983. Respiratory distress syndrome: Diagnosis and management. In *Diagnosis and management of respiratory disorders in the newborn,* edited by L. Stern, 1-13. Menlo Park, CA: Addison-Wesley Publishing Company.

19. Pashley, N. R. T., and L. L. Fan. 1988. Laryngeal injury from endotracheal intubation in the neonate. In *Bronchopulmonary dysplasia,* edited by E. Bancalari and J. T. Stocker, 211-19. Washington, DC: Hemisphere Publishing Corporation.

20. DeLemos, R. A., A. Guajardo, and D. R. Gertsman. 1988. High-frequency ventilation. In *Bronchopulmonary dysplasia*, edited by E. Bancalari and J. T. Stocker, 370-80. Washington, DC: Hemisphere Publishing Corporation.

21. Schellhase, D. E., and L. L. Fan. 1988. Management after the nursery. In *Bronchopulmonary dysplasia*, edited by E. Bancalari and J. T. Stocker, 381-402. Washington, DC: Hemisphere Publishing Corporation.

22. Koops, B. K., and C. Lam. 1988. Outcome in bronchopulmonary dysplasia: Mortality risks and prognosis for growth, neurologic integrity, and developmental performance. In *Bronchopulmonary dysplasia*, edited by E. Bancalari and J. T. Stocker, 403-15. Washington, DC: Hemisphere Publishing Corporation.

23. Bancalari, E. 1988. Pathogenesis of bronchopulmonary dysplasia: An overview. In *Bronchopulmonary dysplasia*, edited by E. Bancalari and J. T. Stocker, 3-15. Washington, DC: Hemisphere Publishing Corporation.

24. Frank, L. 1988. Nutrition: Influence on lung growth, injury and repair, and development of bronchopulmonary dysplasia. In *Bronchopulmonary dysplasia*, edited by E. Bancalari and J. T. Stocker, 78-108. Washington, DC: Hemisphere Publishing Corporation.

25. Gerhardt, T., and E. Bancalari. 1988. Lung function in bronchopulmonary dysplasia. In *Bronchopulmonary dysplasia*, edited by E. Bancalari and J. T. Stocker, 182-91. Washington, DC: Hemisphere Publishing Corporation.

26. Goldberg, R. N., and E. Bancalari. 1988. Respiratory management of infants with bronchopulmonary dysplasia. In *Bronchopulmonary dysplasia*, edited by E. Bancalari and J. T. Stocker, 299-312. Washington, DC: Hemisphere Publishing Corporation.

27. Rosenfeld, W. 1988. Antioxidant therapy. In *Bronchopulmonary dysplasia*, edited by E. Bancalari and J. T. Stocker, 337-44. Washington, DC: Hemisphere Publishing Corporation.

28. Sinkin, R. A., and D. L. Shapiro. 1988. Surfactant replacement therapy. In *Bronchopulmonary dysplasia*, edited by E. Bancalari and J. T. Stocker, 345-55. Washington, DC: Hemisphere Publishing Corporation.

29. Stenmark, K. R. 1988. Steroids. In *Bronchopulmonary dysplasia*, edited by E. Bancalari and J. T. Stocker, 356-65. Washington, DC: Hemisphere Publishing Corporation.

30. Meisels, S. J., J. W. Plunkett, D. W. Rolf, P. L. Pasick, and G. S. Stiefel. 1986. Growth and development of preterm infants with respiratory distress syndrome and bronchopulmonary dysplasia. *Pediatrics* 77:345-52.

31. Simon, B. M., and J. S. McGowan. 1989. Tracheostomy in young children: Implications for assessment and treatment of communication and feeding disorders. *Infants and Young Children* 1:1-9.

32. Mathew, O. P. 1988. Regulation of breathing pattern during feeding: Role of suck, swallow, and nutrients. In *Respiratory function of the upper airway,* edited by O. P. Mathew and G. Sant'Ambrogio, 535-60. New York: Marcel Dekker, Inc.

33. Bosma, J. 1967. Human infant oral function. In *Oral sensation and perception,* edited by J. F. Bosma, 98-110. Springfield, IL: Charles C. Thomas.

Gastroesophageal Reflux

1. Werlin, S. L., W. J. Dodds, W. J. Hogan, and R. C. Arndorfer. 1980. Mechanisms of gastroesophageal reflux in children. *The Journal of Pediatrics* 97:244-49.

2. Shub, M. D., M. H. Ulshen, C. B. Hargrove, G. P. Siegal, P. A. Groben, and F. B. Askin. 1985. Esophagitis: A frequent consequence of gastroesophageal reflux in infancy. *The Journal of Pediatrics* 107:881-84.

3. Danus, O., C. Casar, A. Larrain, and C. E. Pope. 1976. Esophageal reflux: An unrecognized cause of recurrent obstructive bronchitis in children. *The Journal of Pediatrics* 89:220-24.

4. Berquist, W. E., G. S. Rachelefsky, M. Kadden, S. C. Siegel, R. M. Katz, E. W. Fonkalsrud, and M. E. Ament. 1981. Gastroesophageal reflux-associated recurrent pneumonia and chronic asthma in children. *Pediatrics* 68:29-35.

5. Herbst, J. J., 1985. Gastroesophageal reflux in infants. *Journal of Pediatric Gastroenterology and Nutrition* 4:163-64.

6. Carre, I. J. 1959. The natural history of the partial thoracic stomach ("hiatal hernia") in children. *Archives of Diseases in Childhood* 34:344-48.

7. Shepard, R. W., J. Wren, S. Evans, M. Lander, and T. H. Ong. 1987. Gastroesophageal reflux in children: Clinical profile, course and outcome with active therapy in 126 cases. *Clinical Pediatrics* 26:55-60.

8. Basitreri, W. F., and M. K. Farrell. 1983. Gastroesophageal reflux in infants. *The New England Journal of Medicine* 309:790-92.

9. Christie, D. L. 1984. Pulmonary complications of esophageal disease. *Symposium of the Pediatric Airway-Pediatric Clinic of North America* 31:835-49.

10. Orenstein, S. R., and D. M. Orenstein. 1988. Gastroesophageal reflux and respiratory disease in children. *The Journal of Pediatrics* 112:847-58.

11. Malfroot, A., Y. Vandenplas, M. Verlinden, A. Peipsz, and I. Dab. 1987. Gastroesophageal reflux and unexplained chronic respiratory disease in infants and children. *Pediatric Pulmonology* 3:208-13.

12. Mathew, O. P., and F. B. Sant'Ambrogio. 1988. Laryngeal reflexes. In *Respiratory function of the upper airway,* edited by O. P. Mathew and G. Sant'Ambrogio, 259-302. New York: Marcel Dekker, Inc.

13. Herbst, J. J. 1981. Gastroesophageal reflux. *The Journal of Pediatrics* 98:859-70.

14. Hrabovsky, E. E., and M. D. Mullett. 1986. Gastroesophageal reflux and the premature infant. *Journal of Pediatric Surgery* 21:583-87.

15. Sondheimer, J. M. 1988. Gastroesophageal reflux: Update on pathogenesis and diagnosis. *Pediatric Clinics of North America* 35:103-16.

16. Diamant, N. E. 1985. Development of esophageal function. *American Review of Respiratory Disease* 131:S29-S32.

17. Glass, R. P., and L. S. Wolf. 1986. *Clinical management of gastroesophageal reflux: A guide for parents.* Seattle, WA: Children's Hospital and Medical Center.

18. Blumenthal, I., and G. T. Lealman. 1982. Effect of posture on gastroesophageal reflux in the newborn. *Archives of Diseases in Childhood* 57:555-56.

19. Meyers, W. F., and J. J. Herbst. 1982. Effectiveness of positioning therapy for gastroesophageal reflux. *Pediatrics* 69:768-72.

20. Orenstein, S. R., and P. F. Whitington. 1983. Positioning for prevention of infant gastroesophageal reflux. *The Journal of Pediatrics* 103:534-37.

21. Byrne, W. J., A. R. Euler, and M. Campbell. 1982. Body position and esophageal sphincter pressure in infants. *American Journal of Diseases in Childhood* 136:523-25.

22. Nordstrom, D. G. 1988. Cloth sling for treatment of infant gastroesophageal reflux. *American Journal of Occupational Therapy* 42:465-68.

23. Orenstein, S. R., P. F. Whitington, and D. M. Orenstein. 1983. The infant seat as treatment for gastroesophageal reflux. *The New England Journal of Medicine* 309:760-63.

24. Orenstein, S. R. 1990. Effects on behavior state of prone versus seated positioning for infants with gastroesophageal reflux. *Pediatrics* 85:765-67.

25. Boyd, C. W. 1982. Postural therapy at home for infants with gastroesophageal reflux. *Pediatric Nursing* 14:395-98.

26. Ulshen, M. H. 1987. Treatment of gastroesophageal reflux: Is nothing sacred? *The Journal of Pediatrics* 110:254-55.

27. Bailey, D. J., J. M. Andres, G. D. Danek, and V. M. Pineior-Carrero. 1987. Lack of efficacy of thickened feeding as treatment for gastroesophageal reflux. *The Journal of Pediatrics* 110:187-89.

28. Orenstein, S. R., H. L. Magill, and P. Brooks. 1987. Thickening of infant feedings for therapy of gastroesophageal reflux. *The Journal of Pediatrics* 110:181-86.

29. Vandenplas, Y., and L. Sacre. 1987. Milk-thickening agents as a treatment for gastroesophageal reflux. *Clinical Pediatrics* 26:66-8.

30. Orenstein, S. R. 1988. Effect of non-nutritive sucking on infant gastroesophageal reflux. *Pediatric Research* 24:38-40.

---

31. Sutphen, J. L., V. L. Dillard, and M. E. Pipan. 1986. Antacid and formula effects on gastric acidity in infants with gastroesophageal reflux. *Pediatrics* 78:55-57.

32. Machida, H. M., D. A. Forbes, D. G. Gall, and R. B. Scott. 1988. Metoclopramide in gastroesophageal reflux in infancy. *The Journal of Pediatrics* 112:483-87.

33. Euler, A. R. 1980. Use of bathanechol for the treatment of gastroesophageal reflux. *The Journal of Pediatrics* 96:321-24.

34. Giuffre, R. M., S. Rubin, and I. Mitchell. 1987. Antireflux surgery in infants with bronchopulmonary dysplasia. *American Journal of Disease in Children* 141:648-51.

35. Jolley, S. G., J. J. Herbst, D. G. Johnson, M. E. Matlak, and L. S. Book. 1980. Surgery in children with gastroesophageal reflux and respiratory symptoms. *The Journal of Pediatrics* 96:194-98.

Congenital Heart Disease

1. Park, M. K. 1984. *Pediatric cardiology for practitioners.* Chicago, IL: Year Book Medical Publishers.

2. Hans-Heiner, K., F. Majewski, H. J. Trampisch, S. Rammos, and M. Bourgeois. 1987. Malformation patterns in children with congenital heart disease. *American Journal of Diseases in Childhood* 141:789-95.

3. Lynch, M., and A. Sweatt. 1987. Congenital heart disease: Assessment and case-finding by community health nurses. *Home Healthcare Nurse* 5:32-41.

4. Muller, L. 1988. Congenital heart abnormalities. *Nursing RSA Verpleging* 3:16-21.

5. Jordan, S. C., and O. Scott. 1981. *Heart disease in paediatrics,* 2d ed. London: Butterworths.

6. Lees, M. H., and D. H. King. 1987. Cyanosis in the newborn. *Pediatrics in Review* 9:36-42.

7. Panyard, J. L., and M. K. Kaneta. 1988. Hypoplastic left heart syndrome: Clinical manifestations and treatment. *Neonatal Network* 7:17-25.

8. Westerman, G., J. Norton, and S. Van Devanter. 1984. The hypoplastic left heart syndrome. A treatable condition. *The Journal of Arkansas Medical Society* 80:367-70.

9. Watson, D. C., L. M. Bradley, F. M. Midgley, and L. P. Scott. 1986. Costs and results of cardiac operations in infants less than 4 months old. *The Journal of Thoracic and Cardiovascular Surgery* 91:667-73.

10. Le Blanc et al. 1987. PA banding: Results and current indications in pediatric cardiac surgery. *Annals of Thoracic Surgery* 44:628-32.

11. Stewart, S., C. Alexson, and J. Manning. 1988. Long-term palliation with the classic Blalock-Taussig shunt. *The Journal of Thoracic and Cardiovascular Surgery* 96:117-21.

12. Pacifico, A. D., and M. E. Sand. 1987. Advances in the surgical management of congenital heart disease in infants and children. *Cardiovascular Clinics* 17:177-219.

13. Bove, E. L., J. Stark, M. De Leval, F. J. Macartney, and J. F. N. Taylor. 1983. Congenital heart disease in the neonate: Results of surgical treatment. *Archives of Diseases in Childhood* 58:137-41.

14. Gersony, W. M. 1989. Long-term follow-up of operated congenital heart disease. *Cardiology Clinics* 7:915-23.

15. Nadas, A. S. 1984. Update on congenital heart disease. *Pediatric Clinics of North America* 31:153-64.

16. Barkin, R. M. 1986. Congestive heart failure in children. *The Journal of Emergency Medicine* 4:379-82.

17. Pittman, J. G., and P. Cohen. 1964a. The pathogenesis of cardiac cachexia (concluded). *New England Journal of Medicine* 217:453-60.

18. Vanderhoof, J. A., P. J. Hofschire, M. A. Baluff, J. E. Guest, N. D. Murray, W. W. Pinsky, J. D. Kugler, and D. L. Antonson. 1982. Continuous enteral feedings: An important adjunct to the management of complex congenital heart disease. *American Journal of Disease in Children* 136:825-27.

19. Pittman, J. G., and P. Cohen. 1964b. The pathogenesis of cardiac cachexia. *New England Journal of Medicine* 271:403-08.

20. Macrae, M. M., and M. B. Le Boeuf. 1988. Standardized nursing care plan for the open-heart surgery neonate. *Neonatal Network* 7:49-57.

21. Schwarz, S. M., M. H. Gewitz, C. C. See, S. Berezin, M. S. Glassman, C. M. Medow, B. C. Fish, and L. J. Newman. 1990. Enteral nutrition in infants with congenital heart disease and growth failure. *Pediatrics* 86:368-73.

22. Kramer, H. H., F. Majewski, H. J. Trampisch, S. Rammos, and M. Bourgeois. 1987. Malformation patterns in children with congenital heart disease. *American Journal of Diseases in Childhood* 141:789-95.

23. Davenport, S. L. H. 1988. Multiple congenital anomalies: An approach to management. *Pediatrician* 15:37-44.

24. Kaden, G. G., R. J. McCarter, S. F. Johnson, and C. Ferencz. 1985. Physician-parent communication: Understanding congenital heart disease. *American Journal of Diseases of Childhood* 139:995-99.

25. Ferry, P. C. 1987. Neurologic sequelae of cardiac surgery in children. *American Journal of Diseases in Childhood* 141:309-12.

26. Nadas, A. S., and D. C. Fyler. 1972. *Pediatric cardiology.* Philadelphia: W. B. Saunders Co.

Oral-Facial Anomalies

1. Bosma, J. F., J. Lind, and H. M. Truby. 1966. Distortions of upper respiratory and swallow motions in infants having anomalies of the upper airway. *Acta Poediatric Scandinavic* 163:112-28.

2. Shprintzen, R. J. 1988. Pierre-Robin, micrognathia, and airway obstruction: The dependency of treatment on accurate diagnosis. *International Anesthesiology Clinics* 26:64-71.

3. Fletcher, M. M., S. L. Blum, and C. L. Blanchard. 1969. Pierre-Robin syndrome pathophysiology of obstructive episodes. *The Laryngoscope* 79:547-60.

4. Augarten, A., M. Sagy, J. Yahav, and Z. Barzilay. 1990. Management of upper airway obstruction in the Pierre-Robin syndrome. *British Journal of Oral and Maxillofacial Surgery* 28:105-8.

5. Freed, G., M. A. Pearlman, A. S. Brown, and L. R. Barot. 1988. Polysomnographic indications for surgical intervention in Pierre-Robin sequence: Acute airway management and follow-up studies after repair and takedown of tongue-lip adhesions. *Cleft Palate Journal* 25:151-55.

6. Lewis, M. B., and H. M. Pashayan. 1980. Management of infants with Robin anomaly. *Clinical Pediatrics* 19:519-28.

7. Delorme, R., Y. Larocque, and L. Caouette-Laberge. 1989. Innovative surgical approach for the Pierre-Robin anomalad: Subperiosteal release of the floor of the mouth musculature. *Plastic and Reconstructive Surgery* 83:960-64.

8. Clarren, S. K., B. Anderson, and L. S. Wolf. 1987. Feeding infants with cleft lip, cleft palate, or cleft lip and palate. *Cleft Palate Journal* 24:244-49.

9. Haberman, M. 1988. A mother of invention. *Nursing Times* 84:52-53.

10. Campbell, A. N., and M. J. Tremouth. 1987. New feeder for infants with cleft palate. *Archives of Disease in Childhood* 62:1292.

11. Roberts, J. L., W. R. Reed, O. P. Mathew, and B. T. Thack. 1986. Control of respiratory activity of the genioglossus muscle in micrognathic infants. *Journal of Applied Physiology* 61:1523-33.

12. Roberts, J. L., W. R. Reed, O. P. Mathew, A. A. Menon, and B. T. Thack. 1985. Assessment of pharyngeal airway stability in normal and micrognathic infants. *Journal of Applied Physiology* 58:290-99.

13. Cohen, G., and D. J. Henderson-Smart. 1986. Upper airway stability and apnea during nasal occlusion in newborn infants. *Journal of Applied Physiology* 60:1511-17.

14. Razek, M. K. A. 1980. Prosthetic feeding aids for infants with cleft lip and palate. *The Journal of Prosthetic Dentistry* 44:556-61.

15. Markowitz, J. A., R. G. Gerry, and R. Fleishner. 1979. Immediate obturation of neonatal cleft palates. *The Mount Sinai Journal of Medicine* 46:123-29.

16. Balluff, M. A., and R. D. Udin. 1986. Using a feeding appliance to aid the infant with a cleft palate. *Ear, Nose and Throat Journal* 65:50-55.

17. Goldberg, W. B., F. S. Ferguson, and R. J. Miles. 1988. Successful use of a feeding obturator for an infant with a cleft palate. *Special Care in Dentistry* 8:86-89.

18. Balluff, M. A. 1986. Nutritional needs of an infant or child with cleft lip or palate. *Ear, Nose and Throat Journal* 65:44-49.

19. Moss, A. H. L., K. Jones, and R. W. Pigott. 1990. Submucous cleft palate in the differential diagnosis of feeding difficulties. *Archives of Disease in Childhood* 65:182-84.

20. Grady, E. 1977. Breast-feeding the baby with a cleft of the soft palate. *Clinical Pediatrics* 16:978-81.

21. Jones, W. B. 1988. Weight gain and feeding in the neonate with cleft: A three-center study. *Cleft Palate Journal* 25:379-84.

22. Weatherly-White, R. C. A., D. P. Kuehn, P. Mirrett, J. I Gilman, and C. C. Weatherly-White. 1987. Early repair and breast-feeding for infants with cleft lip. *Plastic and Reconstructive Surgery* 79:879-85.

23. Shah, C. P., and D. Wong. 1980. Management of children with cleft lip and palate. *CMA Journal* 122:19-24.

24. Styer, G. W., and K. Freeh. 1981. Feeding infants with cleft lip and/or palate. *Journal of Obstetric, Gynecologic and Neonatal Nursing* 10:329-32.

25. Dunning, Y. 1986. Feeding babies with cleft lip and palate. *Nursing Times* 82:46-47.

26. Heaf, D. P., P. J. Helms, R. Dinwiddie, and D. J. Matthew. 1982. Nasopharyngeal airways in Pierre-Robin syndrome. *The Journal of Pediatrics* 100:698-703.

27. Jones, J. E., L. Henderson, and D. R. Avery. 1982. Use of a feeding obturator for infants with severe cleft lip and palate. *Special Care Dentist* 2:116-20.

28. Morris, S. E., and M. D. Klein. 1987. *Pre-feeding skills*. Tucson, AZ: Therapy Skill Builders.

Tracheoesophageal Fistula/Esophageal Atresia

1. Janik, J. S., J. D. Burrington, and J. Whitfield. 1986. Congenital anomalies of the lower airway. In *Clinical pediatric otolaryngology*, edited by T. J. Balkany and N. R. Pashley, 369-405. St. Louis, MO: C. V. Mosby.

2. Manning, P. B., J. R. Wesley, D. M. Behrendt, R. A. Morgan, T. Z. Polley, M. M. Kirsh, A. G. Coran, and H. E. Sloan. 1986. Fifty years' experience with esophageal atresia and tracheoesophageal fistula. *Annals of Surgery* 204:446-53.

3. Biller, J. A., J. L. Allen, S. R. Schuster, S. T. Treves, and H. S. Winter. 1987. Long-term evaluation of esophageal and pulmonary function in patients with repaired esophageal atresia and tracheoesophageal fistula. *Digestive Diseases and Sciences* 32:985-90.

4. Laks, H., R. H. Wilkinson, and S. R. Schuster. 1972. Long-term results following correction of esophageal atresia with tracheoesophageal fistula: A clinical and cinefluorographic study. *Journal of Pediatric Surgery* 7:591-97.

5. Couriel, J. M., M. Hibbert, A. Olinsky, and P. D. Phelan. 1982. Long term pulmonary consequences of oesophageal atresia with tracheo-oesophageal fistula. *Acta Poediatric Scandinavic* 71:973-78.

6. Andrassy, R. J., R. S. Patterson, J. Ashley, G. Patrissi, and G. H. Mahour. 1983. Long-term nutritional assessment of patients with esophageal atresia and/or tracheoesophageal fistula. *Journal of Pediatric Surgery* 18: 431-35.

7. Smith, J. J., and J. Beck. 1985. Mechanical feeding difficulties after primary repair of oesophageal atresia. *Acta Poediatric Scandinavic* 74:237-39.

8. Holder, T. M., and K. W. Ashcraft. 1981. Developments in the care of patients with esophageal atresia and tracheoesophageal fistula. *Surgical Clinics of North America* 61:1051-61.

9. Ein, S. H., and J. Friedberg. 1981. Esophageal atresia and tracheoesophageal fistula. *Otolaryngologic Clinics of North America* 4:219-49.

10. Adkins, J. C., and W. B. Kiesewetter. 1983. Congenital malformations of the esophagus. In *Pediatric otolaryngology: Vol. II*, edited by C. D. Bluestone and S. E. Stool, 1053-60. Philadelphia, PA: W. B. Saunders.

11. Illingworth, R. J., and J. Lister. 1964. The critical or sensitive period, with special reference to certain feeding problems in infants and children. *The Journal of Pediatrics* 65:839-48.

7 Tools of the Trade: Nipples, Pacifiers, and Bottles

Nipples, pacifiers, and bottles are some of the tools or equipment used by feeding specialists for infant feeding and swallowing treatment. One needs only to take a trip to the local drugstore, supermarket, or toy store to see the myriad nipples, pacifiers, and other paraphernalia available for babies. Each manufacturer touts the superiority of its product over other similar products, often making unsubstantiated claims. Trends in the shape of pacifiers (orthodontic versus traditional) or types of nipples (latex versus silicon) float through the media and the marketplace with incredible speed. Separating the wheat from the chaff to distinguish the important improvements from the newly hyped becomes an awesome task for both parents and feeding specialists.

Therefore, a framework is needed for making a rational, educated decision about which type of nipple or pacifier to use in treating an infant with feeding problems. This will assist the feeding specialist in making decisions about when and why to switch nipples, and in providing parents with guidance in nipple, pacifier, or bottle selection.

Such a framework should be grounded in an understanding of the mechanics, characteristics, and movement components of sucking. The patterns and characteristics of the individual infant's sucking must be clearly understood. These individual sucking components can then be matched with the qualities and features of various nipples, pacifiers, and bottles or the human breast to arrive at an appropriate selection. Choosing one particular style over another based on the interplay between the characteristics of the baby and the characteristics of the feeding equipment insures that the "tools" being utilized will support the desired feeding goals.

Since the availability of feeding products is constantly changing, with familiar products being discontinued and new products emerging, it is imperative to understand the qualities of a product that will make it successful in a particular situation. Therefore, the reader should focus on the qualities of the nipple or pacifier being discussed, rather than on brand names that may be mentioned in this chapter. Despite the large number of products available, the feeding specialist should attempt to keep abreast of changes in product lines. While the selection of "basic" nipples, pacifiers, and bottles will be discussed in this chapter, highly specialized equipment for babies with congenital malformations, such as cleft lip and palate, are covered in chapter 6.

Components of Sucking

The components and characteristics of the sucking process have been described in detail in chapter 1. Pertinent features of sucking will be reviewed briefly to provide a foundation for the rationale that will be suggested for selecting nipples, pacifiers, and bottles.

Movement Components

The tongue, jaw, lips, cheeks, and palate each have specific functions during the sucking process, and their movements are exquisitely integrated. Imaging and pressure studies have provided a picture of the combined movements of these structures during sucking:[1,2,5,7,18,20]

- the tongue forms a trough or central groove to receive the nipple and channel fluid to the oropharynx

- the lips and tongue close around the nipple to form the anterior seal of the oral cavity, though they may relax between sucks; the tongue approximates the lower alveolar ridge and the inside surface of the lower lip

- the posterior portion of the tongue elevates slightly to form a seal with the soft palate

- laterally the cheeks approximate the tongue and help channel the fluid

- the jaw and tongue then work together, the jaw raising and lowering while there is an anterior-posterior peristaltic or wavelike motion of the tongue

- as the jaw raises, the anterior portion of the tongue is elevated and compresses the nipple against the palate, forcing some liquid through the nipple

- as the jaw lowers, the peristaltic wave moves along the tongue, with the posterior position becoming depressed, effectively enlarging the sealed oral cavity and creating negative pressure suction; this draws fluid from the nipple and propels it toward the pharynx.

There is some controversy over whether the movement components of sucking are the same on the breast and the bottle. Clearly, however, there is a major difference in how the infant "latches on" or initiates sucking. In bottle-feeding, the nipple has a predetermined, elongated shape and is placed on the tongue by the feeder. In breast-feeding, the baby is required to draw the nipple into the mouth and form the human nipple into an elongated shape. Once that nipple shape is achieved, the movement patterns of the tongue, lips, jaw, and cheeks are similar on bottle and breast, though it is unclear whether they are identical.[1,2,18]

Pressure

During sucking the infant moves fluid into the mouth by creating changes in pressure. Two types of pressure are found in infant sucking—positive pressure and negative pressure. Positive pressure is created when the infant compresses the nipple between the anterior portion of the tongue and the palate. Negative pressure, or suction, is created when the oral cavity is sealed and then enlarged by the tongue and jaw movements described above.[2,5,18] During bottle-feeding it appears that negative pressure suction may be the key factor in producing effective and efficient feeding. On the other hand, successful breast-feeding may rely on the interplay of these two types of pressure.[8,11]

Normal infants are extremely efficient in generating a wide range of sucking pressures. Not only do they have some control over the type of pressure that is created (suction versus compression), but the amount of pressure can vary widely.[15] Studies have demonstrated suction pressures from -15 mm Hg to -130 mm Hg. The amount of pressure that is produced varies based on the infant's maturation, state and hunger, the characteristics of the fluid, and the characteristics of the nipple or the ease of obtaining fluid.[6,8,14,22]

Impact of Liquid Flow during Sucking

As discussed in detail in chapter 1, during infant feeding there is an intricate interplay and precise coordination between sucking, swallowing, and breathing. One of the key factors that can impact this relationship is the fluid flow during sucking. In particular, the rate of fluid flow affects the relationship between sucking and swallowing—the rate and timing of swallowing—and thus influences respiratory parameters.

In non-nutritive sucking, where no liquid is flowing other than the infant's own secretions, the swallowing rate is low and the respiratory rate remains at baseline levels. The sucking rate may be rapid as there is limited interruption for swallowing.

During nutritive sucking, where there is a flow of liquid, changes in sucking and swallowing rate and alterations to the respiratory pattern will occur. Swallowing generally occurs after every one to two sucks, and respiration is interrupted during each swallow to insure airway protection. This frequently results in an overall decrease in the respiratory rate and other ventilatory parameters during active sucking bursts. For healthy infants, this momentary decrease in respiratory rate is inconsequential and/or the baby is able to recover quickly during sucking pauses. For smaller, sicker infants, however, these decreases in respiratory rate may not be tolerated well and can lead to progressive oxygen desaturation, fatigue, apnea, or bradycardia.

A higher and faster rate of fluid flow will have a greater impact on these functions than a low rate of flow. For example, as the baby's sucking rate increases, the rate of swallowing will also increase, further altering the respiratory rate. Therefore, factors that influence fluid flow during sucking—including infant characteristics such as rate and strength of sucking, as well as nipple characteristics—must be carefully considered in the treatment of certain infant feeding problems to produce well-coordinated and efficient feeding.

Characteristics of Nipples

Human Breast

Many modifications and design features of artificial nipples are developed to try to emulate or imitate the human breast. Understanding the characteristics of the breast during feeding can help determine how successful manufactured nipples are in achieving this goal. Smith et al.[18] used real-time ultrasound to study in vivo the anatomic characteristics of the human nipple during breast-feeding. Their data indicate that the human nipple is extremely elastic, elongating two times its length and narrowing slightly during feeding. With each tongue compression, the nipple height is reduced to 60% of its resting thickness (see figure 7-1). There is little lateral compression, reinforcing the concept that the cheeks act as a stabilizing force and do not put direct pressure on the nipple. The human nipple is not static during feeding but elongates and retracts at a rapid rate during every sucking cycle.

While it is clear that there are many shapes and sizes for the human nipple, its variability in shape and movement during infant feeding is poorly appreciated. Also, little is known about the specific flow characteristics of milk during breast-feeding, though it appears that milk flow varies considerably during the feeding based on the mother's milk ejection, or let-down reflex, as well as the efficiency with which a particular infant removes the milk.

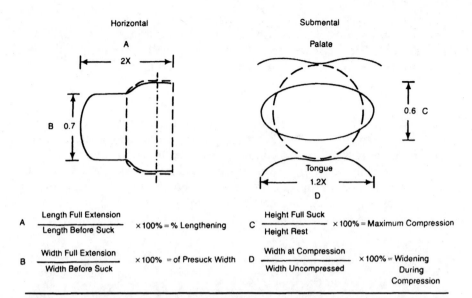

Figure 7-1 Changes in the shape of the human nipple during sucking. Reprinted with permission from: W. L. Smith, A. Erenberg, and A. Nowak. 1988. Imaging evaluation of the human nipple during breast-feeding. *American Journal of Diseases in Childhood* 142:76-78. Copyright 1988, American Medical Association.

Artificial Nipples

While there are many designs for artificial nipples, none precisely mimics the dynamic qualities of the human breast during feeding. There are a number of design variations, however, which relate to feeding treatment. The four primary characteristics that should be considered when selecting a nipple include: shape, size, consistency (compressibility or distensibility), and the size/type of hole.

Nipple shape

In selecting a nipple shape, the feeding specialist should ask, **"Does the shape of the nipple support the oral-motor patterns desired during sucking?"**

While there are many nipple shapes and configurations available, these fall into two basic categories: round cross-section nipples and broad, flat cross-section nipples (see figure 7-2, page 404). Round cross-section nipples may be thought of as traditional nipples. They tend to be straight and gradually taper to a flared base. Most manufacturers have a traditionally shaped nipple in their product line.

Broad, flat cross-section nipples may also be referred to as "orthodontic type" nipples. These nipples generally have bulblike ends that are wider than they are high, and they quickly flare to large, wide bases. The bulblike end may be symmetric or may have a different contour on the tongue and palate sides. This style has been popularized by NUK® brand nipples, but many manufacturers now make similarly shaped nipples.

"Orthodontic" nipples were originally designed to theoretically reflect the shape of the breast nipple during feeding. This claim, however, should be reexamined in light of the recent imaging studies. In the work of Smith et al.[17,18] it seems that the breast typically has a round cross-section, except during compression. It also can be questioned whether the end actually takes on a bulblike configuration during sucking. In any case, at best the broad cross-section nipples may reflect the breast shape during only one small phase of sucking. They certainly do not show the elastic qualities and range of shape that the human nipple takes on during breast-feeding.

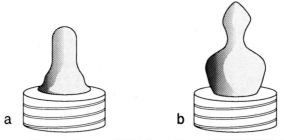

Figure 7-2 Nipples fall into two basic categories: round cross-section nipples (a) and broad, flat cross-section nipples (b).

Nipple size
In selecting a nipple size, the feeding specialist should ask, **"Does the length of the nipple provide adequate contact between the nipple and tongue for effective tongue movements?"**

The most salient characteristic to consider in relation to nipple size is the length of the nipple. Just as in nipple shape, there is a wide range of nipple lengths (see figure 7-3). In determining the size of the nipple, it is important to consider how much of the nipple will actually be in the infant's mouth. As this is limited by the base of the nipple, the type of base and distance from tip to base should be evaluated for each nipple.

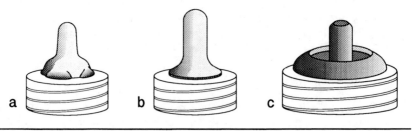

Figure 7-3 Nipple length can vary substantially.

TOOLS OF THE TRADE

The amount of the nipple that is in the mouth will be more variable for nipples with tapered bases. It will reflect the degree of tapering of the base, the strength of the infant's suck, the degree of lip closure around the nipple, and the control the feeder is providing to manage the nipple position. The length of the standard Playtex® nipple (see figure 7-3c) is more dynamic. While the distance between the tip and base of the nipple appears short, as the baby sucks on this nipple it elongates and retracts, much as Smith et al.[18] described for the human breast, although in Smith's study it never became as long as the human nipple.

Consistency

In selecting nipple consistency, the feeding specialist should consider two questions, **"Does the firmness of the nipple provide the appropriate degree of proprioceptive input to the tongue for effective movement?"** and **"Does the consistency match the strength of the infant's suck to support an appropriate flow rate?"**

This characteristic of artificial nipples reflects the firmness, compressibility, or distensibility of the nipple. It describes how much pressure is required to change the shape of the nipple. The type and thickness of material used in manufacturing the nipple, as well as the age of the nipple, can impact the consistency of the nipple. In general, nipples designed for premature infants are softer than those designed for term infants. When other factors are held constant, a soft nipple will have a higher flow rate than a firm nipple. The consistency of the nipple can be assessed only by actually squeezing or pulling the nipple and feeling the amount of resistance that is encountered.

Hole type and size:

In selecting the hole type and size, the feeding specialist should ask, **"Does the hole provide an appropriate flow rate?"**

There are two types of openings found in artificial nipples: holes and crosscuts. Holes are very small openings in the nipple, and always have some measurable diameter. Hole size is felt to be one of the major determinants of flow rate during sucking. While different styles of nipples have different hole sizes (that vary within a small range), there is also wide variability and poor consistency of hole size within each brand of nipple.[13] Relative hole size can be estimated by watching the drip rate from a bottle, though factors such as volume of liquid, tightness of nipple seal, pressure gradients in the bottle, and viscosity of liquid can also influence the drip rate.

A crosscut is a small "X" cut in the tip of the nipple. The tip of the nipple remains essentially closed until compressive pressure is applied to the nipple. Thus the drip rate from a crosscut nipple may be quite low. When the nipple is compressed, however, the crosscut opens and allows fluid to flow. This feature allows quite a large opening for thick or pulpy fluids, but the flow is regulated and occurs only during the portion of each suck when the nipple is compressed.

Hole placement also varies. Most nipples have a single hole located on the tip. Some nipples (such as the Gerber® standard nipple) are designed with several smaller holes at the tip. Ross® standard and premature nipples used in hospitals have both a hole and a small crosscut. While a study by Mathew showed no milk flow through the crosscut[12], this may reflect the lack of compressive pressure during the measurement. Finally, in NUK® nipples the hole is placed so that milk flows out of the top surface of the tip of the nipple. The relative advantages or disadvantages of various placements of nipple holes are not clear.

Considerations in the Selection of Nipples to Support Feeding Treatment

Health professionals are commonly asked, "What is the best nipple for my baby?" The "best" nipple for any baby is one in which the characteristics of the nipple match the qualities of the baby's feeding skills. Most babies are quite flexible in their sucking abilities, so they could feed well with many of the nipples that are available, as well as the human breast.

When feeding problems are identified, however, an initial response is often to change the baby's nipple. While appropriate nipple selection can be a key to achieving the feeding goals for babies with some types of feeding problems, in many cases it is not necessary. The decision to change nipples or other feeding equipment should be carefully considered. The feeding specialist must assess the feeding skills and needs of the infant, consider the attributes of various nipples, then make a selection that reflects an understanding of the interaction between these two parameters. While correct selection of a nipple can enhance the feeding treatment, a mismatch between the infant's abilities and the nipple properties can contribute to dysfunctional feeding. Frequent changes in nipples and feeding equipment can be confusing to the infant and parent, and may obscure the true feeding issues and problems.

There are two basic aspects of feeding function that can be impacted by nipple selection: flow of liquid and sucking mechanics. Each of these will be considered in detail.

Flow of Liquid

As discussed above, the flow of liquid can play an important role in altering the coordination between sucking, swallowing, and breathing. It is also related to the efficiency of feeding. The flow rate depends on the strength of the infant's suck (the amount and type of pressure that is generated), the consistency and hole size of the nipple, and the viscosity of fluid being sucked.

Adjustments in the rate of flow are often used therapeutically to achieve feeding goals. In some situations increased flow may be desirable, though in other cases feeding may be improved by reducing the flow. Caution must be exercised when deciding to increase the flow of liquid. A very rapid flow may contribute to apnea or bradycardia during feeding, particularly in premature and very young infants.[12,13] As the milk flow increases, the number of swallows increases, thereby shortening the time available for breathing. Furthermore, obtaining a very large bolus can lead to coughing and choking, or could potentially stretch mechanoreceptors and trigger a vagally mediated apnea or bradycardia.

Table 7-1 lists some situations where it may be desirable to modify flow during sucking. These situations are discussed in more detail in chapter 5.

Table 7-1

Infants Who May Require Increased Flow of Liquid
- the slow, poky feeder
- the infant with poor endurance
- an infant with a weak suck

Infants Who May Require Slower Flow of Liquid
- the infant with poor coordination of sucking, swallowing, and breathing
- the very fast, eager feeder
- an infant with a particularly strong suck

Nipple selection
Nipple characteristics that can influence fluid flow are the consistency of the nipple and the size of the nipple hole, with hole size playing the larger role.[13] Variations in hole size and consistency among brands of nipples lead to different flow characteristics for different nipples. In two studies, Mathew compared the milk-flow rates of a variety of term and preterm nipple units.[12,13] The number of simulated sucks needed to empty a 120 cc bottle were counted. The fewer simulated sucks needed, the faster the milk flowed. In one study measurements were made at two "sucking pressures" (-60 and -120 cm H_2O), while in the other study flow was carefully related to hole size and nipple thickness.

The nipple units evaluated were: standard term nipples (Ross® Twist-On®, Mead-Johnson® Enfamil® single-hole, Wyeth® SMA® single-hole); preterm standard nipples (same distributors as the term nipples) and orthodontic type nipples (Mead Johnson® Enfamil® Natural nipple®, Wyeth® SMA®, NUK® nipple distributed by Reliance through Ross®).

In general, the standard preterm nipples required fewer simulated sucks than the term standard nipples, but more simulated sucks than the orthodontic type. Therefore, in terms of milk flow, standard term nipples tended to have the slowest flow, preterm nipples were in the middle, and orthodontic type nipples tended to have the fastest flow. There was some variability within these groupings, however; the flow rate of various nipples evaluated in these studies is summarized in table 7-2. While the very small premature nipple (see figure 7-3a, page 404) was not tested, clinically it also appears to have a fast flow rate.

Table 7-2 Comparison of Nipples based on Flow Rate

High Flow	SMA® orthodontic
	Enfamil® premature
	NUK®
Medium Flow	SMA® standard
	Ross® premature
	Enfamil® Natural nipple®
	SMA® premature
Low Flow	Enfamil® standard
	Ross® standard

adapted from Mathew 1988, 1990

One important way, therefore, to influence the flow of liquid during infant sucking is by selecting a nipple with the flow characteristics that are desired. Although the results of Mathew's studies provide a helpful basis for judging the flow characteristics of nipples, these results may not be fully applicable in the clinical setting. Suction was the only pressure component that was evaluated in these studies, so the flow rate may not reflect the actual flow rate in situations where a compression force is also generated. Feeding specialists need to continue to systematically experiment with the numerous nipples available to identify the flow characteristics that may be appropriate for specific babies.

Other options for increasing flow

For a bottle-fed baby, the first step in increasing fluid flow is to select an appropriate manufactured nipple. At times, however, it may be necessary to enlarge an existing nipple hole to increase the fluid flow. This strategy would also be appropriate if the infant's food needed to be thickened and did not flow through a standard size hole, if the infant resisted switching to a high-flow nipple, or if other nipple qualities desired for oral treatment were not found in a high-flow nipple. Enlargement of nipple holes should be done with caution, since small changes in the hole size can lead to substantial increases in flow and the potential associated problems described above.

Two methods of enlarging the hole will produce small increments of change and are fairly easily controlled. The first is boiling the nipple with a toothpick in the hole, which is recommended by many manufacturers. The second method is to pierce the existing hole with a very hot needle.

Another method for enlarging nipple holes is to use a scalpel or thin craft knife to make a slit in the nipple approximately one to three millimeters long. A single slit is generally preferable to a crosscut. The size of the slit is more easily controlled; crosscuts often become too large. With a single slit in the nipple the feeder has some ability to vary the flow by the position of the slit in the baby's mouth. If the nipple is placed in the mouth with the slit perpendicular to the lips, as the baby presses on the nipple with the tongue, the slit will open maximally. If the nipple is inserted with the slit horizontal to the lips, the slit will remain more closed, slowing the flow. Twisting the bottle in the baby's mouth will change the position of the slit and therefore change the flow rate. Monitoring the flow of bubbles while a baby is feeding is important in order to determine the effects of changes made in the nipple hole size. It is best to start with a small enlargement, observe the flow of liquid, then increase the size of the hole only if necessary.

The flow rate can also be affected by the viscosity of the fluid being consumed. When all other variables are held constant, the thinner the liquid, the higher the flow rate. While this could potentially be a treatment approach, generally the infant's nutrient is selected based on nutritional considerations, and "thinner" substitutes may not be available. More often the effect of a thinner liquid on flow rate occurs unintentionally, sometimes magnifying feeding problems. For example, an infant who has subtle difficulties in coordinating sucking, swallowing, and breathing may be feeding reasonably well with formula. However, when glucose water, breast milk, or apple juice (each is slightly thinner than formula) is introduced, significant coughing and choking may be noted as the infant struggles to deal with the increased flow rate.

Other options for decreasing flow rate

A method for reducing the rate of flow, in addition to selecting a nipple with a slower rate of flow, is to alter the viscosity of the liquid. The thicker the liquid, the slower the flow will be. Thickening agents include baby cereals, fruit purees, and commercial thickeners and should be selected with nutritional guidance. Small increases in the viscosity of the fluid, such as adding one tablespoon of rice cereal to two ounces of formula, can have a noticeable effect. The nipple hole may need to be enlarged slightly to accommodate thicker liquid, but this should be done very carefully. Just a slight over-enlargement could actually increase the fluid flow rather than decrease it.

To produce very low rates of fluid flow, devices other than the bottle may be needed. These include the pacifier trainer (described on page 224) and a standard nipple attached directly to a 20-cc syringe. In both of these cases, the syringe creates a closed system where the feeding specialist is able to carefully regulate fluid flow and give the baby single boluses at a time if needed. The slowest rate of flow is obtained by giving droplets of fluid with a soft eyedropper while the infant is sucking on a pacifier.

Sucking Mechanics

To some extent the characteristics of a particular nipple can influence an infant's sucking mechanics. The nipple characteristics most likely to affect oral movements during sucking include nipple shape, size, and consistency.

Using ultrasound, Smith observed the mechanics of sucking on the breast and on Playtex®, Evenflo®, NUK®, and Ross® nipples in 51 full-term babies between 6 to 12 weeks old.[16] Lip, tongue, and jaw movements, reflected in the deformation of the nipple, were similar on the breast and the Playtex®, Evenflo®, and Ross® nipples. While the manufactured nipples did not elongate as much as the human nipple, the Playtex® nipple showed the most elongation. Of those three nipples, the mechanics of sucking on the Playtex® nipple were the most similar to the human breast nipple, though the Playtex® nipple was felt to be too short.

The mechanics of sucking on the NUK® nipple were considerably different than on the other bottle nipples and were also different than on the human nipple. With the NUK® nipple, Smith reports that the tongue used a "squash-pump" action, compressing the bulbous tip of the nipple, which pushed the milk into the infant's mouth. The tongue would relax, the tip of the nipple would refill, and the process would be repeated.

This study suggests that the nipple shape can have a distinct impact on the mechanics of sucking. While the influence of nipple size and consistency

---

on sucking have not been studied in detail, biomechanical and neurosensory principles suggest some indications for the selection of nipples based on these characteristics.

Tongue position and movement: Considering the work of Smith[16], and our clinical experience, it appears that the characteristics of the nipple can impact tongue and lip position and movement during sucking. One of the most frequent reasons, therefore, to choose a particular nipple is that it encourages appropriate tongue movement and position for effective sucking. The qualities of appropriate tongue position include a tongue that sits on the floor of the mouth with tip touching the lower alveolar ridge, has a thin, broad configuration, and has the ability to form a central groove. Chapters 3 and 5 provide further information on normal and abnormal tongue position and movement, as well as treatment strategies.

Tight, bunched, and/or retracted tongues are quite commonly seen in infants with feeding problems. Increased tone may pull the tongue together or back in the mouth, or these patterns may be seen in compensation for low oral tone as the infant works to stabilize the tongue. A tongue with this configuration may not form a central groove well. To minimize bunching and tongue retraction, and to encourage better central grooving, a nipple with a round cross section and firm consistency should be selected. A firm nipple that is narrow provides greater proprioceptive input to the medial portion of the tongue, and can be used to apply additional downward pressure on the tongue, both of which facilitate forward movement and central grooving of the tongue. Broad, flat nipples, such as a standard NUK® nipple, appear to facilitate the "squash-fill" pattern described above, and may interfere with attempts to improve central grooving of the tongue.

If the tongue is retracted, a longer nipple should be selected to allow the greatest contact between the tongue and nipple. We hypothesize that greater anterior-posterior contact between the tongue and nipple facilitates more appropriate tongue movements on the nipple. The standard Playtex® nipple, though it is round, should be used with caution for an infant with a retracted tongue. While this nipple elongates under normal circumstances, its short resting position may not allow adequate tongue contact for appropriate tongue movement and elongation of the nipple. Using the "toddler" size of this nipple, even for small babies, may improve the nipple's length characteristics, if other features of this nipple are beneficial for the baby.

Tongues that are flat and hypotonic may also benefit from a round, firm nipple. If the tongue lacks inherent shape due to decreased tone, the nipple can suggest the appropriate shape and encourage central grooving.

Quick, repeated downward pressure can be supplied through the nipple or pacifier to build tongue tone as needed.

Tongue protrusion and thrusting are problems that can also interfere with effective oral feeding. A broad, flat nipple may provide backward and downward pressure to keep the tongue in the mouth. Considering Smith's findings, however, flat, broad nipples may actually encourage the use of a pushing or protrusion pattern during sucking. A protruding or thrusting tongue often lacks an appropriate central groove and/or anterior-posterior peristaltic movement. Therefore, a firm, round cross-section nipple may be most effective in improving this type of sucking pattern.

Lip position and movement: The shape of the nipple, in particular the base, can impact lip control. A narrow base will encourage more active lip seal. Infants with poor lip control may suck more effectively from a nipple with a wide, bulb-type end. The wide base might form a functional seal with the lips, but it would be a passive seal and therefore might not contribute to improvement in lip control. A wide bulb-type base might be desired, however, if the baby needed to develop better lip flanging for breast-feeding.

Mouth size: The size of the nipple relative to the size of the infant's mouth can impact sucking mechanics. The amount of contact between oral surfaces and the nipple can affect tongue movements and may influence the stability of the nipple in the mouth. While most standard commercial nipples will fit the mouth of any full-term infant, the question of nipple size often arises in feeding small premature infants.

A very short nipple is available in hospitals from several manufacturers for small premature infants (see figure 7-3a, page 404). The vast majority of premature infants who are sufficiently mature to feed orally, however, have mouths that are big enough to accommodate the standard size nipple. It is the rare premature baby who is ready to feed but cannot use a typical length nipple, though it may be of "premature" consistency. In many cases the short, small premature nipples do not allow adequate contact between the tongue and nipple for effective sucking. In addition, since the premature baby has relatively less subcutaneous fat and contact between oral structures (that is, decreased positional stability), a larger, standard size nipple may actually help to fill the oral cavity and provide a point of internal stability.

The final consideration in the relationship between mouth size and nipple size is the sensitivity of the gag response. If the infant demonstrates a hypersensitive gag reflex that is triggered by the nipple on the posterior portion of the tongue, the nipple may be too long. A shorter nipple may be selected, or a standard-length nipple may be used and not placed fully in the infant's mouth. In either case, the need to decrease the gag response must be balanced with the infant's need for adequate tongue-nipple contact for effective sucking. Additional treatments to integrate the gag response should also be included in the feeding program.

Strength of sucking: To promote efficient sucking, the consistency or firmness of the nipple should match the strength of the infant's suck. The infant with a weak suck will usually perform better with a soft nipple. If the nipple is too firm, minimal fluid may be obtained and each suck is less efficient. This effect can be mediated to some degree when the nipple hole is larger. The infant with a strong suck, on the other hand, should have a nipple with a firm consistency. If a nipple with a soft consistency is used with this infant, the nipple will frequently "collapse," stopping fluid flow.

Pacifiers

Pacifiers are typically used to meet an infant's innate desire to suck. Sucking, whether on a nipple, pacifier, or the infant's own hand is one of the infant's first methods of self-quieting and self-regulation. For infants who are non-orally fed, sucking takes on added importance in maintaining appropriate oral-motor patterns and tactile responses, which will help in the return to oral feeding. Pacifiers, like nipples, vary considerably in terms of shape, size, and consistency (see figure 7-4). Therefore, for the infant with feeding difficulties, some thought should go into the selection of a pacifier if one is used.

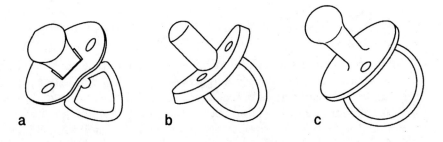

Figure 7-4 Pacifiers are available in many designs.

Orthodontic versus Conventional Pacifiers

Characteristics often emphasized by manufacturers are the "orthodontic" qualities of the pacifier (see figure 7-4a, page 413). Many manufacturers claim that orthodontic pacifiers have a positive influence in shaping the mouth or teeth. At least one study has evaluated the validity of this claim. Bishara et al. measured the various maxillary and mandibular dental arch parameters in 122 infants over an 18-month period.[4] The infants were either breast- or bottle-fed and used either a conventional or functional ("orthodontic") nipple and/or pacifier. Six groups of infants were compared: (1) breast-fed, no pacifier; (2) bottle-fed, conventional nipple, no pacifier; (3) breast-fed, functional pacifier; (4) functional nipple and pacifier; (5) conventional nipple and pacifier; and (6) a residual group who switched between feeding methods and pacifier groups. At 18 months of age, the researchers found no significant differences in absolute or percentage changes of dental arch parameters between the pacifier and no-pacifier groups, between the two types of pacifiers, or between the method of feeding and pacifier used. Thus this study suggests that feeding specialists can select a pacifier based on the qualities of shape, size, and consistency, without concern for the "orthodontic" qualities.

Pacifier Selection

In general, guidelines for selecting pacifiers are the same as those used in selecting a nipple to influence sucking mechanics. In other words, if it appears that an infant will benefit from a straight, firm, round cross-section nipple to facilitate central grooving and tongue movement, a pacifier with similar qualities should be selected (see figure 7-4b, page 413). Feeding specialists should not assume that the same brand of pacifier and nipple always have the same qualities. While a Playtex® nipple and pacifier look similar, the pacifier is quite a bit longer than the resting nipple. Similarly, the NUK® nipple and pacifier have different shapes. If a nipple and pacifier of the same brand do not both have the desired qualities, varying brands of nipple and pacifier can be quite successful.

There are other factors that should also be considered in pacifier selection. Pacifiers with "balls" at the tip (see figure 7-4c, page 413) should be avoided for infants with many types of feeding problems. While the large tip may help keep the pacifier from falling out of the infant's mouth, the infant can maintain the pacifier in the mouth with weak lick-suck motions using very little functional sucking activity. Pacifiers with a firm, curved shield around the baby's lips need not be selected for their "orthodontic" qualities, but this type of pacifier may help to encourage lip seal by the strong proprioceptive input of continuous pressure to the lips.

Pacifier Use with Non-orally Fed Infants

In infants who are non-orally fed, the selection and use of a pacifier are particularly important. The benefits of non-nutritive sucking (NNS) on a pacifier for premature infants who are receiving gavage feeding are well documented.[3,9] These include more rapid transition to oral feeding, greater weight gain, and shorter hospitalizations. If the infant will have a long period where oral feeding is not possible, use of a pacifier becomes crucial. Non-nutritive sucking is the link that will facilitate potential return to oral feeding. Clinical experience indicates that while not all non-orally fed infants who continue NNS will return quickly to nutritive sucking and oral feeding when medically advisable, it is rare for the infant who does not have NNS to return to oral feeding by sucking.

For the infant who is non-orally fed, the oral-motor and sucking characteristics that are desired should again be considered in selecting the pacifier. The pacifier should resemble a nipple from which liquid can be obtained. Many non-orally fed infants become "hooked" on one particular type of pacifier. They consider this to be the only safe item to suck on and refuse to suck on a standard nipple. As most pacifiers are substantially different from their nipple counterparts, a discriminating, hypersensitive baby may reject the nipple when bottle-feeding is introduced. Another approach is to encourage the infant to suck on a variety of pacifiers during the period of non-oral feeding. One style of pacifier might be used for recreational NNS, with another style chosen for sucking done in conjunction with the non-oral feeding. The infant then maintains greater flexibility and is less likely to refuse a bottle nipple simply because it feels different.

Home-made pacifiers: In attempting to find pacifiers with qualities that are the same as bottle nipples, it is tempting to fabricate pacifiers by plugging a manufactured nipple. This is an unsafe practice, as there have been several infant deaths related to aspiration of baby-bottle nipples that were used as pacifiers.[10] Manufacturers are beginning to see this need, however; the Soother™ distributed by Ross® now has a shape that is identical to the Ross® bottle nipples.

Bottles

The variety of bottles available for babies is also increasing. New bottles are designed to facilitate self-feeding, to prevent air swallowing and colic, and for decorative reasons. When selecting a bottle, the feeding specialist should consider two questions: **Does the bottle allow appropriate infant head position?** and **Is the bottle comfortable in the feeder's hand so that oral facilitation techniques are possible?**

Influence of Bottle on Head Position

The infant's head position during feeding is an important consideration, as discussed in detail in chapters 3 and 5. A neutral or slightly forward-flexed position is desired for many babies, especially those with swallowing dysfunction or excessive extensor tone. During feeding, the liquid must cover the outlet of the nipple or the baby will suck in air and milk, making air swallowing likely. For some feeders it may be difficult to achieve a flexed head position and keep the nipple filled with fluid when using a standard eight-ounce bottle. Better results may be achieved using a short bottle such as a two-ounce Volu-feed® (distributed by Ross®), which is available in hospital nurseries (see figure 7-5b). Angled-neck bottles are also available. They are designed to facilitate an upright, chin-tucked position during feeding. The Corecto® feeding bottle (Corecto® Products Company, PO Box 1014, Atlanta, GA 30301) and the Degree® bottle (Degree® Baby Products, Inc., West Hills, CA 91307) are examples of bottles with angled necks (see figure 7-6).

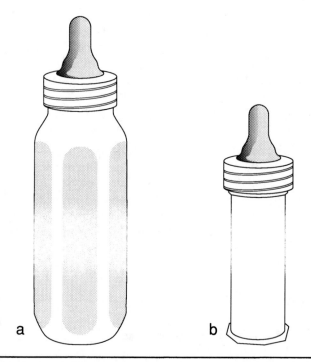

a   b

Figure 7-5 Note the difference in size between a standard eight-ounce bottle (a) and a two-ounce Volu-feed® (b).

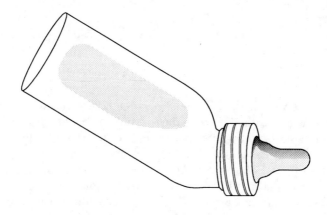

Figure 7-6 An angled-neck bottle.

Ease of Providing Oral Facilitation

Ease of hand and finger positioning for oral facilitation is another important consideration in bottle selection. The diameter of the neck of the bottle,
length, and weight of the bottle when full will affect how easily a feeder
can use the fingers for oral control. Again the small Volu-feed® is an
excellent treatment tool (see figure 7-5b). This bottle is small enough to fit in
the feeder's thenar web space, freeing the other fingers to provide input such
as simultaneous facilitation to the jaw and cheeks. The less complex oral
facilitation techniques, such as providing simple jaw support, can generally
be accomplished while holding a standard 4- or 8-ounce bottle.

Monitoring Flow

The ability to monitor the flow of the liquid is another factor to consider
when selecting bottles for treatment. Observing the rate of flow (expressed
as the return of bubbles into the bottle) gives the feeder a sense of the pace
and efficiency of the feeding. It also provides the feeding specialist with
valuable feedback about the baby's response to intervention techniques.
Clear or slightly translucent bottles are best for observing flow. Bottles with
bags inside to hold the liquid make it impossible to monitor small increments of liquid flow. In addition, with this type of bottle, it is very difficult
to measure intake accurately without making pre- and post-feeding measurements in a separate container.

Air Swallowing

A final consideration in selecting a bottle is the issue of air swallowing. Several manufacturers state that certain design features of their bottles minimize air swallowing. To evaluate these claims one must consider what is known about how air swallowing occurs.

In a standard bottle, if the nipple is completely covered with liquid, the bubbles observed inside the bottle during sucking occur as air rushes into the bottle to equalize the low pressure created when liquid flows out into the mouth. The air bubbles in the bottle are not reflective of air going into the infant's stomach, but are simply a response to changing pressures within the bottle. Although bubbles in the bottle do not reflect air swallowing, all babies do swallow air to varying degrees while feeding, on both the bottle and breast. There are several factors that seem to be related to the amount of air that is swallowed. These include bolus size, head/neck position, and timing of swallowing and breathing.

On radiologic evaluation, Ardran et al. noted that the harder it was for the baby to obtain the liquid, the more air was swallowed.[2] During ultrasonographic examination of sucking on the breast and bottle, Smith et al. observed air leaking into the oral cavity when the lip seal was poor.[18] Potentially, air that has entered the mouth from any route (lips, pharynx, an unsealed cleft in the palate), and is present as the bolus is moved into the pharynx, can be swallowed. Neck extension during feeding may adversely affect a baby's ability to maintain adequate lip seal and thereby increase the likelihood of air swallowing.

The efficiency with which babies remove air from their pharynxes prior to the swallow may also be an important factor in how much air a particular baby swallows, and is related to the baby's ability to coordinate swallowing with breathing. Several researchers have documented the presence of a "swallow-breath" that occurs at the onset of swallowing in infants.[19,21] When swallowing interrupted inspiration, there was a brief continuation of inspiratory effort against a closed airway. It has been hypothesized that the function of this "swallow-breath" is to clear the pharynx of air prior to the swallowing so that air swallowing does not occur. As the timing of the events of the "swallow-breath" are exceedingly precise, slight deviations in the timing between swallowing and breathing could increase the likelihood of air swallowing. For some infants, air swallowing is a maturational problem that improves with increasing age.

Therefore, when choosing treatment materials and techniques for an infant who swallows excessive amounts of air, the feeding specialist must consider the infant's head position, lip control, and the rate of liquid flow, as well as the coordination of swallowing and breathing.

References

1. Ardran, G. M., F. H. Kemp, and J. Lind. 1958a. A cineradiographic study of breast-feeding. *British Journal of Radiology* 31:156-62.

2. _____. 1958b. A cineradiographic study of bottle-feeding. *British Journal of Radiology* 31:11-22.

3. Bernbaum, J. C., G. R. Pereira, J. B. Watkins, and G. J. Peckham. 1983. Non-nutritive sucking during gavage feeding enhances growth and maturation in premature infants. *Pediatrics* 71:41-45.

4. Bishara, S. E., A. J. Nowak, F. J. Kohout, D. A. Heckert, and M. M. Hogan. 1987. Influence of feeding and non-nutritive sucking methods on the development of the dental arches: Longitudinal study of the first 18 months of life. *Pediatric Dentistry* 9:13-21.

5. Colley, J. R. T., and B. Creamer. 1958. Sucking and swallowing in infants. *British Medical Journal* 2:422-23.

6. Crook, C. K., and L. P. Lipsitt. 1976. Neonatal nutritive sucking: Effects of taste stimulation upon sucking rhythm and heart rate. *Child Development* 47:518-22.

7. Dreier, T., and P. H. Wolff. 1972. Sucking, state, and perinatal distress in newborns. *Biology of the Neonate* 21:16-24.

8. Ellison, S. L., D. Vidyasagar, and G. C. Anderson. 1979. Sucking in the newborn infant during the first hour of life. *Journal of Nurse-Midwifery* 24:18-25.

9. Field, T., E. Ignatoff, S. Stringer, J. Brennan, R. Greenberg, S. Widmayer, and G. C. Anderson. 1982. Non-nutritive sucking during tube feedings: Effects on preterm infants in an intensive care unit. *Pediatrics* 70:381-84.

10. Hubbell, K. 1986. Makeshift pacifiers. *MCN* 11:240.

11. Lawrence, R. A. 1989. *Breast-feeding: A guide for the medical profession.* St. Louis, MO: C. V. Mosby Company.

12. Mathew, O. P. 1988. Nipple units for newborn infants: A functional comparison. *Pediatrics* 81:688-91.

13. _____. 1990 Determinants of milk flow through nipple units: Role of hole size and nipple thickness. *American Journal of Diseases in Childhood* 144:222-24.

14. Pollitt, E., B. Consolazio, and F. Goodkin. 1981. Changes in nutritive sucking during a feed in two-day and thirty-day-old infants. *Early Human Development* 5:201-10.

15. Sameroff, A. J. 1968. The components of sucking in the human newborn. *Journal of Experimental Child Psychology* 6:607-23.

16. Smith, W. L. 1989. Breast-feeding: Beyond the basics. Presentation at Swedish Hospital and Medical Center. Seattle, WA.

17. Smith, W. L., A. Erenberg, and A. Nowak. 1988. Imaging evaluation of the human nipple during breast-feeding. *American Journal of Diseases in Childhood* 142:76-78.

18. Smith, W. L., A. Erenberg, A. Nowak, and E. A. Franken. 1985. Physiology of sucking in the normal term infant using real-time ultrasound. *Radiology* 156:379-81.

19. Thach, B. T., and A. Menon. 1985. Pulmonary protective mechanisms in human infants. *American Review of Respiratory Diseases* 131:S55-S58.

20. Weber, F., M. W. Woolridge, and H. D. Barum. 1986. An ultrasonographic study of the organization of sucking and swallowing by newborn infants. *Developmental Medicine and Child Neurology* 28:19-24.

21. Wilson, S. L., B. T. Thach, R. T. Brouillette, and Y. K. Abuosba. 1981. Coordination of breathing and swallowing in human infants. *Journal of Applied Physiology: Respiratory Environmental and Exercise Physiology* 50:851-58.

22. Wolff, P. H. 1972. The interaction of state and non-nutritive sucking. In *Oral sensation and perception: The mouth of the infant,* edited by J. F. Bosma, pp. 293-312. Springfield, IL: Charles C. Thomas.

8 *Breast-Feeding*

As stated by the World Health Organization, "Breast-feeding is an integral part of the reproductive process, the natural and ideal way of feeding the infant, and a unique biological and emotional basis for child development."[1] Breast milk is known to be the "ideal" food for human infants, specifically designed to meet their unique and changing nutritional needs. It is most easily digestible, protects against infection, and minimizes allergic responses. In addition, the process of breast-feeding promotes maternal-infant bonding, which is important for the provision of ongoing care to the infant.

Unfortunately, the process of breast-feeding may be disrupted by illness or hospitalization of the infant or by lack of success in an otherwise healthy infant. As these feeding problems may come to the attention of feeding specialists working with infants, it is crucial that they clearly understand the breast-feeding process. This will allow feeding specialists to support breast-feeding and aid in the diagnosis and remediation of breast-feeding problems.

Physiology of Breast-Feeding

For breast-feeding to be effective there must be controlled delivery of milk to the infant, in the correct amount and at appropriate intervals. The establishment and maintenance of such a system is determined by several factors. First, the anatomical structure of the human mammary tissue and development of alveoli, ducts, and nipple must be adequate. This provides a storage system, exit channels, and a prehensile appendage. Second, secretion of milk must be initiated and maintained. Third, milk must be ejected or propelled from the alveoli to the nipple. Finally, there must be a receptor for the milk that provides ongoing stimuli for further secretion and ejection of milk.[2,3]

Anatomic Structures

Anatomically, the breast is a modified exocrine gland, composed of glandular tissue and surrounded by adipose tissue. Alveoli, composed of secretory cells, are the location of milk production. They open into progressively larger ductules, lactiferous ducts, and lactiferous sinuses, which have dual functions as exit channels and vessels where milk is pooled. These converge and exit through the nipple. Surrounding the nipple is the areola. Both contain erectile tissue that facilitates prehension of the nipple by the infant[2,4] (see figure 8-1).

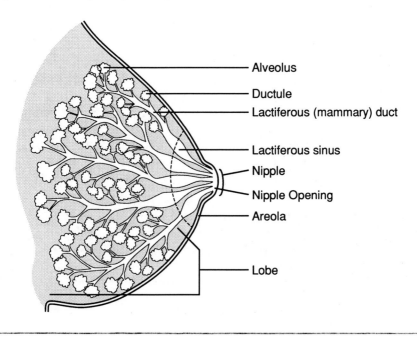

	Alveolus
	Ductule
	Lactiferous (mammary) duct
	Lactiferous sinus
	Nipple
	Nipple Opening
	Areola
	Lobe

Figure 8-1 Anatomy of the lactating breast.

Milk Production

Breast milk is a secretion of the mammary gland. Milk is produced by the secretory cells of the alveoli after stimulation from high levels of prolactin; a response that is mediated by the hypothalamus. Prolactin levels increase after birth and with stimulation to the breast by nursing. This plays a key role in the sensitive supply-demand response, which provides the correct amount of milk for the infant's changing needs.[2,4]

Milk Ejection

Milk does not passively flow from the alveoli to the nipple but is ejected. Excitation of the posterior pituitary gland, again mediated by the hypothalamus, leads to release of oxytocin. This in turn stimulates contraction of the myoepithelial cells surrounding the alveoli, whereby milk is expelled into the ducts and is readily available to the infant. This response is referred to as the let-down or milk ejection reflex and may occur multiple times in each breast during feeding. Once the reflex is elicited, rhythmic milk ejection continues uninterrupted until sucking ends.[5] This reflex has a key function in the success of breast-feeding. If milk is produced but not excreted, further milk production will be suppressed.

The most efficient stimulation to trigger this reflex is sucking on the breast. The relative roles of tactile and pressure stimuli in eliciting the milk ejection reflex during sucking are not clear, although this is under investigation.[5] Emotional state also has a clear influence on the let-down reflex. It may be triggered by the infant's crying or thoughts of the infant, and it may be inhibited by pain, stress, and mental anguish.[2,4]

Sucking Responses during Breast-Feeding

The infant's role in the breast-feeding process is equally important. As just described, the infant's sucking is crucial to providing the appropriate stimulus for milk production and ejection. The infant also creates a receptacle for the milk and assists in withdrawing it. The development and mechanics of sucking are described in chapter 1, although for technical reasons most studies have examined bottle-feeding. Some research, however, has focused specifically on sucking responses during breast-feeding.

Sucking Mechanics

The mechanics of sucking during breast-feeding were initially described by Ardran and colleagues in 1958 using cineradiographic films.[6] Similar observations of bottle-feeding allowed comparison.[7] They found that as the baby sucked the breast into the mouth an elongated teat was formed from the nipple and areola. Elevation of the jaw and tongue compressed the teat, with pressure beginning at the gum ridges and progressing back along the palate. The teat then shortened and became thicker, the jaw was lowered, and the sequence was repeated.

More recent studies utilizing real-time ultrasound imaging have provided similar but enhanced descriptions. It is now observed that the lateral margins of the tongue "cup" around the nipple, forming a central groove.[8] The nipple elongates to twice its resting length during sucking, is compressed to half its height between the tongue and palate, and maintains its dimension in width[9] (see figure 7-1, page 403). Whether the tongue moves primarily in an anterior-posterior peristaltic wave, or an up-and-down pistonlike movement in conjunction with the mandible and hyoid, remains a controversial question. Both patterns have been described in breast-feeding.[8,9]

Many breast-feeding authorities describe differences in the action of the tongue during breast- and bottle-feeding, though they fail to substantiate these observations.[2,4] "Nipple confusion," which is described as a difficulty switching between bottle and breast, is generally attributed to these differences in tongue movements. Reviewing studies using imaging techniques, however, the differences in oral movements between breast- and bottle-feeding are less clear. In the pioneering work by Ardran, Kemp, and Lind, no differences were noted in tongue movements between breast and bottle.[6,7] Weber describes a rolling, peristaltic movement of the tongue on the breast and a pistonlike squeezing on the bottle. Smith reports that tongue movements are similar on the breast and standard bottle nipples but notes that a different tongue movement is used on the Nuk® nipple.[10]

Some infants are observed to have difficulty changing between bottle nipples of different designs, so the phenomenon of nipple confusion may not be limited to differences between bottle nipples and the breast. This observation suggests that tactile and proprioceptive qualities of an object may influence the infant's oral movements and acceptance. It is possible that the primary motoric difference between sucking from the breast and from the bottle is in initiating sucking. This area, however, has not been fully studied. While the rigid bottle nipple is inserted into a partially open mouth and placed on the tongue, the mouth must be opened wide to accept the breast and the baby must actively draw it in to form a teat. In addition, differences in sucking mechanics on the breast and bottle may also be due to variations in rate of flow of milk from different mothers and different types of manufactured nipples.

The role of negative-pressure suction and positive-pressure compression of the nipple in breast-feeding has been investigated. It appears that the infant uses suction to draw the nipple into the mouth and maintain it there. Positive pressure of the tongue against the nipple and areola, coupled with the ejection of the milk by the milk ejection reflex, evacuates the milk. Lawrence feels that suction facilitates refilling of the sinuses and ducts.[2] Smith et al., on the other hand, observe that milk ejection occurs later than maximal nipple compression, in conjunction with jaw and tongue depression, and suggest that negative pressure may play a larger role in evacuating the milk.[9] In actuality it is likely that both compression and suction play a role; as milk can be expelled strictly by compression such as by manual (hand) expression or solely by suction created by mechanical breast pumps.

Sucking Patterns and Milk Flow

The rate and pattern of sucking at the breast have also been studied. While there is a distinct difference between nutritive sucking rate on the bottle and non-nutritive sucking rate (NS = 1 suck/second, NNS = 2 sucks/second),[11] continuous variation is seen during breast-feeding. Sucking rate (within the sucking burst) is high for the first one to three minutes (similar to NNS) until the let-down reflex occurs.[12] Then a slower rate (similar to NS on a bottle) is noted, though the rate gradually increases over the feeding.[13] This pattern is repeated on the second breast. A linear relationship between milk flow and sucking rate helps to explain this observation: sucking rate is high before a let-down and the beginning of milk flow; it is lower following a let-down when milk flow is high; then it increases as milk flow diminishes at the end of a feeding.[14] The pattern may repeat if a mother has more than one let-down per breast.

Lucas and colleagues report that approximately 50% of the milk is taken from each breast during the first two minutes of productive sucking, with 80% to 90% taken by four minutes.[15,43] Milk flow is high early in the feeding and diminishes substantially in the second half. Milk volume is reported to be 0.14 ml/suck early in the feeding, yet only 0.01 ml/suck at the end, also supporting the concept of higher milk flow and greater intake early in the feeding.[12] In addition, early in the feeding sucking bursts are long in duration, with short, infrequent pauses. As the feeding progresses, sucking bursts become shorter, with more frequent and longer pauses.[13] The smaller percentage of time spent in sucking as the feeding progresses would also contribute to decreased intake later in the feeding. Woolridge et al. report that for each mother-infant pair there is a characteristic rate of milk transfer.[48] This is determined by both the rate of milk release by the mother and the rate of milk demand by the baby.

The duration of sucking time at the breast also is not necessarily related to intake. Although infants may spend equal time sucking at each breast, some infants take consistently less milk from the second breast. Satiation may play a role in this finding, but milk availability does not; intake will be less at the second breast even when the remaining milk supply is abundant.[16] Infants appear to have a high degree of self-regulation with regard to milk intake. In the DARLING study, the amount of milk not taken (residual milk) was not significantly different between "low" and

---

"average" intake feeders at 3 months. Thus, infants with lower intake left just as much milk unconsumed as infants with higher intake.[49]

Butte and colleagues also report that daily milk intake is not correlated significantly with feeding duration or the number of feedings per day.[17] It appears that the breast-feeding infant may spend a considerable portion of time at the breast engaged in non-nutritive or minimally nutritive sucking. The role of this NNS at the breast in maintaining maternal milk supply or in facilitating infant well-being is poorly understood. Additionally, little is known about changes in sucking pressure during a typical feeding and how they relate to milk flow.

Some maturational changes in duration of sucking time at the breast have been described.[17] Over the first four months the duration and number of feedings decline, yet total intake remains fairly constant. Each feeding is therefore larger and the infant must be more efficient to take in a greater volume in less time. Possible explanations include more effective emptying of the breast, more expedient let-down reflexes, and a decreased need for non-nutritive sucking.

Breast-Feeding Problems in the Nonhospitalized Infant

Although breast-feeding is a natural biologic process, it is neither instinctive nor simple.[45] Numerous factors can interfere with the success of breast-feeding. In conjunction with national goals to increase the number of mothers who breast-feed their infants,[18] lactation specialists are increasingly available. They can educate mothers on the benefits of breast-feeding and are trained to assist with difficulties in establishing or maintaining breast-feeding. Common problems include engorgement, breast pain or infection, sore or cracked nipples, inadequate milk supply and/or let-down, and maternal concern regarding the relationship of the infant's behavior to breast-feeding. Current management strategies for problems such as these are well described,[2,4,19,42] and will not be addressed in this text, though they should be familiar to those working with mother-infant pairs on breast-feeding.

Although the main focus when breast-feeding difficulties arise may be on attributes of the mother (nipples, breasts, diet, handling of the infant, feeding schedules, emotional state, etc.), breast-feeding is an interaction between the mother and the infant. The infant feeding specialist is particularly well trained to evaluate the *infant's* participation and can make a unique contribution to the evaluation of breast-feeding problems. The problem-solving orientation presented throughout this text continues to be applicable. Based on a thorough understanding of the processes involved, the subcomponents and their potential role in the problem can be evaluated. At that point a meaningful treatment plan can be developed.

Many general problems in breast-feeding are successfully handled by lactation specialists, nurses, and lay specialists such as those trained by La Leche League. The problems of nonhospitalized babies that are referred to infant feeding specialists generally fall into two groups: (1) infants who are failing to thrive, where an "infant cause" is suspected, and (2) infants felt to be sucking inadequately on the breast and at risk for failing to thrive if maintained solely on the breast.

Lawrence has developed a flow chart (figure 8-2) that should serve as a background to evaluation of such infants.[2] It helps depict the complex nature of breast-feeding problems when weight gain is poor. When there is any type of problem in breast-feeding, the interrelated nature of the dyad requires attention to the physical and emotional/behavioral status of both the mother and the infant (figure 8-3). Should a problem develop in one aspect of the breast-feeding process, other aspects are affected quickly and thus may become additional problems. For this reason, while the infant feeding specialist may focus on difficulties with the infant's oral and sucking skills, it is important to consider whether this is the primary problem or a secondary problem. Interventions may also be necessary in the related areas of milk supply and the mother's emotional status.

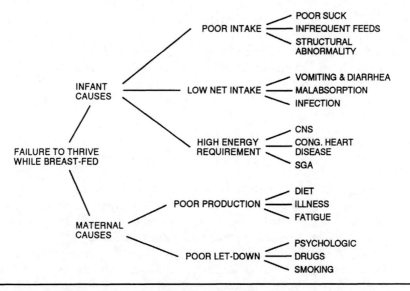

Figure 8-2 Diagnostic flow chart for failure to thrive. Reprinted with permission from: R. A. Lawrence. 1989. *Breastfeeding: A guide for the medical profession.* St. Louis, MO: C. V. Mosby Company.

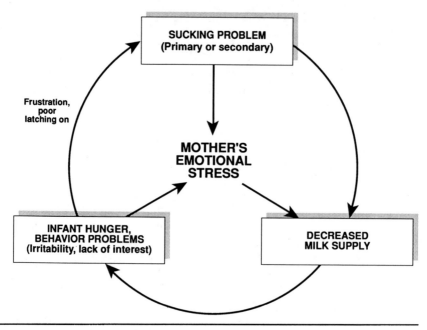

Figure 8-3 The interrelated nature of the breast-feeding dyad.

Common "Infant Causes" for Breast-Feeding Problems

Many of the infant causes for breast-feeding problems are also potential problems in bottle-feeding. Evaluation and treatment strategies discussed in chapters 3 and 5 are generally applicable in both feeding methods and will be referred to below. With a thorough understanding of the breast-feeding process and the problem at hand, creativity is called for in modifying these techniques and developing new treatments to maximize the potential for breast-feeding success.

Tongue-tip elevation: When the infant shows strong tongue-tip elevation, nipple placement is difficult (see page 114). The tongue provides a physical barrier to nipple insertion. Attempts to use the breast nipple to stroke the tongue tip and encourage it to descend are often unsuccessful. The tissue of the breast is soft and provides minimal proprioceptive input to the tongue to help it descend. Preparatory activities such as those on page 237 are appropriate to facilitate improved tongue position. In addition, when very wide mouth opening is facilitated prior to nipple insertion, the tongue will more likely move with the mandible and break its attachment to the palate. The breast-feeding mother should become aware of the sensation of the tongue movement under the breast nipple and the degree of suction that is produced when the tongue is properly positioned.

Tongue retraction: In this abnormal tongue position, the tongue tip is well behind the alveolar ridges. Tongue retraction is described in detail in chapter 3 (see page 114). At rest the breast nipple is often shorter than a bottle nipple. Therefore, when the breast is placed in the mouth there is limited contact between it and the retracted tongue. The lack of contact between nipple and tongue may hinder the development of suction and the ability to draw the nipple further into the infant's mouth. Even if some suction is created to lengthen the nipple, the tongue may not be positioned correctly below the nipple to create adequate pressure on the breast for ongoing milk ejection. Preparatory treatment strategies (see page 235) may involve firm pressure to the tongue before or during feeding. The soft consistency of the breast nipple may not provide the firm pressure needed to help maintain a more forward tongue position, so activities should utilize the feeder's finger to bring the tongue forward. As above, the mother should become aware of the sensation and amount of suction when the tongue is adequately positioned. If adequate contact between tongue and breast still cannot be achieved, use of a nipple shield may be considered to create a longer "nipple." This should be done with caution, however, as described in the next section.

Poor central grooving of the tongue: When the tongue does not spontaneously create a central groove during sucking, abnormal tongue movements may develop in compensation as the infant searches for a means of stabilizing the nipple and producing milk flow. Tongue protrusion and strong compression or "chewing" on the nipple are common. Sucking is often ineffective, with minimal negative-pressure suction generated (see pages 18 and 114). Preparatory treatment strategies are described on page 236. This type of tongue generally needs firm pressure along the midline to facilitate improved grooving. The breast nipple may be too soft to provide the degree of proprioceptive sensory input needed during feeding.

When the limited proprioceptive properties of the breast appear to interfere significantly with eliciting the proper tongue movements, and other oral treatment methods have not been successful, the use of a nipple shield may be considered. This is particularly true if an appropriate sucking pattern can be elicited on a finger or artificial nipple but not on the breast. The nipple shield is a thin latex or silicone device that resembles a "sombrero." It is placed over the breast nipple and, although flexible, makes the nipple slightly more rigid and sometimes longer, thereby providing greater proprioceptive input.

The decision to utilize a nipple shield should be made with caution, as drawbacks do exist. First, an infant often becomes "attached" to the nipple shield, and it can be difficult to wean the baby from it. If other

---

techniques are not successful, however, a mother may decide that even prolonged use of such a device would be satisfactory. Unfortunately, nipple shields also reduce the amount of milk received by the infant. The thinnest shields have the least effect on milk transfer but also provide the least proprioceptive input. The sucking rate and time spent resting may also increase, indicating that the infant must work harder to obtain milk with a shield in place.[2] Reductions in milk transfer may contribute to decreased intake and may ultimately interfere with milk supply. Therefore, use of a nipple shield would be contraindicated for infants with limited strength and endurance and for those mothers with tenuous milk supply. If this strategy is utilized, careful monitoring of the infant's weight and mother's milk supply would be required.

Small or recessed jaw: The effects of this problem are often seen in tongue position or movement (see page 118). If the tongue is also retracted or shows poor central grooving, techniques discussed above on each of these topics may be appropriate. When the jaw is recessed, the tongue may not be able to physically come forward adequately to be positioned properly below the breast nipple.

In addition, the lower jaw may not be positioned correctly to compress the areola for effective milk ejection. It has been suggested that mothers hold the jaw and provide a forward traction during nursing to obtain maximal forward positioning of the jaw and the best tongue position possible. If tongue retraction is associated with intermittent airway obstruction during feeding, position changes may be required. Possibly prone or semiprone positioning may allow gravity to draw the jaw and tongue forward. Another option is a very upright sitting position. It may be easiest to achieve this position by using a modified "football hold," bringing the infant into an upright position while sitting next to or straddling the mother's thigh.

Excessive jaw excursion: This may lead to inefficient sucking on the breast, loss of suction, and frequent need to "re-latch." Factors in need of evaluation are found on page 118. Treatment strategies are similar to those described on page 241. Careful attention should be given to head and neck positioning, with the optimal position maintained through steady head support. Jaw and/or cheek control may also be provided at the breast, with hand position as illustrated in figure 8-4.[44]

Inadequate mouth opening: Full mouth opening is essential to proper attachment to the breast. Factors to consider in facilitating mouth opening are discussed on page 239. Marmet and Snell also describe a technique whereby gentle downward pressure is provided to the chin prior to and during nipple insertion.[20]

Mouth-breast "mismatch": Although there are numerous designs available in artificial nipples, each with its own attributes (see chapter 7), there is far greater variation in human nipples. The mother's nipples and the infant's sucking characteristics therefore may present a "mismatch" that must also be addressed. For example, a slightly retracted tongue position may not impact breast feeding if the mother has long and well-defined nipples, but it may have a more serious impact if the mother has inelastic breast tissue and short nipples that do not elongate well. Therefore, in addition to evaluating and treating the oral-motor characteristics of the infant, the characteristics of the mother's nipples must be considered. Information on such assessment and intervention is available,[2,4,19] and the infant feeding specialist not familiar with these techniques should consult additional references and/or a lactation specialist for assistance in this area.

Behavior and state: Evaluation techniques and treatment strategies would be similar to those described in chapters 3 and 5. Barnes et al. describe five categories of infant temperament during breast-feeding: barracudas, excited ineffectiveness, procrastinators, gourmets or mouthers, and resters.[46] Such differences should be kept in mind when providing state and behavioral interventions. Therefore, infants with some feeding styles may benefit from these activities, while others may ultimately do better without such interventions, even if feeding proceeds at a rate that is faster or slower than "typical."

Energy and endurance: Again, evaluation and treatment strategies are similar to those discussed in chapters 3 and 5. Supplementation may be necessary, and options specific to breast-feeding are discussed below.

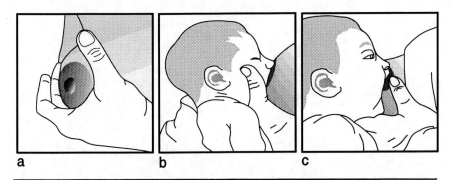

a   b   c

Figure 8-4 Hand position for providing jaw and cheek support at the breast is shown. Cupping the breast in the ulnar portion of the palm (a) frees the thumb and fingers for cheek support (b) and/or chin support (c).

Methods of Supplementing Breast-Feeding Intake

When breast-feeding problems exist, the infant may not receive adequate intake from the breast. Although reduced volume may be acceptable in some infants for short periods while breast-feeding modifications are attempted, supplemental methods of providing nutrition are often necessary since appropriate weight gain is crucial to all aspects of infant development. When supplementation is needed, it is important to encourage the mother to pump as much as is feasible, so that the baby can continue to receive the nutritional benefits of breast milk and the mother can maintain or increase her milk supply. Three methods that might be considered in the infant with some sucking ability, along with strengths and limitations, are described below. Non-oral methods are also a possibility when more serious problems exist or during the transition to complete breast-feeding. These methods have been discussed in detail in chapter 5.

Feeding tube devices: These include commercially available appliances such as the Lact-aide, Medella® Supplemental Nursing System (SNS), and similar devices that are fabricated from medical tubing and syringes[21] (see figure 8-5). In all of these devices, a reservoir holds the nutrient (often expressed breast milk), which flows through a small tube to the tip of the breast nipple as the baby sucks. Care is taken so that the fluid does not flow by gravity but is received, along with any breast milk that is present, only when the baby sucks at the breast. As the baby becomes more efficient at sucking on the breast, the amount of milk extracted from the reservoir will gradually decrease.

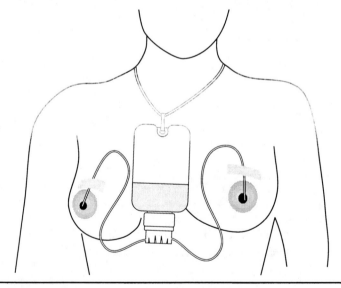

Figure 8-5 A commercially available feeding-tube device.

Strengths:

- Oral-tactile, proprioceptive, and motoric experiences are only at the breast. There is less opportunity to develop nipple confusion.

- Ongoing practice of the specific sucking mechanics of breast-feeding occurs.

- The mother's nipples receive stimulation to enhance milk production.

Limitations:

- The mother may reject the use of equipment to breast-feed her infant.

- The equipment may be "finicky," resulting in difficulty establishing the proper flow rate.

- Some particularly sensitive infants may notice the tube and reject the breast with the tube.

- Proper breast-feeding positioning and techniques and proper tube placement are crucial to success. If positioned improperly, these devices can actually encourage inappropriate sucking patterns or magnify the infant's original problem. For example, if the tube extends past the end of the nipple, the infant may suck the tube rather than take the whole nipple and areola into the mouth. Although milk may be received (like sipping through a straw), the infant will be practicing inappropriate breast-feeding skills. This also provides poor stimulation to the mother's milk supply.

Finger feeding: This technique is often suggested for the infant who has difficulty establishing sucking on the breast and is not successful with supplementation at the breast as described above. It is introduced with the hope that it will produce less nipple confusion for the infant than using a bottle. A commercial lactation supplementation device is taped securely to the mother's finger. The infant then sucks the mother's finger and receives nourishment through the tube. The size of the tubing and height of the reservoir may be adjusted to provide the correct flow rate. Alternately, a small-diameter catheter may be taped to the mother's finger and attached at the other end to a syringe filled with milk.

Strengths:

- Skin-to-skin contact between the infant's mouth and the finger is advocated by some as perhaps reducing nipple confusion and aiding in the transition to the breast.

- The firm proprioceptive input of the finger in the mouth and on the tongue may assist in developing more appropriate tongue movements during sucking.

Limitations:

- The finger, though skin covered, is much firmer than the breast, providing markedly different proprioceptive input. The finger has a predetermined shape, may be placed directly in the correct position on the tongue, and does not change shape with sucking. The infant does not have to actively elongate the finger nor maintain its position in the mouth. While these factors may aid in establishing tongue movements, the infant may become reliant on such proprioceptive cues to the tongue, hindering the return to the breast with its softer consistency, limited proprioceptive qualities, and deformation during sucking.

- To position the mouth correctly on the breast, maximal mouth opening is required. In contrast, minimal mouth opening is required to insert the finger. Poor mouth opening, resulting in inappropriate tongue and jaw movements, may have been the factor contributing to inadequate nursing. Many mothers using this technique may inadvertently overlook the need to encourage wide mouth opening as practice for returning to the breast. Lack of experience in mouth opening may also then make returning to the breast more difficult.

- Because of the finger's rigid nature, the baby does not develop the skill of drawing the nipple into the mouth. These skills are needed in latching on to the breast.

Bottle-feeding: This is often recommended by medical practitioners as an easy and effective method of providing adequate nutrition. Many infants who are having trouble establishing breast-feeding will have little or no difficulty taking a bottle, though the reasons for this phenomenon are not clearly understood. Conversely, breast-feeding specialists generally feel that the bottle should be a last resort, as it produces nipple confusion and may reduce the motivation of the infant and the mother to work toward successful breast-feeding.

Strengths:

- It may appear "easier" for the infant to obtain nourishment from the bottle.

- There is a large variety of nipple shapes available. A nipple should be chosen that will support the necessary feeding components to return to breast-feeding. For example, if wider mouth opening is desired, a nipple with a broad base should be selected. If it is necessary to facilitate central grooving of the tongue, a firm, straight nipple would be appropriate.

Limitations:

- The ease of bottle-feeding may diminish motivation of mother and infant to continue breast-feeding attempts. Although expressed breast milk may initially be given by bottle, work involved to pump and bottle-feed may soon lead to cessation of pumping and use of commercial formula.

Breast-Feeding and the Hospitalized Infant

There are very few conditions for which the provision of breast milk is contraindicated. Conversely, there are a number of medical conditions for which breast milk actually limits the disease process or aids in recovery.[2] In some circumstances, however, putting the infant to the breast for feeding is not possible. These typically involve hospitalization and include the presence of mechanical ventilation, immaturity such that the coordination of sucking and swallowing is not adequate for oral feeding, and feeding intolerance. In other conditions that interfere with oral feeding ability, breast-feeding may not be contraindicated, but the potential for success may be marginal. Anomalies of the oral area (cleft lip and palate, etc.), neurologic impairment (secondary to hypoxia or intracranial hemorrhage), and motor dysfunction (such as cranial nerve palsy) are examples.

One of the early decisions facing families of a hospitalized neonate is whether to provide breast milk for the infant's nutrition. This decision is often made at a time when the infant is not receiving any enteral nutrition. The shock of dealing with the infant's overall health status is typically overwhelming, and nutritional considerations may be of low priority. In addition, resources to discuss the potential benefits of providing breast milk may be limited.

While breast milk provides many benefits to the healthy infant, these benefits may become even more important to the hospitalized infant. In particular, breast milk may provide protection against infection for the infant who is exposed to the many organisms in the hospital environment. The ease of digestion of breast milk may improve feeding tolerance in an infant with an immature or ailing gastrointestinal tract. A reduced incidence of gastrointestinal disorders in babies receiving breast milk is another benefit. Most of the beneficial qualities of breast milk are maintained during storage while awaiting the infant's readiness for milk feedings. Providing the special qualities of breast milk to a compromised infant may also give the mother feelings of satisfaction and reward.[2]

Gathering Milk through Breast Pumping

When an infant cannot be put to the breast to receive breast milk, some method of expression must be used. The details of that process, including the type of equipment used, the mother's emotional investment, and the mother's rigor in carrying out the program of milk expression, will determine the level of success in supplying the infant with breast milk. Feeding specialists counseling mothers about breast milk collection should have a thorough knowledge of these techniques. Following is a brief synopsis of key considerations.[2,23]

- Inducing and maintaining an adequate milk supply will be most successful if a good breast pump is used. Manual expression or use of battery-operated pumps is possible for occasional collection but is rarely adequate for long-term use. Electric pumps with alternating suction are recommended, and mothers should be encouraged to rent a pump for home use.

- Pumping should commence as soon after birth as possible. It should occur at least five times per day for a total of at least 100 minutes. An uninterrupted sleep period of at least six hours may be included.

- A pump that allows simultaneous pumping of both breasts will save time and produce greater milk volume than pumping each breast individually for the same length of time.

- The pumping milieu and the mother's routine should promote the let-down reflex and development/maintenance of the milk supply.

- Clear guidelines for collection and storage of human milk should be developed by each center. There is controversy regarding the safest collection and storage techniques, so guidelines should take into account current research, as new information is reported frequently. Factors to consider include infection-control procedures during milk collection, the type of containers to use for collection and storage, time lines for storage, labeling, and thawing or heating procedures. Periodic culturing for contamination may be instituted. Although refrigerated milk should be used within 24 hours of collection, milk collected for the mother's own infant may be stored longer by freezing.[22]

The benefits of breast milk are considered so great for infants with special needs that in some regions milk banks have been developed for the processing, storage, and distribution of donor milk. More detailed guidelines are necessary for collection, processing, and storage of this milk.[2]

Preterm Infants

One of the largest groups of hospitalized infants that must delay breast-feeding is preterm infants. Increasingly, medical personnel are becoming aware of the many benefits of nourishing these infants with breast milk. The infection-protective qualities of human milk are extremely valuable in this group, which is prone to infections such as necrotizing enterocolitis, sepsis, viral infections, and meningitis.[23] Research is beginning to support the hypothesis that preterm and low-birth-weight infants who are fed breast milk have lower rates of infection than those fed commercial formulas.[24,25] Early feedings of colostrum by breast or gavage tube may contribute to protection from infection.[2]

Human milk is also relatively more digestible than cow's milk formula. Amino acid and fat absorption are superior, and the initial phase of digestion occurs more quickly. Utilizing human milk allows optimal nutrition to promote growth, without imposing significant metabolic stress on these small infants.[2,26]

There are qualitative differences in the milk of mothers of premature infants when compared to term infants.[23] Generally these differences are consistent with the specific nutritional needs of the low-birth-weight infant. Larger amounts of nitrogen and protein are found. There are more calories per ounce, which makes this milk a higher energy source. Lactose values are lower, perhaps aiding digestion in the immature gut. Some nutrients, such as calcium and phosphorus, may not be present in adequate quantities for the very small premature infant. Even though quantities of protein are higher than in milk of mothers of term infants, protein still may be inadequate.[23] For this reason nutritional supplementation is often provided to the preterm infant nourished by mother's milk, most often for infants less than 1500 grams. Powdered supplements may be added to the mother's breast milk (e.g., Enfamil® human milk fortifier). Liquid supplements (e.g., Similac Natural Care®) designed for use in conjunction with human milk may be provided when supply is inadequate.[2,26]

Feasibility and Effects of Breast-Feeding the Preterm Infant

Many hold the view that breast-feeding is too stressful for the preterm infant who is initiating oral feedings. It is often felt that feeding at the breast requires more "work" and thus more energy than bottle-feeding, potentially compromising tenuous weight gain in these infants. Therefore, a typical progression is to move from gavage feeding to bottle-feeding. Then, if desired, breast-feeding is introduced once bottle-feeding is established and occurring without difficulties.

Bottle-feeding has some advantages to the medical staff caring for the premature infant in the hospital. Primarily, exact intake is easily quantifiable, and it is easily accomplished in the mother's absence. Following a sequence that mandates effective bottle-feeding prior to breast-feeding, however, may inadvertently undermine the potential for the infant to breast-feed successfully. Breast-feeding may not be introduced until close to the time of hospital discharge, leaving little time for the mother and baby to practice in the supportive nursery environment where experienced nurses are available to guide this process. In addition, the infant has become skilled at obtaining food from a bottle and may not have the patience or flexibility to adjust to the differences of taking the breast. These differences primarily include the necessity of latching on and drawing the breast nipple into the mouth and maintaining non-nutritive sucking while awaiting the let-down reflex. Whether different tongue movements are required during sucking remains a controversial question.

Meier and colleagues have carried out research designed to evaluate the ability of young preterm infants to breast-feed, as well as the physiologic impact of early breast-feeding.[27-29] Summarizing their findings, breast-feeding was initiated successfully in infants as young as $32\frac{1}{2}$ weeks gestation and 1,220 grams. While gestational age and maturity were felt to play a role in readiness for breast-feeding, weight was not. All infants who were studied, however, did demonstrate coordination of sucking and swallowing prior to initiation of *any* oral feeding. Each infant had at least one bottle prior to being put to the breast, though some had been given bottle-feedings for as long as nine days. Length of time of bottle-feeding before introduction of the breast appeared to be related to ease of establishing breast-feeding skills. Although infants who had taken the bottle occasionally for three to four days had few problems initiating breast-feeding, the transition to breast-feeding appeared more difficult for those who had taken the bottle exclusively for longer periods. Interestingly, once breast-feeding was initiated, regular inclusion of bottle-feeding did not seem to interfere with the infant's ability to maintain breast-feeding skills. These observations may vary with individual mother-infant pairs.

In these studies, characteristics of sucking varied between breast and bottle. All infants needed repeated assistance attaching to the breast during the first few feedings. During the earliest feedings a more clear burst-pause pattern was noted on the breast when compared to the bottle, with infants demonstrating independent pacing of sucking bursts and pauses on the breast. As their age increased, infants showed longer and smoother burst-pause patterns on both the breast and bottle. Although during breast-feeding infants showed no signs of distress (i.e., bradycardia, tachycardia, color change, or gagging), while bottle-feeding, episodes of burping, gagging, and bradycardia were noted. Mean feeding times ranged from 9 to 19 minutes on the bottle and 16 to 31 minutes at the breast. This was attributed to consistent nutritive sucking on the bottle, with non-nutritive sucking and increased mother-infant interaction interspersed during breast-feeding.

In regard to physiologic measures, Meier et al. found that the pattern of transcutaneous PO_2 (tcPO$_2$) was quite dissimilar between bottle- and breast-feeding.[29] During breast-feeding, minimal fluctuation was seen above and below baseline values, even during sucking bursts. During bottle-feeding, tcPO$_2$ dropped during periods of sucking, increased to baseline values when sucking ceased, plateaued during prolonged rests such as burping, and gradually declined during the 10 minutes after the feeding was completed.

These findings, while descriptive of a limited number of premature infants, suggest that breast-feeding is possible for the young premature infant who is showing feeding readiness. Breast-feeding did not appear to cause additional physiologic stress, and in fact may cause less physiologic stress than bottle-feeding. In this age group, coordination of sucking, swallowing, and breathing may be more successful at the breast than at the bottle. Speculation regarding the mechanisms underlying these observations focuses on two factors: ventilatory interruption and milk flow. Previous studies have found similar patterns of drops in tcPO$_2$ during bottle-feeding,[30,31] and it is felt that these observations may reflect the interruption of ventilation during swallowing.

Mathew has studied ventilatory patterns during breast- and bottle-feeding.[32] His results suggest that ventilatory patterns remain closer to baseline values during breast-feeding than during bottle-feeding. While his use of mothers in the early stages of lactation (when milk availability is questionable) limits comparison, it is tempting to speculate that differences in ventilatory pattern at the breast might be responsible for the limited changes in tcPO$_2$ reported by Meier and colleagues.[27-29] Mathew attributes the differences in ventilatory pattern he found between breast and bottle to differences in milk delivery and flow rate.[32] Less flow per suck on the breast, leading to a reduced swallowing rate, may minimize feeding-related oxygen desaturation by increasing the time available for breathing.

Although Mathew suggests that the differences he has found might disappear as lactation is well established, Meier's work suggests this might not be the case. She also speculates that infants may be able to modify sucking pressures and/or milk flow at the breast to facilitate organized feeding in a way they are not able to do with the bottle. Further study is obviously called for to solidify our understanding of the interrelationship of feeding method and physiologic responses in both term and preterm infants. This research, however, should encourage health care providers to attempt breast-feeding in the early stages of initiating oral feeding, even in younger premature babies.

Transition to Breast-Feeding

As Lawrence states, "The risks of starving a premature infant while he adapts to nursing at the breast are real."[2] Thus, this process must be accomplished with care and forethought to accomplish a trio of goals: (1) maintaining the infant's nourishment and growth, (2) developing the infant's skills at obtaining milk from the breast, and (3) maintaining/building the mother's milk supply so that it is adequate to meet the infant's needs. A possible progression, along with many considerations for implementation, is presented below. Further details regarding some aspects of this process are found elsewhere.[23,33,34,44] There is no "recipe for success" in this process; it must be individualized to each mother-infant pair. Characteristics of premature infants that might interfere with this process, such as state, behavior, and posture (see chapters 3 and 6) should be considered, along with the potential oral difficulties that were discussed earlier in this chapter.

1. **Non-nutritive sucking (NNS):** Enteral tube feedings are the common method of providing nourishment to the infant who is not yet mature enough for oral feeding. The benefits of providing NNS during such feedings are well demonstrated.[35-37] NNS appears to aid digestion, assist in state control, and promote weight gain, earlier transition to oral feeding, and earlier hospital discharge.

   When NNS is possible, the mother-infant pair planning for breast-feeding should initiate NNS at the breast.[2] This can be accomplished by the mother prepumping and emptying her breast. Beginning the transition process with NNS at the breast has several advantages. First, it allows the infant to begin practicing the mechanics of breast-feeding at an earlier age. In particular, the infant can develop skill in latching on to the breast. The environment during this practice may also be less stressful for the mother and the infant. The mother does not need to worry about the success of feeding and attends only to the sucking process. The infant should not be overly hungry and thus may be more patient in learning this new skill, and may be satisfied solely by the sucking activity. NNS at the breast can be done in conjunction with gavage feedings or at other times when the infant's state is appropriate. If necessary, part of the gavage feeding can be given prior to putting the baby to the breast to alleviate hunger. Even after bottle-feeding has been initiated, NNS at the breast can be a helpful method of beginning the transition to the breast.

2. **Beginning oral feeding:** As discussed in detail in earlier sections, when an infant appears ready for oral feeding, there are generally no contraindications to introducing breast-feeding. Simultaneous introduction of breast and bottle has been successful, with ongoing use of both methods not appearing to compromise breast-feeding success.[27-29]

Many clinicians worry that nipple confusion will develop when the baby is taking both breast and bottle. It would seem, however, that nipple confusion may be more problematic if bottle-feeding has been the sole oral feeding method for more than a week prior to the introduction of breast-feeding.[27] On the other hand, if an infant has difficulty maintaining physiologic stability on the bottle, bottle-feeding may be discontinued, and breast-feeding continued, awaiting further maturation.[29]

Measurement of intake is also a consideration during breast-feeding. Meier and colleagues advocate not terminating breast-feeding sessions based on imposed rules, but continuing as long as mother and infant are comfortable.[27-29] In the hospital, nursing staff members are available to monitor clinical and physiologic change and help the mother determine if these factors should lead to termination of the feeding. Early breast-feeding may be limited to one breast. Daily weighing is suggested to monitor growth. If this method of monitoring intake is not acceptable, the baby can be weighed pre- and post-feeding. The use of a special electronic scale that takes multiple readings in rapid succession and provides an averaged value will be required to obtain reliable measurement.[47]

The atmosphere and degree of support for the mother during early breast-feeding attempts should be carefully considered. A private and relaxing atmosphere will facilitate the mother's and baby's responses. Assistance should be available at the level needed and desired by the mother.

3. **Maintaining milk supply:** Although putting the infant to the breast should provide additional stimulation for milk production, complete emptying must also be maintained. Therefore, in the early phases of transition to breast-feeding, the mother should pump after each feeding session. In addition to providing the complete emptying that will stimulate maintenance of milk supply, pumping may help the mother determine approximate intake without weighing the infant at each feeding. Post-breast-feeding pumping should be tapered off gradually until the infant is fully feeding by breast.[41]

4. **Supplementary nutrition:** The process of moving to total breast-feeding may take several weeks to several months. During this time the infant will need additional nourishment. Supplemental bottles may be given at certain feedings, providing known quantities of nourishment. A method called "triple timing" may be used. First, the mother nurses the baby. Next, the baby is fed previously expressed breast milk by bottle. Lastly, the mother pumps to express the maximal amount of milk for that feeding so it can be used at subsequent feedings. Complementary bottles of formula, to top off a feeding, should be avoided as

they may lead to lactation failure.[2] Use of a feeding tube device (see page 432) may also be useful to ensure adequate nutrition during this transition period. In some cases, gavage feeding may continue until breast-feeding is completely established.[33]

5. **Transition to home:** Being at home with the infant should facilitate breast-feeding, as the mother and baby have constant access to each other. Success may depend on the amount of breast-feeding experience the mother and infant have had in the hospital and the mother's knowledge of what to expect during the transition process. Frequent feeding during the first few days is suggested to aid in making this transition.[33,34] Since some breast-feeding problems or questions are likely to occur, a source of follow-up contact should be established. A study by Howard links self-perceived success in breast-feeding a premature infant to factors such as higher motivation and fewer breast-feeding difficulties.[38] Lack of success was related to maternal problems with milk supply, let-down, and pumping, as well as difficulties getting the infant to suck on the breast. Establishing successful breast-feeding before discharge from the hospital is certainly the best way to ensure success at home. In lieu of that, greater success in breast-feeding preterm infants may be achieved by providing more resources to assist mothers with breast-feeding difficulties after hospital discharge.

Hospitalized Infants with Other Medical Problems

Hospitalized infants with a variety of other health problems may also have difficulty initiating breast-feeding. These would include babies with Down syndrome, those with neurologic insult from asphyxia or intracranial hemorrhage, and those with oral-facial anomalies. Such infants tend to have general feeding problems related to abnormal oral-motor characteristics. Assessment of overall feeding skills would proceed as outlined in chapter 3. The relation of specific oral problems to the breast-feeding process should be considered as described earlier in this chapter. Parent training material is available on techniques relevant to breast-feeding when certain medical conditions exist.[39,40] The amount of maternal support and teaching that occurs during the initiation of breast-feeding, when the greatest number of problems exist, seems to be related to the ultimate success of breast-feeding.

Other infants will have adequate oral-motor skills but medical limitations that interfere with breast-feeding. Much of the information presented in this chapter in reference to preterm infants may be applicable to infants with limited endurance secondary to congenital heart defects and other similar problems. When an infant has prolonged feeding intolerance and highly specialized formulas are required, use of a feeding tube device may be necessary. The information on transition to the breast (presented above) may also be applicable to infants with other medical problems. Breast-feeding the child with oral anomalies such as cleft lip and palate is discussed separately (see chapter 6).

Attitudes and Decision Making regarding Breast-Feeding

There are times when it may unfortunately appear that medical profession-als working with infants fall into two divergent camps regarding the issue of breast-feeding: those who support breast-feeding to the exclusion of other options, and those who see little reason to encourage it, particularly if conditions arise that might make it more difficult. When such messages do not fit with a parent's attitudes, desires, or experience, confusion, and/or guilt can ensue. Therefore, in counseling parents regarding breast-feeding a sense of balance must be found that couples enthusiastic support for breast-feeding with realistic expectations.

Although breast-feeding offers many potential benefits to the mother and child, not all mothers want to breast-feed. Whatever their reasons, they should be accepted without judgment. In addition, it must be acknowl-edged that breast-feeding is not always successful, even in the healthy full-term infant.[41] These cases must be quickly identified and care taken to insure that the mother does not feel like she or her baby have "failed" at this endeavor. On the other hand, when an infant is sick or premature and the mother has planned to breast-feed, it is an injustice to simply brush her plans aside. Many mothers of sick or premature infants decide to at least provide their infant with breast milk. This is a contribution only the mother can make and she should be fully supported even if this is the only component of the breast-feeding experience that she has with her infant.

When an infant is sick or breast-feeding is not fully successful, making decisions regarding breast-feeding becomes a difficult process. As mothers and families struggle to make the decisions that are right for them in these stressful circumstances, they deserve thorough and unbiased information on breast-feeding options and the benefits and limitations of breast-feeding in their situation.[34] They also deserve support and encouragement toward complete breast-feeding if at all possible. This would include:

Options for breast-feeding: Most parents assume that breast-feeding means exclusively putting the infant to the breast to obtain nourish-ment. Depending on the infant's circumstances, pumping to obtain mother's milk to be given by an alternate route should be presented as an option. The availability of feeding tube devices as a primary or adjunct method of breast-feeding may also be recommended. Each of these should be considered a method of "breast-feeding." Parents should be aware that while termination of lactation may be difficult to reverse, once the mother has developed a milk supply, any plans for lactation or breast-feeding (including pumping or using a feeding-tube device) can always be changed if they are not meeting the parent's or infant's needs.

Nutritional benefits: These should be addressed as they relate to the specific infant. The benefits of breast milk will be particularly relevant for some infants. Other infants grow normally and have no additional complications from commercial formula.

Emotional considerations: While numerous emotional benefits are attributed to breast-feeding, at times these benefits may be outweighed by the difficulties surrounding breast-feeding. When feeding at the breast is not immediately possible, or is not going well, the emotional benefits will be delayed. Mothers should always be reassured that there are many ways to establish a strong emotional bond with their infant, even if they are not successful or choose not to put the infant to the breast. Providing pumped breast milk may be one method, though many options unrelated to breast-feeding exist; these include the mother's physical presence, touching, holding, talking to, and rocking the infant.

It should also be acknowledged that breast-feeding may be difficult to establish in some infants, and that this is not the "fault" of the mother. During the process of establishing breast-feeding in an infant who is having difficulties, the mother may feel like she is on an emotional roller coaster that depends on the success of each feeding. This can add a significant stress to the developing mother-infant relationship. In addition, mothers of sick infants may fear for their baby's outcome and be hesitant to participate in activities that require an emotional investment.

Practical benefits and limitations: Parents should be aware that when breast-feeding is well established and working smoothly, it is an easy and convenient method of feeding their infant. Milk is readily available, with no preparation necessary. Even when working smoothly, however, it does require a commitment from the mother to be present and available at feeding times.

For the hospitalized infant or the infant having difficulty establishing breast-feeding, the commitment of time and energy may be much greater. Pumping must be done faithfully to maintain the milk supply. This is often in addition to hospital visits. Pumping may be necessary even when the infant is nursing at the breast, increasing the time spent in feeding-related activities. If feeding tube devices are used, the equipment must be cleaned and set up with each feeding.

Once the family has been provided with the information described above, they should consider two questions: what feeding method is best for the baby nutritionally and emotionally? and what feeding method is best for the mother emotionally and practically? At times the answers to these questions may not fit together neatly. Only the family can determine the relative weight given to maternal versus infant needs. Families deserve healthy encouragement of their ability to make the decisions that are correct for them, when they are given adequate information. They also deserve professional support for whatever decisions they make. This would include emotional support as well as technical assistance from persons trained or experienced in management of breast-feeding problems. When there are obstacles to breast-feeding success, a mother who decides to pursue breast-feeding should be assured that if it ultimately is not successful, any level of breast-feeding she can achieve with her infant will be beneficial for the baby. The ability or inability to establish full nutrition at the breast should not be taken as a reflection of her ability to "mother" her infant.

Decision making in these conditions is often difficult. Providing adequate information and support should allow the process to proceed without adding additional stress to the family, either during the decision-making process or later from feelings of having had inadequate information to make appropriate decisions.

References

1. Houston, M. J. 1981. Breast-feeding: Success or failure. *Journal of Advanced Nursing* 6:447-54.

2. Lawrence, R. A. 1989. *Breast-feeding: A guide for the medical profession.* St. Louis, MO: C. V. Mosby Company.

3. Worthington-Roberts, B. S. 1989. *Nutrition in pregnancy and lactation.* St. Louis, MO: Times Mirror/Mosby College Publishing.

4. Riordan, J., and B. A. Countryman. 1983. The anatomy and psychophysiology of lactation. In *A practical guide to breast-feeding*, edited by J. Riordan. St. Louis, MO: C. V. Mosby Company.

5. Luther, E. C., J. C. Arballo, N. L. Sala, and J. C. Cordero Funes. 1974. Suckling pressure in humans: Relationship to oxytocin-reproducing reflex milk ejection. *Journal of Applied Physiology* 36:350-53.

6. Ardran, G. M., F. H. Kemp, and J. Lind. 1958. A cineradiographic study of breast-feeding. *British Journal of Radiology* 31:156-62.

7. Ardran, G. M., F. H. Kemp, and J. Lind. 1958. A cineradiographic study of bottle-feeding. *British Journal of Radiology* 31:11-22.

8. Weber, F., M. W. Woolridge, and J. D. Baum. 1986. An ultrasonographic study of the organization of sucking and swallowing by newborn infants. *Developmental Medicine and Child Neurology* 28:19-24.

9. Smith, W. L., A. Erenberg, and A. Nowak. 1988. Imaging evaluation of the human nipple during breast-feeding. *American Journal of Diseases in Children* 142:76-78.

10. Smith, W. L. 1989. Breast-feeding: Beyond the basics. Conference presented in Seattle, WA.

11. Wolff, P. H. 1968. The serial organization of sucking in the young infant. *Pediatrics* 42:943-55.

12. Woolridge, M. W., T. V. How, R. F. Drewett, P. Rolfe, and J. D. Baum. 1982. The continuous measurement of milk intake at a feed in breast-fed babies. *Early Human Development* 6:365-73.

13. Drewett, R. F., and M. Woolridge. 1979. Sucking patterns of human babies on the breast. *Early Human Development* 3/4:315-20.

14. Bowen-Jones, A., C. Thompson, and R. F. Drewett. 1982. Milk flow and sucking rates during breast-feeding. *Developmental Medicine and Child Neurology* 24:626-33.

15. Lucas, A., P. J. Lucas, and J. D. Baum. 1979. Pattern of milk flow in breast-fed infants. *The Lancet* 8133:57-59.

16. Drewett, R. F., and M. Woolridge. 1981. Milk taken by human babies from the first and second breast. *Physiology and Behavior* 26:327-29.

17. Butte, N. F., C. Wills, C. A. Jean, E. O. Smith, and C. Garza. 1985. Feeding patterns of exclusively breast-fed infants during the first four months of life. *Early Human Development* 12:291-300.

18. Report from the surgeon general's workshop on breast-feeding and human lactation. Publication no. HRS-D-MC 84-2, Department of Health and Human Services, 1984.

19. Jolley, S. 1988. *Breast-feeding triage tool*. Seattle, WA: Seattle-King County Department of Public Health.

20. Marmet, C., and E. Shell. 1984. Training neonates to suck correctly. *MCN (Maternal and Child Nursing)* 9:401-07.

21. Riordan, J., and E. R. Cerutti. 1983. Pediatric health problems and breast-feeding. In *A practical guide to breast-feeding*, edited by J. Riordan. St. Louis, MO: C. V. Mosby Company.

22. Meier, P., and S. Wilks. 1987. The bacteria in expressed mother's milk. *MCN (Maternal and Child Nursing)* 12:420-23.

23. Lemons, P., M. Stuart, and J. A. Lemons. 1986. Breast-feeding the premature infant. *Clinics in Perinatology* 13:111-22.

24. Narayanan, I., et al. 1980. Partial supplementation with expressed breast milk for prevention of infection in low birth weight infants. *Lancet* 2:561-63.

25. Stevenson, D. K., C. Yang, J. A. Kerner, and A. S. Yeager. 1985. Intestinal flora in the second week of life in hospitalized preterm infants fed frozen breast milk or a proprietary formula. *Clinics in Pediatrics* 24:338-41.

26. Steichen, J. J., S. K. Krug-Wispe, and R. C. Tsang. 1987. Breast-feeding the low weight preterm infant. *Clinics in Perinatology* 14:131-71.

27. Meier, P., and E. J. Pugh. 1985. Breast-feeding behavior of small preterm infants. *MCN* 10:396-401.

28. Meier, P., and G. C. Anderson. 1987. Responses of small preterm infants to bottle- and breast-feeding. *MCN* 12:97-105.

29. Meier, P. 1988. Bottle- and breast-feeding: Effects on transcutaneous oxygen pressure and temperature in preterm infants. *Nursing Research* 37:36-41.

30. Mathew, O. P. 1988. Respiratory control during nipple feeding in preterm infants. *Pediatric Pulmonology* 5:220-24.

31. Sivpuri, C. R., R. J. Martin, W. A. Carlo, and A. A. Fanaroff. 1983. Decreased ventilation in preterm infants during oral feeding. *The Journal of Pediatrics* 103:285-89.

32. Mathew, O. P., and J. Bhatia. 1989. Sucking and breathing patterns during breast- and bottle-feeding in term neonates. *American Journal of Diseases in Childhood* 143:588-92.

33. Boggs, K. R., and P. K. Rau. 1983. Breast-feeding the premature infant. *American Journal of Nursing* (October, 1983):1437-39.

34. Meier, P., and J. Riordan. 1983. Breast-feeding support in the high-risk nursery and at home. In *A practical guide to breast-feeding*, edited by J. Riordan. St. Louis, MO: C. V. Mosby Company.

35. Measel, C. P., and G. C. Anderson. 1979. Non-nutritive sucking during tube feedings: Effect on clinical course in premature infants. *Journal of Obstetric, Gynecologic and Neonatal Nursing* 8:265-72.

36. Bernbaum, J. C., G. R. Pereira, J. B. Watkins, and G. J. Peckham. 1983. Non-nutritive sucking during gavage feeding enhances growth and maturation in premature infants. *Pediatrics* 71:41-45.

37. Field, T., E. Ignatoff, S. Stringer, J. Bremman, R. Greenberg, S. Widmayer, and G. C. Anderson. 1982. Non-nutritive sucking during tube feedings: Effects on preterm neonates in an intensive care unit. *Pediatrics* 70:381-84.

38. Howard, M. M. 1986. Factors associated with the success of breast-feeding the premature infant. Master's thesis, University of Washington.

39. Danner, S. C., and E. R. Cerutti. 1984. *Nursing your baby with Down's syndrome.* Rochester, NY: Childbirth Graphics Ltd.

40. Danner, S. C., and E. R. Cerutti. 1984. *Nursing your neurologically impaired baby.* Rochester, NY: Childbirth Graphics Ltd.

41. Neifert, M. R., and J. M. Seacat. 1987. Lactation insufficiency: A rational approach. *Birth* 14:182-90.

---

42. Frantz, K. B. 1983. Slow weight gain. In *A practical guide to breast-feeding*, edited by J. Riordan. St. Louis, MO: C. V. Mosby Company.

43. Lucas, A., P. J. Lucas, and J. D. Baum. 1981. Differences in the pattern of milk intake between breast and bottle-fed infants. *Early Human Development* 5:195-99.

44. McBride, M. C., and S. C. Danner. 1987. Sucking disorders in neurologically impaired infants: Assessment and facilitation of breast-feeding. *Clinics in Perinatology* 14:109-30.

45. Naylor, A., and R. Wester. 1987. Providing professional lactation management consultation. *Clinics in Perinatology* 14:33-38.

46. Barnes, G. R., A. N. Lethin, E. B. Jackson, and N. Shea. 1953. Management of breast-feeding. *Journal of the American Medical Association* 151:192-99.

47. Drewett, R. F., M. W. Woolridge, V. Greasley, C. N. Mcleod, J. Hewison, A. F. Williams, and J. D. Baum. 1984. Evaluating breast-milk intake by test weighing: A portable electronic balance suitable for community and field studies. *Early Human Development* 10:123-26.

48. Woolridge, M.W., J. D. Baum, and R. F. Drewett. 1982. Individual patterns of milk intake during breast-feeding. *Early Human Development* 7:265-72.

49. Dewey, K. G., M. J. Heinig, L. A. Nommsen, and B. Lonnerdahl. 1991. Maternal versus infant factors related to breast-milk intake and residual milk volume: The DARLING study. *Pediatrics* 87:829-37.

Index

Acidity of esophagus, 80, 81, 82, 83
Acyanotic heart disease, 350-351
AIDS, effects on swallowing, 33
Air flow
    monitoring, 68-70
    role in respiration, 37, 38
Air pressure changes, role in respiration, 38
Air swallowing, 360, 418
Airway defense reflexes, 40-43, 105
Airway disease, reactive
    as a cause of wheezing, 133
    as a cause of respiratory compromise, 259
    as a complication of bronchopulmonary dysplasia, 325
    associated with gastroesophageal reflux, 336
    in respiratory compromise model, 188
Airway maintenance (patency), 40, 43-45
    relationship to head and neck position, 101
Airway obstruction
    as cause of apnea, 70, 131
    as cause of bradycardia, 140
    associated with Pierre-Robin malformation sequence, 361-362
    due to pooling of secretions, 127
Airway patency. *See* Airway maintenance
Airway resistance, impaired, associated with bronchopulmonary dysplasia, 322
Airway stability, 43
    effect of neck position on, 44-45
Airway-constricting forces, 43-44
Airway-dilating forces, 43, 44
Airways, lower, evaluation of, 83
Airways, role in respiration and feeding, 3
Airways, upper,
    evaluation of, 83
    instability or spasms of, role in respiratory failure, 47

structural narrowing of, role in respiratory failure, 47
Alveoli
    role in respiration, 35, 36
    role in respiratory failure, 48, 299, 320
Amniotic fluid, maternal-fetal imbalance, effect on development of swallowing, 24
Amniotic fluid, too much. *See* Polyhydramnios
Anastomosis, used to treat tracheoesophageal fistula/esophageal atresia, 378
Anatomic defects. *See also* Cleft lip and palate; Heart disease, congenital; Pierre-Robin malformation sequence; Tracheoesophageal fistula
    effect on sucking, 23
    effects on swallowing, 33
    use of bronchoscopy in identifying, 83
Anatomy and physiology of the suck/swallow/breathe triad, 3-53
Anemia, associated with gastroesophageal reflux, 346
Antireflux surgery, used to treat gastroesophageal reflux, 346
Aortic body, role in respiration, 38
Aortic stenosis, 353-354
Apnea, 70, 130-131, 139
    as an indication of a feeding problem, 165, 170-179
    as a cause of bradycardia, 140
    as an indication of swallowing dysfunction, 126, 128-129
    associated with aspiration, 230
    associated with gastroesophageal reflux, 43, 71, 336, 337, 338, 346
    associated with retracted tongue, 117
    effect of maturation on, 52-53
    effect on respiration rate, 141

---

types of pressure involved, 16-18
Breast-feeding problems, infant causes for, 428-431
Breast milk
  benefits of, 435, 437
  guidelines for the collection and storage of, 436
  maintaining supply of, 441
Breast milk banks, 436
Breast pumping, 436
Breathing. *See* Respiration
Bronchi, 35, 47
Bronchioles, 35, 47
Bronchiolitis, 47
Bronchitis, 47
Bronchoconstriction
  as a cause of wheezing, 133
  role in airway defense, 42, 43
Bronchopulmonary dysplasia (BPD), 319-335
  abnormal oral-motor patterns associated with, 329-330
  associated with gastroesophageal reflux, 339
  associated with learned behaviors that interfere with feeding, 331-332
  associated with oral-tactile hypersensitivity, 330-331
  associated with reduced endurance, 146, 258, 327-328
  associated with respiratory compromise, 48, 144, 259, 265
  clinical course and complications of, 324-326
  criteria for diagnosis of, 319
  feeding-related problems seen in, 326-335
  in premature infants, 297, 300, 313
  in respiratory compromise model, 188
  medical treatment and management of, 144, 323-324
  poor coordination of sucking, swallowing, and respiration associated with, 328-329
  pulmonary changes in, 36, 320-323
  risks of feeding to infant with, 142
  swallowing problems associated with, 330-331
Bronchoscopy, 83
Bronchospasm, 47, 337
Bronchospasm, reflex, associated with gastroesophageal reflux, 337
Bulbar palsies. *See* Palsies
Bundling, 255. *See also* Swaddling
Button, gastrostomy, 271
Calming, techniques for, 213-215
Carbon dioxide, 35, 36, 37, 38, 70
Cardiac function, role in infant feeding, 37, 138-140

Cardiac surgery, in feeding-related apnea model, 175
Cardiac system, congenital defects of, 347-359, 378
Cardiologist, role in assessment and treatment of feeding problems, 162-163
Cardiorespiratory (CR) monitor, 64-65, 139-141
  use in clinical feeding evaluation of infants, 88, 170, 176
Caregiver, interview of for clinical feeding evaluation of infants, 86, 89
Carotid body, 38
Central grooving of tongue, 9, 18, 19, 114, 117
  in breast-feeding, 424, 428
  treating problems with, 236-237
Central hypoventilation syndrome, 47
Central rhythm generator (CRG), 15
  role in respiration, 38, 40
Cerebral palsy
  due to intracranial hemorrhage, 318
  effect on sucking, 23
  effect on swallowing, 33
  in feeding problem model, 180
  related to feeding-induced apnea, 136
Cervical compression, in feeding problem model, 181
Cervical nerves, role in sucking, swallowing, and respiration, 10-14, 27, 29, 30
CFEI. *See* Clinical feeding evaluation of infants
CHARGE, associated with congenital heart disease, 358
CHD. *See* Heart disease, congenital
Cheek stability, poor, treatment of, 244-245
Cheeks
  anatomy of, 5, 6
  changes with maturation, 10
  effect of prematurity on, 301
  evaluation of role in sucking, 113, 119-121
  hypotonic, 233
  innervation of, 24
  position and movement of, 120
  role in bolus formation, 120
  role in sucking, 18, 19, 400
  support of during breast-feeding, 428
Chemoreceptors
  role in airway defense, 40-43
  role in respiration, 35, 39
Chewing, references regarding, 233
Chilled formula, as treatment for delayed swallow, 222-223, 290
Choanal atresia, 47
Choking, 138
  as a sign of stress, 145

definition of, 165
diagnostic tests and procedures for, 63-83
diagnostic versus problem-oriented approach to evaluation and treatment of, 297
gathering information for clinical feeding evaluation of infants, 86
identifying, 164-166
preparation for the treatment of, 209-211
Feeding problems, assessment of, 85-157, 159-206
use of teams for, 159-164
problem-driven models for, 166-205
reasons to begin early, 165
Feeding problems, treatment of, 207-293
carry-over from feeding specialist to other caregivers in, 286-288
combination of techniques for, 288-290
consideration of whole baby in, 209
developing new techniques for, 292
medical techniques for, 209
modification of program for, 290-292
use of therapeutic techniques in, 209
Feeding schedule, role in feeding history, 91
Feeding skills, oral, critical period for the acquisition of, 112, 248
Feeding specialist
qualifications of, 164
role in assessment and treatment of feeding problems, 163-164
Feeding specialists, disciplines, 1
Feeding teams, use of for assessment and treatment, 159-164
Feeding tube. See Gastrostomy; Gavage feeding; Jejunal tube; Nasogastric tube; Orogastric tube; Tube feeding
Feeding tube device, 432-433
Feeding-induced apnea. See Apnea, feeding-induced
Feeding-related apnea. See Apnea, feeding-related
Finger feeding, as a means to supplement breast-feeding, 433-434
Fistula, tracheoesophageal. See Tracheoesophageal fistula
Flow of liquid
ability to monitor using different bottles, 417
associated with feeding-related apnea, 312
factors determining rate of, 407
impact of in sucking, 401-402
impact on swallowing ratio, 51-52
in breast-feeding, 425-426
increasing to treat weak suck, 240
methods to modify, 406-410
rate during sucking, 22

relationship to nipple type, 405-406, 407-410
role in feeding, 406-407
situations requiring modification of, 407
Flow of liquid, slowing of, as possible treatment for abnormal sucking, swallowing, and respiration, 87
Flow of liquid, too fast, as possible reason for arching during feeding, 104
Fluid overload, associated with bronchopulmonary dysplasia, 319
Food types and textures, inability to handle, associated with tracheoesophageal fistula/esophageal atresia, 382
Foreign bodies, effects on swallowing, 33
Foreign-body impaction, as a complication of tracheoesophageal fistula/esophageal atresia, 380
FTT. See Failure to thrive
Full-term and older infants, feeding-related apnea in, 305
G-tube. See Gastrostomy tube; Tube feeding
Gag reflex, 107, 108-109
Gag reflex
associated with inability to suck, 290
consideration of in nipple selection, 412-413
Gag reflex, hyperactive, associated with tube feeding, 270
Gagging
as a hypersensitive or aversive response, 111, 247
as a sign of stress, 145
associated with clefts, 360
associated with early satiety, 356
associated with the use of a gavage tube, 270, 275
Gas exchange, impaired, associated with bronchopulmonary dysplasia, 322
Gasping
as a sign of stress, 145
as indication of swallowing dysfunction, 128-129
in feeding problem model, 184
Gastric emptying, evaluation of, 73
Gastric retention of feedings, as a sign of necrotizing enterocolitis, 313
Gastroenterologist, role in assessment and treatment of feeding problems, 162-163
Gastroesophageal reflux. See Reflux, gastroesophageal
Gastrointestinal discomfort, as possible reason for arching during feeding, 104
Gastrointestinal tract, congenital defects of, associated with tracheoesophageal fistula/esophageal atresia, 378

Hoarseness, as indication for bronchoscopy, 83
Hospitalization, prolonged
    and infant trust, 332
    in bronchopulmonary dysplasia, 324
HSV lesions, effect on sucking, 23
Hunger/satiation cycles, normalization of, in transition from to oral feeding, 284
Hyaline membrane disease (HMD). *See* Infant respiratory distress syndrome
Hydrocephalus
    as an outcome of intracranial hemorrhage, 318
    effects on swallowing, 33
    in feeding problem model, 181
Hyoid,
    anatomy of, 5, 6, 7
    changes with maturation, 10
    role in feeding, swallowing, and respiration, 7-8
    role in pharyngeal phase of swallowing, 27
Hypersensitivity, oral-tactile
    as impediment to discontinuing non-oral feeding, 283
    assessment of, 109-111
    associated with bronchopulmonary dysplasia, 330-331
    associated with inability to suck, 290
    associated with tube feeding, 270
    causes of, 247-249
    description of, 111, 247
    treatment of, 247-252
Hypersensitivity, oral-tactile, extreme, indication for use of full non-oral feeding, 274
Hypertonia, as a causal factor in oral-motor problems, 117, 119, 120-121
Hypertonia, oral-facial, treatment of, 234-235
Hypertonicity. *See also* Muscle tone; Tone
    associated with excessive jaw movement, 242
    associated with tongue retraction, 235
Hypoglossal nuclei, role in swallowing and respiration, 14
Hypopharynx, anatomy of, 5, 6
Hypoplastic left heart syndrome (HLHS), 353
Hypothalamus
    role in breast-feeding, 422, 423
    role in swallowing reflex, 25
Hypothermia, avoidance of in arousing baby, 213
Hypotonia. *See also* Muscle tone; Tone
    associated with inadequate jaw movements, 119, 241
    associated with inadequate tongue movement, 116, 117, 237, 238

associated with poor lip seal, 120, 243
Hypotonia, oral-facial
    associated with poor cheek stability, 120, 245
    treatment of, 233-234
Hypoxia, 143
    as a result of airway defense mechanisms, 40
    associated with bronchopulmonary dysplasia, 322, 323, 325
    associated with congenital heart disease, 352
    in infant respiratory distress syndrome, 299
ICH. *See* Intracranial hemorrhage
Illness, as a cause of hypersensitive/aversive responses, 112, 248
INFANIB, 98
Infant respiratory distress syndrome (IRDS), 298-300
    as a cause of reduced endurance, 258, 312-313
    as a cause of respiratory failure, 48, 259
    as a complication of prematurity, 297, 298, 312
    associated with bronchopulmonary dysplasia, 319
    impact of on feeding, 300
    in feeding-related apnea model, 172
    in respiratory compromise model, 188, 189, 196
    risks of feeding an infant with, 142
Infections, congenital, effects on swallowing, 33
Intake, relationship to sucking time in breast-feeding, 425-426
Intercostal muscles, role in respiration, 36
Intracranial hemorrhage (ICH)
    associated with bronchopulmonary dysplasia, 321
    effect of on sucking, 23
    in premature infants, 297, 300, 318-319
    role in respiratory failure, 47
Intubation
    as a cause of abnormal palate formation, 122
    as a cause of hypersensitive/aversive responses, 112, 248
    associated with bronchopulmonary dysplasia, 320, 323, 324, 329, 330
    associated with neck hyperextension, 98
Intubation, difficult, as indication for bronchoscopy, 83
Intubation, prolonged, and infant trust, 332
IRDS. *See* Infant respiratory distress syndrome

Mandible. *See* Jaw
Manometry, esophageal, 83
Maturation
    changes in mechanics of sucking with, 19
    effect on feeding and respiration, 9-10
    effect on sucking and respiration, 52-53
Maturation, anatomic, in premature infants, 301
Mechanoreceptors, role in respiration, 35, 37, 39
Medical evaluation
    in poor weight gain model, 198, 199, 200, 202
    in respiratory compromise model, 194, 196
Medical history. *See* Feeding history
Medulla
    role in esophageal phase of swallowing, 30
    role in respiration, 38, 39
    role in sucking, swallowing, and respiration, 14, 15
    role in swallowing, 31, 32, 33
Meningomyelocele
    in feeding problem model, 180, 181
    role in respiratory failure, 47
Metabolic problems, in poor weight gain model, 198, 199
Micrognathia, 119, 361-366, 370-373
    associated with tongue retraction, 235
    comparison of medical and surgical management strategies for airway obstruction secondary to, 363
    effect on airway maintenance, 44
    effect on sucking, 23
    effect on swallowing, 33
    role in respiratory failure, 47
Midbrain. *See* Medulla
Milk. *See* Breast milk
Milk flow. *See* Flow of liquid
Moebius syndrome, effects on swallowing, 33
Monitoring of physiologic functions, 64-83, 138-144
Mother-child interaction
    in clinical feeding evaluation of infants, 90
    in poor weight gain model, 199, 200, 201, 204, 205
Motor control
    as a system in infant feeding, 160
    assessment of as possible cause of inadequate suction, 125
    in clinical feeding evaluation of infants, 85, 97-104
    of esophageal phase of swallowing, 30
    of nerves in sucking, swallowing, and respiration, 10-15
    of oral phase of swallowing, 24-26

of pharyngeal phase of swallowing, 27, 29
Motor control, deficits in
    as indication for use of full non-oral feeding, 274
    due to intracranial hemorrhage, 99, 318
Motor-oral control. *See* Oral-motor control
Mouth. *See also* Oral cavity
    as a cause of breast-feeding problems, 430
    as infant's sensorium, 105
Mouth opening, lack of spontaneous, treatment of, 239-240
Mouth size, effect of prematurity on, 301
Mouth size, relative to nipple size, impact on sucking, 412-413
Movement
    observation of in clinical feeding evaluation of infants, 97-104
    use for arousal, 212-213
    use for calming, 215
    use to treat abnormal tone, 218-219
Movement Assessment of Infants (MAI), 98
Mucociliary clearance, role in airway defense, 41, 43
Mucus secretion, role in airway defense, 42
Muscle tone, as an element of neuromotor control, 97, 98. *See also* Tone
Muscles
    role in esophageal phase of swallowing, 30, 31
    role in feeding, swallowing, and respiration, 7, 8
    role in pharyngeal phase of swallowing, 26, 27, 28, 29
Muscular development, immature, associated with weak suck, 240
Muscular weakness, as a cause of reduced endurance, 258
Musculoskeletal anomalies, as a cause of respiratory compromise, 259
Myopathy
    as a cause of reduced endurance, 258
    associated with oral-facial hypotonia, 233
    associated with weak suck, 240
    in feeding problem model, 180
    role in respiratory failure, 48
NA. *See* Nucleus ambiguous
Narcotics, role in respiratory failure, 47
Nasal breathing in infants, 45-47
Nasal cavity
    anatomy of, 4
    role in respiration and feeding, 3
Nasogastric tube, 268-271. *See also* Tube feeding
    in feeding problem model, 183
    associated with gastroesophageal reflux, 340

Nissen fundoplication, used to treat gastroesophageal reflux, 346
NNS. *See* Sucking, non-nutritive
Noise, effect on feeding, 210-211
Noise, reduction of, used to treat disorganized sucking, 255
Noisy respiration
  as an indication of aspiration after swallow, 227
  with delayed swallow, 223
Non-oral and supplemental feeding methods, 266-286
Non-oral feeding. *See* Feeding, non-oral
Nose
  role in airway defense, 40, 42
  role in respiration, 3, 35, 37, 39
Nose, congestion of, and difficult breathing during feeding, 129
Nose, obstruction of, role in respiratory failure, 47
NS. *See* Sucking, nutritive
NTS. *See* Nucleus tractus solitarius
Nucleus ambiguous (NA)
  role in swallowing, 32, 33
  role in swallowing and respiration, 14
Nucleus tractus solitarius (NTS)
  role in respiration, 38
  role in swallowing, 32, 33
  role in swallowing and respiration, 14
Nurses, role in assessment and treatment of feeding problems, 162, 163
Nutrition, poor, as a cause of reduced endurance, 258
Nutrition, supplemental
  methods of, 266-276
  during transition to breast feeding, 441-442
Nutrition, total parenteral, 268
Nutritional assessment, in poor weight gain model, 198, 199, 200, 202, 204
Nutritional supplements, used to treat reduced endurance, 259
Nutritional support, in transition from to oral feeding, 284
Nutritionist, role in assessment and treatment of feeding problems, 161, 163
Observation, importance in the evaluation of feeding problems, 85
Obstructive heart defects, 353-354
Occupational therapists, role in assessment and treatment of feeding problems, 161, 163
OG tube. *See* Orogastric tube
Oral and facial musculature, effect of prematurity on, 301

Oral cavity
  anatomy of, 5, 6
  changes with maturation, 10
  in oral phase of swallowing, 24-25
  role in feeding and respiration, 3, 6
  role in respiration, 35
  role in sucking, 16-18, 22
Oral cavity, defects of, effects on swallowing, 33
Oral cavity, obstruction of, role in respiratory failure, 47
Oral exploration, used in oral-tactile normalization, 251-252
Oral feeding. *See* Feeding, oral
Oral infections, effect on sucking, 23
Oral pain, effect on sucking, 23
Oral prostheses. *See* Palatal obturators
Oral reflexes. *See* Reflexes, oral
Oral stimulation, minimizing negative or aversive, 317. *See also* Oral-tactile normalization
Oral therapy
  used to maintain oral skills in infant with necrotizing enterocolitis, 314-317
  used to maintain oral-motor skills, 230
Oral therapy program
  primary features of, 276-277
  use of sham feedings in, 317
  used in infants with micrognathia and the Pierre-Robin sequence, 371
Oral trauma, effect on sucking, 23
Oral-facial anomalies, 359-377
Oral-facial anomalies
  achievement of oral feeding in infants with, 376-377
  characteristics of bottle-feeding in infants with, 365-366
  comparison of feeding components and feeding methods for infants with, 364
  feeding modifications and devices used for infants with, 373-376
  impact of surgical repair on oral feeding in, 377
  role of supplementary non-oral feedings in infants with, 377
Oral-facial hypertonia, treatment of, 234-235
Oral-facial hypotonia, treatment of, 233-234
Oral-motor control
  in clinical feeding evaluation of infants, 85, 113-122
  in feeding problem model, 180, 182, 183
  in poor weight gain model, 198
  relationship to tone, state, physiologic control, 215-216
  treatment of, 233-247

Oral-motor control, impaired, as indication for continuing non-oral feeding, 280

Oral-motor control, poor, as cause of short sucking bursts, 136-137

Oral-motor patterns, abnormal, associated with bronchopulmonary dysplasia, 329-330

Oral-motor skills, maintaining for non-orally fed infant through oral therapy, 276

Oral-tactile experiences, unpleasant, as a cause of hypersensitive/aversive responses, 248

Oral-tactile hypersensitivity
associated with bronchopulmonary dysplasia, 330-331
treatment of, 247-252

Oral-tactile normalization
modalities used in, 250-252
to treat hypersensitive/aversive responses, 249-250

Organizational abilities, as a system in infant feeding, 160

Orogastric, tube, 268-271. *See also* Tube feeding

Oropharynx
anatomy of, 5, 6
role in nasal versus oral breathing, 46

Osteopenia, as a complication of bronchopulmonary dysplasia, 326

Otolaryngologist, role in assessment and treatment of feeding problems, 162-163

Oximeters, 66, 67, 143

Oximetry, 66-68
in feeding-related apnea model, 172, 176, 178
in respiratory compromise model, 188, 189, 194, 197
use of to determine need for supplemental oxygen, 261

Oxygen saturation
definition of, 143
evaluation of, 138, 142, 143-144
in feeding-related apnea model, 170, 172, 174, 176, 178
in respiratory compromise model, 188, 194, 196
monitoring of, 64, 66, 67, 68, 70

Oxygen, decreased
as a cause of bradycardia, 140
as a result of sucking pattern, 133-136, 252-256
as a result of apnea, 131
as a result of respiratory compromise, 260
as a result of periodic respiration, 131
as a result of feeding-related apnea, 253

comparison of between breast-feeding and bottle feeding, 435
due to pooling of secretions, 127
in premature infants, 305, 306, 311

Oxygen, supplemental
assessment of infant's response to, 261-262
in feeding-related apnea model, 177
in respiratory compromise model, 196, 197
used to treat bronchopulmonary dysplasia, 319, 323, 324
used to treat respiratory compromise, 261, 292

Oxygen therapy
determining effectiveness of, 66
used as treatment for respiratory distress, 300

PA banding. *See* Pulmonary artery banding

Pacifier trainer, 410
use of to treat delayed swallow, 224

Pacifiers
orthodontic versus conventional, 414
selection of, 413-415
use of to stimulate swallow reflex, 223
use with non-orally fed infants, 145, 284, 371

Pacifiers, home-made, cautions regarding, 415

Pacifiers, nipples, and bottles, selection of, 399-418

Pacing, external
as possible treatment for abnormal sucking, swallowing, and respiration, 87, 253, 262-263
in feeding-related apnea model, 170, 179
in feeding problem model, 185

Palatal movement, poor, treatment of, 246-247

Palatal obturators, for infants with oral-facial anomalies, 375, 368-369

Palatal training appliance (PTA)
used to assist palatal movement, 227-228, 247
used to treat poor palatal movement, 247

Palate
anatomy of, 4, 5, 6
evaluation of role in sucking, 113, 121-122, 125
role in oral phase of swallowing, 25
role in sucking, 18, 19, 400

Palate, cleft. *See* Cleft lip and palate

Palate, defects of, effects on swallowing, 33

Palate, soft
changes with maturation, 10
control of, 76
role in feeding, swallowing, and respiration, 8-9

PTA. *See* Palatal training appliance

Pulmonary artery banding (PA banding), used to treat congenital heart disease, 354

Pulmonary compliance, decreased, associated with bronchopulmonary dysplasia, 322

Pulmonary evaluation, in respiratory compromise model, 188, 189, 190, 192, 194, 196, 197

Pulmonary status, evaluation of relative to aspiration, 229

Pulmonary stenosis, 353-354

Pulmonary stretch receptors (PSRs), role in respiration, 37, 38

Pulmonary vasculature, role in respiratory failure, 47

Pulmonologist, role in assessment and treatment of feeding problems, 162-163

Pyloroplasty, used to treat gastroesophageal reflux, 346

RAD. *See* Reactive airway disease

Radiologic procedures for monitoring physiologic function, 71-80

Radiologist, role in assessment and treatment of feeding problems, 162

Reactive airway disease. *See* Airway disease, reactive

Recurrent laryngeal nerve (RLN). *See also* Cranial nerves
  role in esophageal phase of swallowing, 31
  role in swallowing, 32

Reflex activity, as an element of neuromotor control, 97, 98

Reflexes, oral
  definition of, 105
  evaluation of, 105

Reflexes, oral, adaptive, 105, 106

Reflexes, oral, protective, 105, 107

Reflexes, tactile, *See* Touch, reflexes to

Reflux, gastroesophageal (GER), 336-347
  as a complication of bronchopulmonary dysplasia, 326
  as a complication of tracheoesophageal fistula/esophageal atresia, 381, 383
  as a component of asthma, 128
  as a factor in aspiration, 229, 230
  as cause of apnea, 70, 131
  associated with feeding problems, 138, 289, 292
  associated with gastrostomy tube, 272
  associated with respiratory compromise, 260
  association with respiratory symptoms, 81
  causes of, 336
  definition of, 336

dietary management of, 343-345

evaluation of, 71, 72, 73, 74, 75, 80, 81, 82, 83

feeding-related problems associated with, 346-347

in feeding-related apnea model, 170, 171, 172, 173, 176

in poor weight gain model, 199

in respiratory compromise model, 188, 189, 192, 193

medical management of, 345

positional management of, 340-343

respiratory disease as a causal factor in, 338-340

surgical management of, 346

Regurgitation, nasal, associated with clefts, 360

Respiration
  anatomy and physiology of, 35-48
  brain-stem control of, 38-40
  changes in pattern of, 130-131
  effect of feeding on, 139
  effect of heart function on, 37
  effect of swallowing on, 48-50
  effect on sucking, 50-51
  in infants with oral-facial anomalies, 364, 365, 366, 367, 371
  monitoring, 70
  nasal vs. oral in infants, 45-46
  neural control of, 10-15, 38-40
  over-suppression of with prolonged sucking, 136
  poor coordination with sucking and swallowing, 255, 289, 292
  protective mechanisms and reflexes in, 40-45
  relationship to sucking and swallowing, 3
  rhythmic patterns in, 15

Respiration, cessation of, role in airway defense, 40

Respiration, coordination with sucking and swallowing, evaluation of, 122-138

Respiration, depth of, 36

Respiration, distress during, as cause of different sucking rhythms, 137

Respiration, dysrhythmic, and effect on coordination between sucking, and swallowing, 132

Respiration, irregular, as a sign of stress, 145

Respiration, noisy, 132-133
  as indication of swallowing dysfunction, 126, 127-128
  associated with feeding problems, 289
  in feeding problem model, 183
  in respiratory compromise model, 192

Respiration, periodic, 132

Respiration, quality of during feeding, evaluation of, 129-133

Respiration, sucking, and swallowing. *See also* Sucking, swallowing, and respiration

assessment of in relationship to feeding, 122-138

Respiration, sucking, and swallowing, coordination of, 48-53

effect of maturation on, 52

Respiration, sucking, and swallowing, poor coordination of

in feeding problem model, 183, 184, 188

in feeding-related apnea model, 170

in poor weight gain model, 198

Respiration, work of, 36, 129-130, 137

Respiration and drive to breathe, 37

Respiration and swallowing, timing of, 129

Respiration rate, 36

decrease during sucking, 257

evaluation of, 138, 141-143

in respiratory compromise model, 188, 189, 196, 197

monitoring, 64, 65, 68

Respiratory rate, increased

dealing with, 260-261

in feeding-related apnea model, 174

Respiration rate, rapid, with short sucking bursts, 137

Respiration rhythm, in respiratory compromise model, 195

Respiratory compromise

in premature infants, 312

treatment of, 257, 259-266

Respiratory compromise model for the assessment of infant feeding problems, 167, 188-197

Respiratory control during feeding, in premature infants, 304-306

Respiratory control problems, in feeding problem model, 181

Respiratory disease

as a cause of gastroesophageal reflux, 336-338, 338-340

as a symptom of gastroesophageal reflux, 71

associated with gastroesophageal reflux, 346

effect on respiration, 36

Respiratory disorders

as a cause of reduced endurance, 258

associated with bronchopulmonary dysplasia, 319, 321

Respiratory distress, in feeding problem model, 186

Respiratory distress syndrome, infant. *See* Infant respiratory distress syndrome

Respiratory effort

as indication for continuing non-oral feeding, 279

associated with gastroesophageal reflux, 339

Respiratory endurance problems, associated with weak suck, 240

Respiratory evaluation, role in feeding problem model, 181

Respiratory failure

etiologies of, 47-48

retractions as sign of, 130

Respiratory function

impact of indwelling nasogastric tubes on, 271

role in infant feeding, 160

Respiratory illness

associated with aspiration, 230, 231, 232

in the premature infant, 298-300

Respiratory infections, as indication of swallowing dysfunction, 126, 128

Respiratory infections, upper, in respiratory compromise model, 188, 189, 192, 194

Respiratory insufficiency, events leading to, associated with prematurity, 299

Respiratory muscle weakness, role in respiratory failure, 48

Respiratory pauses, as signs of stress, 145

Respiratory problems

as possible response to arching during feeding, 104

associated with disorganized sucking, 255

association with short sucking bursts, 255

good position for feeding infant with, 221

Respiratory status, evaluation of relative to aspiration, 229

Respiratory support, when to consider, 265

Respiratory symptoms, association with acid reflux, 81

Respiratory syncytial virus (RSV)

associated with gastroesophageal reflux, 339

in respiratory compromise model, 188, 194

Reticular formation, role in swallowing, 32, 33

Retractions, as indication of increased work of breathing, 129-130, 300

Retrognathia, 361

Rhythm, sucking, 124

Rhythmic movements in sucking, 19

Rhythmic patterns in sucking, swallowing, and respiration, 15, 19

---

in poor weight gain model, 200, 201
in response to touch, 103
Stress, motoric, 99-101
Stress, state-related, 96
Stricture formation
  as a complication of tracheoesophageal fistula/esophageal atresia, 380
  associated with gastroesophageal reflux, 336
Stridor, 133
  as indication for bronchoscopy, 83
  associated with gastroesophageal reflux, 337, 339
  associated with tracheomalacia, 380
  in feeding problem model, 180, 181
  with delayed swallow, 223
Subglottic stenosis, role in respiratory failure, 47
Submucous cleft, 247, 360, 365-370
Suck:breathe ratio, 134
Suck:swallow ratio, 20, 21-22, 51, 134
Suck:swallow:breathe ratio, 133-138
Suck-swallow reflex, 106
Sucking
  anatomy and physiology of, 15-23
  biomechanics of, 16-19, 400, 401
  characteristics of, 20-22
  characteristics of, in breast-feeding versus bottle-feeding, 19, 401, 424, 425, 438-439
  continuous, without respiration, in feeding-related apnea model, 178
  continuous, without respiration, in feeding-induced apnea, 134-136, 140, 253-254
  definition of, 15
  effect of respiration on, 50-51
  evaluation of, 123-125
  flow during, 22
  in premature infants, 301-304, 311
  in utero, 15-16
  relationship to swallowing and respiration, 3
  relationship to swallowing pattern, 20-21, 51-52
  role in the life of the young infant, 15
  role of compression in, 16-19, 22
  role of suction in, 16-19, 22
Sucking, abnormalities of, etiologies of, 23
Sucking, disorganized, 137
  treatment of, 255-256
Sucking, inefficient, associated with bronchopulmonary dysplasia, 329
Sucking, initiation of, 123, 125
  poor, 245-246
  poor, in feeding problem model, 181

Sucking, mechanics of
  during breast-feeding, 423-425
  in relationship to nipple characteristics, 410-413
Sucking, neural control of, 10-15
Sucking, non-nutritive (NNS)
  advantages of in premature infants, 306
  characteristics of, 20-22
  definition of, 20
  effect on gastroesophageal reflux, 345
  evaluation of, 123-125
  impact of lack of flow on, 51, 52, 401
  importance of accompanying tube feedings, 306, 315, 415, 440
  in premature infants, 301-302
  on the breast, 426, 440
  selecting pacifier for, 251, 414-415
  used to maintain oral skills in infant with necrotizing enterocolitis, 314-317
Sucking, nutritive (NS)
  characteristics of, 20-22
  definition of, 20
  evaluation of, 123-125
  evaluation of rhythm during, 133-134
  in premature infants, 302-304
  rhythm of, 20-21, 124, 134, 137-138
  role of flow in, 51, 52, 402
Sucking, short bursts of, 135, 136-137
  associated with bronchopulmonary dysplasia, 328
  treatment of, 254-255
Sucking, signature, 20
Sucking, swallowing, and respiration, coordination of, 48-53
  effect of maturation on, 52
  in premature infants, 303-306
  treatment of, 252-256
Sucking, swallowing, and respiration, coordinating evaluation of, 133-138
Sucking, swallowing, and respiration, pacing of, 253
Sucking, swallowing, and respiration, poor coordination of
  associated with prematurity, 311-312
  associated with bronchopulmonary dysplasia, 328-329
Sucking, weak, treatment of, 240-241
Sucking pads. See Cheeks
Sucking pressure, 16-18, 22, 123, 124, 125
  control by infant, 52
  role of state and behavior on, 22
Sucking rate, 20, 124
Sucking rate and pattern of in breast-feeding, 425-426
Sucking reflex, 105, 106
Sucking rhythm, 20-21, 124, 134, 137

in feeding problem model, 180, 183, 184, 186, 188
in poor weight gain model, 198
in respiratory compromise model, 188, 195
treatment of, 252-256
Swallowing center, 31-33
afferent (sensory) level of, 31, 32
efferent (motor) level of, 31, 32-33
Swallowing dysfunction. *See also* Swallowing problems
Swallowing function, monitoring, 75, 77, 79
Swallowing problems
associated with bronchopulmonary dysplasia, 330
etiologies of, 33, 34, 222
in poor weight gain model, 198
in respiratory compromise model, 189
position for feeding an infant with, 220
related to sucking and respiration, 3, 252-256
treatment of, 222-232
Swallowing reflex, 25, 26
effect of medical status changes, 25
role of sensory information, 26
Swallows, multiple, as indication of swallowing dysfunction, 126, 127
Sweat chloride test, in poor weight gain model, 202
Syndromes
associated with congenital heart disease, 358
associated with oral-facial anomalies, 361
Tachycardia, 140. *See also* Heart rate
Tachypnea, 142. *See also* Respiration
as a sign of respiratory distress, 300
associated with decreased endurance, 355
associated with feeding problems, 290
associated with hypoplastic left heart syndrome, 353
associated with patent ductus arteriosus, 351
Tachypnea, transient of the newborn, in feeding problem model, 184
Tactile input. *See* Touch
Tactile reflexes. *See* Touch, reflexes to
Technetium scan, 71-73
in feeding-related apnea model, 171, 172, 173, 177
in respiratory compromise model, 192, 193
TEF. *See* Tracheoesophageal fistula
Temperature, cold, use in treating swallowing problems, 222
Temperature, cool, use for arousal, 213
Temperature, effect on feeding, 211
Temporomandibular joint, role in supporting oral function, 9-10

Term infants, sucking and respiratory patterns in. *See* Respiration
Tetralogy of fallot (TOF), 352
TGA. *See* Transposition of the great arteries
Theophylline
effect on gastroesophageal reflux, 340
in feeding-related apnea model, 177
use to treat central apnea, 173
Thermal stimulation, as treatment for delayed swallow, 222-223
Thickened liquid
as possible treatment for abnormal sucking, swallowing, and respiration, 87, 254
in respiratory compromise model, 191, 193
relationship to decreased flow rate, 409-410
use of to treat aspiration, 226, 232
use of to treat delayed swallow, 224
use of to treat disorganized sucking, 256
use of to treat gastroesophageal reflux, 343
Thoracic cage, reduction of movement, role in respiratory failure, 48
Thoracic cage, role in respiration, 36
Thrush, effect on sucking, 23
Tidal volume, in respiration, 36
TOF. *See* Tetralogy of fallot
Tone. *See also* Hypertonia; Hypotonia
changes of as treatment for oral motor problems, 233-247
evaluation and interpretation of in clinical feeding evaluation of infants, 97-104, 113-122
relationship to state, physiologic control, and oral-motor control, 215-216
role in treatment of feeding problems, 215-221
Tone, abnormal
and feeding position, 102
as possible cause of arching during feeding, 104
Tongue
abnormal movement and rhythm, 118
abnormal tone of, 115, 117
anatomy of, 5, 6
asymmetries of position or movement, 117
characteristics of movement of, 115-116
characteristics of position of, 114
decreased tone of, 117
deviations of position of, 114-115
differences in action of during breast- and bottle-feeding, 424
effect of prematurity on, 301
evaluation of role in sucking, 113, 114
formation of central groove, 9, 18, 19, 114
inability to form and hold bolus, 117

increased tone of, 115, 116, 117
lack of rhythm of movements, 116
lack of shape definition of, 117
role in bolus formation, 114
role in feeding, swallowing, and respiration, 8-9
role in nasal vs. oral respiration, 46
role in oral phase of swallowing, 24
role in pharyngeal phase of swallowing, 27, 28, 29
role in sucking, 16, 18, 19, 400
role in suction and compression, 114
Tongue, control of
assessment of as possible cause of inadequate suction, 125
effect on feeding, 233
Tongue, inability to form central groove, 117
treatment of, 235-237
Tongue, large. See Macroglossia
Tongue, mass in. See Hemangioma
Tongue movements, abnormal
associated with excessive jaw movement, 242
associated with poor lip seal, 243
Tongue movements, poorly coordinated, associated with bronchopulmonary dysplasia, 328
Tongue, poor central grooving of, as a cause of breast-feeding problems, 429
Tongue position, abnormal, associated with micrognathia and Pierre-Robin malformation sequence, 361
Tongue, position and movement
changes with maturation, 10
impact of nipple characteristics on, 411-412
Tongue, posteriorly placed. See Micrognathia
Tongue, protrusion of, 117
treatment of, 238-239
Tongue, retracted, 117
good position for feeding infant with, 220
as a cause of breast-feeding problems, 429
treatment of, 235-236
Tongue thrust, 116, 117, 119, 122
Tongue-tip elevation
as a cause of breast-feeding problems, 428
associated with sucking difficulty in premature infants, 311
treatment of, 237-238
Tongue-to-lip adhesion, used to treat micrognathia and Pierre-Robin malformation sequence, 361, 363, 371
Toothbrush trainer, used in oral-tactile normalization, 251
Total parenteral nutrition (TPN), 268, 314
Touch, as a stimulus
in esophageal phase of swallowing, 31

in pharyngeal phase of swallowing, 30
in respiration, 38
Touch
aversive responses to, 111-112
behavioral responses to, 109-113
hypersensitive responses to, 111
hyposensitive responses to, 110-111
type, 110
used for calming, 214-215
used for arousal, 213
Touch, infant's response to, role in clinical feeding evaluation of infants, 105-113
Touch, problems with, as cause of different sucking rhythms, 137
Touch, reflexes to, role in feeding, 105
Touch to face, 109
Touch/pressure, used in oral-tactile normalization, 250
TPN. See Total Parenteral nutrition
Trach collar, 333
Trachea
anatomy of, 5, 6
compression of as a cause of stridor, 133
role in feeding and respiration, 3
role in respiration, 35
Trachea, extrathoracic, obstruction of, role in respiratory failure, 47
Trachea, intrathoracic, obstruction of, role in respiratory failure, 47
Tracheoesophageal fistula, as indication for bronchoscopy, 83
Tracheoesophageal fistula/esophageal atresia, 378-385
associated with gastroesophageal reflux, 383
classification of, 378
effects on swallowing, 33
feeding-related problems seen in, 381-385
in feeding problem model, 180
in feeding-related apnea model, 170, 178
surgical repair of, 378-379
Tracheomalacia
as a cause of stridor, 133
as a complication of tracheoesophageal fistula/esophageal atresia, 380
associated with gastroesophageal reflux, 339
identification of, 83
role in respiratory failure, 47
Tracheostomy, 333-335
relationship to feeding, 334-335
used in infants with micrognathia and the Pierre-Robin sequence, 372
used to treat bronchopulmonary dysplasia, 324, 328

Tracheostomy, long-term, indication for gastrostomy, 273
Transposition of the great arteries (TGA), 352
Trauma, effects on swallowing, 33
Treatment of feeding problems. *See* Feeding problems, treatment of
Treatment of infant feeding problems. *See* Feeding problems, treatment of
Treatment techniques, evaluation of response to, 76, 77, 79
Trigeminal nuclei, role in swallowing and respiration, 14
Triple timing, 441. *See also* Breast-feeding, methods of supplementing intake
Trisomy 13, associated with congenital heart disease, 358
Trisomy 21, associated with congenital heart disease, 358
True vocal folds, 5, 7
Trust, effect on oral feeding, 332
Tube feeding, 268-274. *See also* Feeding, non-oral; Gastrostomy; Gavage tube; Jejunal Tube; Nasogastric tube; Orogastric tube
  as a means to supplement breast-feeding, 432-433, 442
  deciding on type of tube, 273
  in infants with micrognathia and the Pierre-Robin sequence, 371
  in poor weight gain model, 203
  in premature infants, 306
  in respiratory compromise model, 191, 195
  role of non-nutritive sucking in, 251, 306, 415, 440
  strengths and limitations of different types, 269-273
  use of to treat delayed swallow, 224
Tube feeding, transition from to oral feeding, 276-286
  assessing child's readiness for, 277-278
  assessing parents' readiness for, 277, 282-286
  barriers to, 278
  importance of child's medical condition in, 278-279
  importance of child's oral-motor control in, 279-280
  importance of child's swallowing ability in, 280-281
  treatment for, 284-286
Tumor, brain-stem, in feeding problem model, 180
Tumors, identification of, 83
Turner's syndrome, associated with coarctation of the aorta, 353
Vagus nerve. *See also* Cranial nerves

  role in esophageal phase of swallowing, 30, 31
  role in respiration, 38, 39
Valleculae, anatomy of, 5, 6
Vascular accident, effects on swallowing, 33
Vascular ring
  as a cause of stridor, 133
  effects on swallowing, 33
  identification of, 83
VATER
  associated with congenital heart disease, 358
  associated with tracheoesophageal fistula/esophageal atresia, 378
Velopharyngeal closure, assessment of as possible cause of inadequate suction, 125
Ventilation, mechanical. *See also* Intubation
  used as a treatment for respiratory distress, 300
  mechanical, with bronchopulmonary dysplasia, 324, 328
Ventilation, positive pressure, associated with bronchopulmonary dysplasia, 319, 320
Ventral respiratory group (VRG), role in respiration, 38, 40
Ventricular septal defect (VSD), 350
  in feeding problem model, 186, 187
VFSS. *See* Videofluoroscopic swallowing study
Vibration, used in oral-tactile normalization, 250-251
Videofluoroscopic swallowing study (VFSS), 75-80
  in feeding problem model, 181, 182, 183
  in feeding-related apnea model, 171, 176, 177
  in respiratory compromise model, 189, 190, 191
  indications of need for, 75-80
  involvement of parents in, 80
  personnel involved in, 78
  protocol used for, 78
  relationship to clinical feeding, 78-79
  risks of for infant with inability to handle secretions, 127
  use of, 126, 128, 222, 228
Viscera, effect of feeding on, 139
Vision problems, due to intracranial hemorrhage, 318
Visual stimuli, effect on feeding, 210
Vocal cord, anomalies or paralysis of, role in respiratory failure, 47
Vocal cord paralysis
  as a cause of stridor, 133